Glycosaminoglycans and Proteoglycans

Special Issue Editor
Barbara Mulloy

MDPI • Basel • Beijing • Wuhan • Barcelona • Belgrade

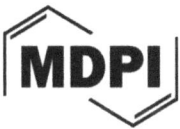

MDPI

Special Issue Editor
Barbara Mulloy
UK

Editorial Office
MDPI
St. Alban-Anlage 66
Basel, Switzerland

This edition is a reprint of the Special Issue published online in the open access journal *Pharmaceuticals* (ISSN 1424-8247) from 2017–2018 (available at: http://www.mdpi.com/journal/pharmaceuticals/special_issues/glycosaminoglycans_proteoglycans).

For citation purposes, cite each article independently as indicated on the article page online and as indicated below:

Lastname, F.M.; Lastname, F.M. Article title. *Journal Name* **Year**, *Article number*, page range.

First Edition 2018

ISBN 978-3-03842-835-0 (Pbk)
ISBN 978-3-03842-836-7 (PDF)

About the Special Issue Editor

Barbara Mulloy, Prof. Dr. Before her retirement, Barbara Mulloy worked for over 30 years at the UK's National Institute for Biological Standards and Control, where she specialized in the physicochemical analysis of complex biological medicines such as the glycosaminoglycan heparin. Her research interests are in the field of structural glycobiology, with special emphasis on glycosaminoglycans and their interactions with proteins. She is Visiting Professor at the Institute of Pharmaceutical Sciences, King's College London, and at the Glycosciences Laboratory in the Department of Medicine, Imperial College.

Preface to "Glycosaminoglycans and Proteoglycans"

1. Introduction

This short article is intended to provide a brief introduction to the structures of glycosaminoglycans (GAGs) and proteoglycans (PGs) to set the articles in this special issue of *Pharmaceuticals* on "*Proteoglycans and Glycosaminoglycans*" into context. The class of glycosylated proteins known as PGs is represented in the pharmaceutical world chiefly by its carbohydrate constituents. These are polysaccharides known as GAGs, such as heparin (Hp) [1] and chondroitin sulfate (CS) [2]. When attached to their native protein cores these polysaccharides form the glycoconjugates known as PGs. Whole PGs are less often proposed as therapeutic agents, though recently, particularly in the context of regenerative medicine, the concept of PG mimetics, 'neoproteoglycans', is becoming more familiar [3]. The development of PG- and GAG-based medicines is beginning to take into account the way the GAGs are organized and presented by attachment to their PG cores, as well as the sequences and covalent structures of the compounds themselves. In this special issue, contributed articles will cover the current pharmaceutical uses of GAGs and their mimetics, with others describing the involvement of GAGs in processes, such as cell growth and differentiation, morphogenesis, inflammation, and healing; all of which are likely to give rise to future therapeutic uses of GAGs and PGs.

2. Glycosaminoglycans

2.1. Structural Features

GAGs are linear and heterogeneous sulfated glycans. Although they are structurally complex, the backbones of these polysaccharides are simply made up of repeating disaccharide building blocks composed of alternating uronic acid (UA) and hexosamine units. The UA units can be either β-D-glucuronic acid (GlcA) or its C5 epimerized version, α-L-iduronic acid (IdoA). The amino sugars can be either glucose (Glc)-based (α-D- or β-D-glucosamine, GlcN) or galactose (Gal)-based, as N-acetyl-β-D-galactosamine (GalNAc). The permutation of these monosaccharide units within the GAG backbones gives rise to different GAG families, such as the GlcN-containing heparan sulfate (HS) and Hp [4,5], and the GalNAc-containing CS and dermatan sulfate (DS) [6]. Keratan sulfate (KS) alternates N-acetyl-glucosamine (GlcNAc) with Gal, and does not contain UA [7,8]; hyaluronan or hyaluronic acid (HA) alternates GlcNAc with GlcA, and does not have a protein core [9].

The disaccharides of HS and Hp are both composed of alternating 4-linked UA and 4-linked α-GlcN units [4,5]. Structurally, HS and Hp differ only in the relative proportions of their monosaccharide and disaccharide substructures. HS has β-D-GlcA as its major UA type while Hp has α-L-IdoA. GlcA in HS usually alternates with GlcNAc units, but lower amounts of N-sulfated glucosamine (GlcNS) and rare amounts of unsubstituted GlcN can also occur. Hp is conversely predominantly composed of 2-sulfated IdoA units (IdoA2S) together with N,6-di-sulfated GlcN units (GlcNS6S). These disaccharides are reflected in the three-dimensional structures of HS/Hp tetrasaccharides shown in Figure 1A,B. They are experimental structures from the Protein Databank (PDB), and clearly adopt fairly linear shapes, though in solution they may twist and fold to varying extents depending on the exact monosaccharide sequence [10].

Rarely, 3-O-sulfation at the GlcNS6S units can also occur (GlcNS3S6S) in both HS and Hp but is more common in the Hp chains; a pentasaccharide containing this unusual monosaccharide residue confers high affinity for antithrombin and, thereby, high anticoagulant activity, on Hp [1].

Since the length of GAG chains can vary widely, both among different GAG types and among chains of the same GAG type, the range of MWs in GAGs is very broad, ranging from a few kDa to over a hundred kDa. It is also true that manufacturing processes can alter the molecular weight (MW) of

GAGs; for example, unfractionated heparin (UFH) and low-molecular weight heparin (LMWH) have chains whose average MWs are respectively ~15 kDa (~25 disaccharide units) and less than 8 kDa (~12 disaccharide units or fewer). The measurement of MWs for LMWH is not straightforward, as Hp consists of a mixture of sequence types as described above, each occurring in domains with particular hydrodynamic and conformational properties. The contribution of Jian Liu and co-workers, introducing the concept of homogeneous structurally defined MW markers for Hp is a real step forward [11].

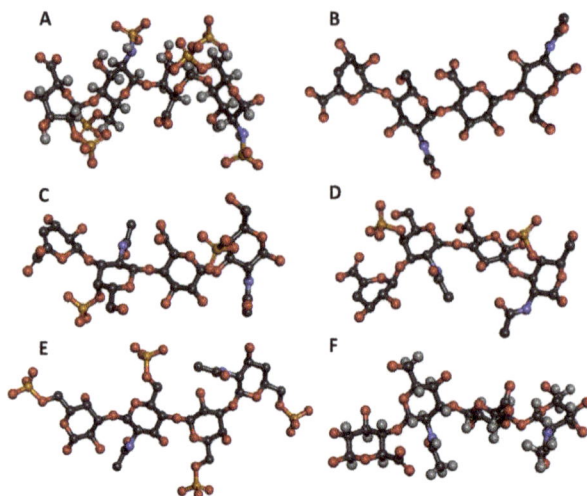

Figure 1.   Three-dimensional tetrasaccharide representations, taken from files in the PDB as indicated, of: (**A**) Heparin [IdoA2S(α1→4)GlcNS6S(α1→4)IdoA2S(α1→4)GlcNS6S] from 1HPN; (**B**) heparan sulfate [GlcA(β1→4)GlcNAc(α1→4)GlcA(β1→4)GlcNAc] from 3E7J; (**C**) chondroitin 4-sulfate [GlcA(β1→3)GalNAc4S(β1→4)GlcA(β1→3)GalNAc4S] from 1OFM; (**D**) dermatan sulfate [IdoA(α1→3)GalNAc4S(β1→4)IdoA(α1→3)GalNAc4S] from 1OFL; (**E**) keratan sulfate [Gal6S(β1→4)GlcNAc6S(β1→3)Gal6S(β1→4)GlcNAc6S] from 1KES; and (**F**) hyaluronan [GlcA(β1→3)GlcNAc(β1→4)GlcA(β1→3)GlcNAc] from 2BVK. The atoms in the ball-stick representations are carbon (grey), nitrogen (blue), hydrogen (light grey); oxygen (red) and sulfur (yellow). A and F are NMR solution structures, and non-exchangeable protons are shown; the others are crystal structures so are shown without protons.

CS disaccharides are essentially composed of alternating 4-linked β-D-GlcA and 3-linked GalNAc units. Various CS subtypes exist; for example, CS-A is mostly 4-sulfated at the GalNAc units (Figure 1C), while CS-C is predominantly 6-sulfated. CS-B, widely known as DS (Figure 1D), has α-L-IdoA units rather than β-D-GlcA. The IdoA units in DS may occasionally bear 2-sulfation while the GalNAc units are mostly 4-sulfated [6]. The MWs of CS-A, CS-B, and CS-C are around 20–60 kDa. Thus, approximately 35–130 disaccharide units for CS-A, CS-B, and CS-C calculated based on the MWs of their commonest disaccharide structures.

KS disaccharides are composed of alternating 3-linked β-D-Gal and 4-linked β-D-GlcNAc units [8]. These KS disaccharides can bear sulfation at the 6-position of either unit (Figure 1E), although sulfation at GlcNAc occurs more often [7,8]. The typical average MW of KS is around 20 kDa, thus, around 45 disaccharide units assuming the MW of the commonest structure. HA is the only GAG type which is not sulfated; it is composed of repeating disaccharide units of alternating 4-linked β-D-GlcA and 3-linked β-D-GlcNAc (Figure 1F) [9], and has the longest chain among all GAG types. The MW of HA is usually above 100 kDa and the degree of polymerization of HA is, therefore, in the range of at least

255 disaccharide units/chain, ranging upwards to MW of several million [12]. This very high MW polysaccharide has high viscosity at low concentration [12].

The structures of all these GAG families are represented in Figure 1. The GAG structural variations and heterogeneities associated with their high sulfation content (except HA) and their common occurrence at the extracellular matrix (ECM) or at the surface of cells are all contributing factors to the diversity of their biomedical roles because they give GAGs the capacity of binding to multiple extracellular proteins [13,14] whose actions are spread in various pathophysiological events (Figure 2).

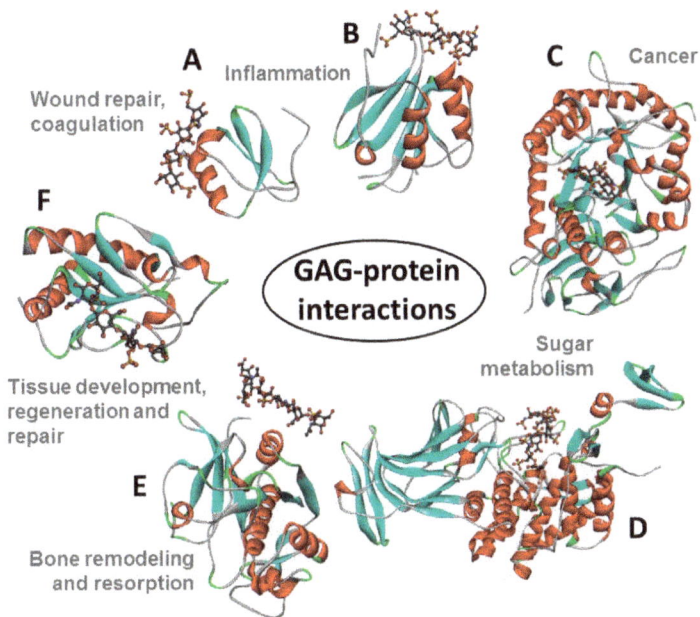

Figure 2. Structural representations from the crystal structures of some illustrative GAG-protein complexes in PDB: (**A**) macrophage inflammatory protein 1-alpha (CCL3) monomer + Hp 4-mer (from 5D65); (**B**) platelet factor 4 (CXCL4) dimer + fondaparinux (antithrombin-high affinity Hp 5-mer) (from 4R9W); (**C**) human heparanase complex + Hp tetrasaccharide (from 5E9C); (**D**) D-glucuronyl C5-epimerase + Hp 6-mer (from 4PXQ); (**E**) cathepsin K monomer + DS 6-mer (from 4N79); and (**F**) Sonic Hedgehog (Shh) monomer + CS-A 4-mer (from 4C4M). The atoms of the GAG ligands represented in the ball-stick view are carbon (grey), nitrogen (blue), hydrogen (light grey); oxygen (red) and sulfur (yellow). In the proteins, the alpha-helices, beta-sheets, loops, and random coils are represented, respectively, in red, blue, green and grey. The pathophysiological systems in which these complexes play a role are indicated by grey fonts in the panel.

2.2. Pharmaceutical Applications of GAGs and PGs

GAGs interact with proteins in many biological systems, and as a consequence they have numerous biological and therapeutic functions [15–21]. In fact, GAGs can be considered the most exploited carbohydrates in the pharmaceutical market [14]. The use of GAGs as therapeutic agents is dominated by the potent anticoagulant and antithrombotic GAG Hp [1], isolated from mast-cell rich tissues such as intestinal mucosa of pigs and cattle [22]. Hp is the by far the most widely used GAG type and perhaps the most common therapeutic carbohydrate worldwide [23]; it is used in treatments and prophylaxis of thromboembolic disorders [1,24,25]. The pharmaceutical analysis of Hp preparations is rarely simple; in this issue, a radical new approach to molecular weight measurements using synthetic calibrant and computational extrapolation [11] is proposed. The potent anticoagulant activity of Hp occasionally requires an antidote in clinical use. Hogwood and co-workers address the use of protamine to neutralize Hp from different species and tissues [26]. The heterogeneity of Hp, and other consequences of its origins as a natural mammalian product, has led to the development of synthetic and semi-synthetic Hp mimetics, as described by Mohamed and Coombe in this issue [27].

CS [2] and HA [28] are also exploited as pharmaceutical ingredients. CS can be used as an alternative therapeutic in cases of osteoarthritis [29], and sometimes even osteoporosis [30], because of its essential roles in cartilage and other connective tissues, though some degree of caution in interpretation of trials may be wise [30,31]. The beneficial use of CS in arthritic disease is usually associated with the use of GlcN, another key constituent of cartilage tissues. Santos and coworkers have in this issue described a systematic process based on electrophoresis, liquid-chromatography and NMR for assessment and control of pharmaceutical preparations of CS combined with GlcN [32]. KS can be employed as active ingredient in eye drops for treatment of certain visual dysfunctions; KS is one of principal functional components in cornea [7,8]. The best-known physicochemical property of HA is its capacity of forming gels in solution. This property enables HA to be used as a vehicle to make specific hydrogel formulations for regenerative medicine [33,34]. HA-based medium can be employed in cosmetics to soften and smooth skin owing to its inherent regenerative and hydrating properties; HA is an important functional component of the ECM of skin [35,36].

3. Proteoglycans

There are fewer than 50 distinct PG genes, though many more proteins due to alternative splicing [37]. Fewer than 20 distinct mammalian HS-PG core proteins have so far been identified [38]. This apparently limited repertoire of structures is responsible for numerous structural and functional properties of animal cells and ECM. Though many PGs are also glycoproteins, bearing N- and O-glycans, the defining type of glycosylation for PGs is the presence of one or more—sometimes many more—O-linked GAG chains. These GAGs make their contribution to the biological functions of PGs in many ways, and in some extreme cases the protein core may simply act as a scaffold for the presentation of the biologically-active GAG.

Most PGs act predominantly in the extracellular space, either as structural elements or as ligands for the many small protein growth factors, cytokines, chemokines, and morphogens that regulate embryonic development, inflammatory responses to pathogens and injury, and communication between cells [16,37]. PGs are often large proteins, heavily glycosylated and attached to membranes at the cell surface or in the ECM.

Descriptions of PGs have often used simple schematic diagrams, such as those shown in Figure 3 and in [39] depicting cartoon schematics for two major cell-surface PGs, syndecan, and glypican, and several PGs of the ECM (aggrecan and the small leucine rich PGs (SLRPs) such as decorin, lumican and biglycan). They are useful to show the rough relative sizes of PGs, with number and approximate attachment sites of GAG chains. These simple diagrams can give a clue as to function; where GAG chains are closely spaced they are likely to have a space-packing function, in the extracellular matrix in the case of aggrecan, and in the mast cell secretory granules in the case of serglycin. Where the GAG chains are less dense, such as on the cell surface attached to glypican or syndecan, their role is more likely to be in signaling, or in tissue organization. In this short article we will introduce only a few of the best known PGs; more comprehensive descriptions can be found elsewhere [37].

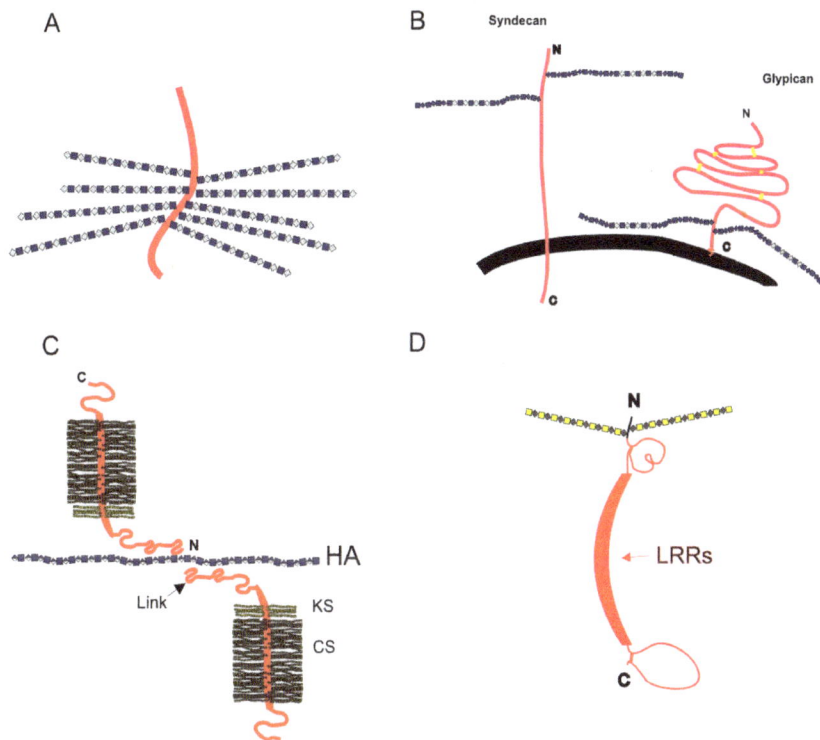

Figure 3. Schematic cartoon images (not to scale) for PGs on the cell surface and in the ECM. Protein chains are shown as red ribbons, and GAG chains are depicted in a simplified form of the symbology recommended by the Consortium for Structural Glycomics [40]; (**A**) the intracellular PG serglycin, bearing closely packed Hp (or oversulfated chondroitin) chains, on a small peptide core; (**B**) cell-surface PGs syndecan and glypican; the cell membrane is shown in black; (**C**) the complex between aggrecan and HA, mediated by Link protein, that forms the structural basis for cartilage elasticity; and (**D**) a generic diagram of a SLRP, such as biglycan or decorin. Between the globular regions near the N- and C-termini the leucine-rich repeats (LRRs) form a curved structure; the dimers can form by interaction between the two offset concave faces of monomers.

3.1. Intracellular Proteoglycans

The PG from which Hp is derived is called serglycin [41], and it is unusual as a PG in that it is found only in the granules of mast cells and related cell types, not, like other PGs, in the ECM or on the cell surface. The narrowly spaced Hp chains on the small peptide backbone of serglycin accommodate positively charged proteins, such as the proteolytic enzymes found in mast cell secretory granules, allowing much closer packing by neutralizing their charge [42]. Hp is partially depolymerized on degranulation of mast cells, to give the MW distributions characteristic of Hp sodium in clinical use [43]. Further deliberate depolymerization gives rise to the range of LMWH products, such as enoxaparin, described by Arnold et al. in this issue [11].

3.2. Cell Surface PGs: Syndecans and Glypicans

The cell-surface PG groups of glypicans are modulators of morphogens such as Wnt, bone morphogenetic proteins (BMPs), fibroblast growth factors (FGFs) and Sonic Hedgehog (Shh) [44]. There are six mammalian glypican genes, giving rise to core proteins glypican-1 to glypican-6, all of them attached to the outer surface of the cell membrane by a C-terminal glycosylphosphatidylinositol (GPI) anchor [44]. The 'cartoon' schematics shown in Figure 3 depict the glypicans as globular proteins, with an extended sequence containing HS attachment sites between the globular region of the protein and the GPI anchor [45]. The glypican-1 protein measures about 120 Å along its long axis [46], whereas a 50–100 residue long HS chain could extend to 200–400 Å. The HS attachment site is a few amino acid residues away from the globular protein core, with more than 50 amino acids between it and the GPI anchor, allowing considerable freedom in the orientation of protein and GAG [46], both of which may be available for interactions with extracellular proteins simultaneously.

By contrast, the four mammalian syndecans [45,47] hold their GAG side-chains out further from the cell surface, around 200 amino acids from the cell surface, though we have no information on the 3D structure of syndecan ectodomains. Syndecans have a transmembrane domain, and a cytodomain that interacts with kinases and the actin cytoskeleton [47].

Cell-surface GAGS attached to these PGs play a part in the early stages of viral invasion of the host cell. As an example, Kim and co-workers in this issue describe the recognition of cell surface GAGs by the envelope proteins of Flaviviruses, including dengue and yellow fever viruses [17]. In addition, viral carbohydrates are involved in interaction with the cell surface receptor dendritic cell-specific ICAM-grabbing non-integrin, DC-SIGN [17].

GAGs are also involved in the cell uptake of potentially useful drug-delivery systems. Takechi-Haraya and associates have in this issue described the contribution of GAGs in the non-endocytic direct cell membrane translocation of arginine-rich cell-penetrating peptides by studying the cell-permeation of octaarginine monitored through real-time in-cell ^{19}F NMR spectroscopy [21].

Damage to the cell surface glycocalyx, of which GAGs form an important part, is a feature of disease states of the vascular endothelium. Wodicka and coworkers have developed a PG mimetic designed to bind to inflamed endothelium and prevent platelet binding to create a more quiescent endothelial state [20].

3.3. Extracellular Matrix Proteoglycans

3.3.1. Aggrecan in the Extracellular Matrix

The most abundant PG in ECM rich tissues such as cartilage is aggrecan, which forms very large aggregates with HA, mediated by the link protein [18]. These aggregates are held in a collagen network to form strong but elastic articular cartilage structure, a target tissue for regenerative medicine due to the ubiquity of osteoarthritis in the aging population [18]. The close packing of CS chains attached to the aggrecan core gives the molecule a 'bottle-brush' appearance, not only in the simplified diagram in Figure 3C, but also in atomic force microscopy images [48].

3.3.2. Perlecan at the Basement Membrane

No 3D structure has been published for the large, multi-domain PG perlecan, found at the basement membrane and in the pericellular space. As an HS-bearing PG in the space between cells, perlecan can act as an extracellular storage device for growth factors such as FGFs and is involved in angiogenesis through its interactions with vascular endothelial growth factor (VEGF) [49].

3.3.3. Small Leucine-Rich Proteoglycans

The SLRPs exemplified by decorin have ordering functions in tissues; decorin in tendons appears to wrap round the D-band of collagen fibrils forming a ring-mesh of GAG [50]. SLRPs are also important for the structure of cornea, for which transparency requires an absolutely regular structure. The SLRP lumican is substituted with three *N*-linked KS chains [51] and its absence leads to a loss of order in the array of collagen fibrils, resulting in opacity of the cornea [52]. The importance of the SLRPs and their DS chains provides the focus of Mizumoto and coworkers, who, in this issue, have described mutations in human genes encoding the glycosyltransferases, epimerases, and sulfotransferases responsible for the biosynthesis of DS chains and their effects on connective tissue disorders, including some forms of Ehlers-Danlos syndrome [19].

4. The Context of Glycosaminoglycans, Proteoglycans, and Their Pharmaceutical Uses in the Special Issue *"Glycosaminoglycans and Proteoglycans"*

This special issue on *"Glycosaminoglycans and Proteoglycans"* contains a diverse collection of articles, illustrating the range of biological systems in which GAGs and PGs operate and can be considered in the design of pharmaceutical interventions. They range from the analysis of GAG pharmaceutical products [32] and Hp neutralization [26] through Hp mimetics [27], GAG-mediated uptake of cell penetrating peptides [21], to the development of PG mimics for endothelial repair [20]. Review articles cast a new light on regenerative medicine [18], chemokine-GAG interactions [16], the DS-PG related human genetic disorders, and Flavivirus interactions with host cells [17].

Some puzzles, vital to the progress of GAG and PG pharmaceuticals research, remain. The complex substitution patterns that GAGs are capable of displaying allow a remarkably large repertoire of structural motifs for recognition by proteins at the cell surface and between cells. We know that HS epitopes vary through processes of stem cell differentiation and embryonic development [18], and that the fine structure of GAGs adds to the intricacies of interactions between chemokines and their receptors [16]. We still, however, have no clear strategy to determine the exact preference of a protein for a specific sequence within a GAG polysaccharide chain, as we are hampered by a lack of experimental tools for the task. The development of synthetic GAG mimetics [27] may, in the future, offer libraries of homogenous GAG-like compounds that will allow detailed identification of protein ligand motifs within long GAG chains, leading to the possibility of the rational design of a whole new class of pharmaceuticals.

Conflicts of Interest: The authors declare no conflict of interest.

Vitor H. Pomin and Barbara Mulloy

Special Issue Editors

References

1. Mulloy, B.; Hogwood, J.; Gray, E.; Lever, R.; Page, C.P. Pharmacology of Heparin and Related Drugs. *Pharmacol. Rev.* **2016**, *68*, 76–141. [CrossRef] [PubMed]
2. Mantovani, V.; Maccari, F.; Volpi, N. Chondroitin Sulfate and Glucosamine as Disease Modifying Anti-Osteoarthritis Drugs (DMOADs). *Curr. Med. Chem.* **2016**, *23*, 1139–1151. [CrossRef] [PubMed]
3. Weyers, A.; Linhardt, R.J. Neoproteoglycans in tissue engineering. *FEBS J.* **2013**, *280*, 2511–2522. [CrossRef] [PubMed]
4. Sasisekharan, R.; Venkataraman, G. Heparin and heparan sulfate: Biosynthesis, structure and function. *Curr. Opin. Chem. Biol.* **2000**, *4*, 626–631. [CrossRef]
5. Rabenstein, D.L. Heparin and heparan sulfate: Structure and function. *Nat. Prod. Rep.* **2002**, *19*, 312–331. [CrossRef] [PubMed]
6. Sugahara, K.; Mikami, T.; Uyama, T.; Mizuguchi, S.; Nomura, K.; Kitagawa, H. Recent advances in the structural biology of chondroitin sulfate and dermatan sulfate. *Curr. Opin. Struct. Biol.* **2003**, *13*, 612–620. [CrossRef] [PubMed]
7. Pomin, V.H. Keratan sulfate: An up-to-date review. *Int. J. Biol. Macromol.* **2015**, *72*, 282–289. [CrossRef] [PubMed]
8. Funderburgh, J.L. Keratan sulfate: Structure, biosynthesis, and function. *Glycobiology* **2000**, *10*, 951–958. [CrossRef] [PubMed]
9. Almond, A. Hyaluronan. *Cell Mol. Life Sci.* **2007**, *64*, 1591–1596. [CrossRef] [PubMed]

10. Khan, S.; Fung, K.W.; Rodriguez, E.; Patel, R.; Gor, J.; Mulloy, B.; Perkins, S.J. The Solution Structure of Heparan Sulfate Differs from That of Heparin: Implications for Function. *J. Biol. Chem.* **2013**, *288*, 27737–27751. [CrossRef] [PubMed]

11. Arnold, K.M.; Capuzzi, S.J.; Xu, Y.; Muratov, E.N.; Carrick, K.; Szajek, A.Y.; Tropsha, A.; Liu, J. Modernization of Enoxaparin Molecular Weight Determination Using Homogeneous Standards. *Pharmaceuticals* **2017**, *10*, 66. [CrossRef] [PubMed]

12. Cowman, M.K.; Schmidt, T.A.; Raghavan, P.; Stecco, A. Viscoelastic Properties of Hyaluronan in Physiological Conditions. *F1000Research* **2015**, *4*, 622. [CrossRef] [PubMed]

13. Gandhi, N.S.; Mancera, R.L. The structure of glycosaminoglycans and their interactions with proteins. *Chem. Biol. Drug Des.* **2008**, *72*, 455–482. [CrossRef] [PubMed]

14. Pomin, V.H. A Dilemma in the Glycosaminoglycan-Based Therapy: Synthetic or Naturally Unique Molecules? *Med. Res. Rev.* **2015**, *35*, 1195–1219. [CrossRef] [PubMed]

15. Volpi, N. Therapeutic applications of glycosaminoglycans. *Curr. Med. Chem.* **2006**, *13*, 1799–1810. [CrossRef] [PubMed]

16. Proudfoot, A.E.I.; Johnson, Z.; Bonvin, P.; Handel, T.M. Glycosaminoglycan Interactions with Chemokines Add Complexity to a Complex System. *Pharmaceuticals* **2017**, *10*, 70. [CrossRef] [PubMed]

17. Kim, S.Y.; Li, B.; Linhardt, R.J. Pathogenesis and Inhibition of Flaviviruses from a Carbohydrate Perspective. *Pharmaceuticals* **2017**, *10*, 44. [CrossRef] [PubMed]

18. Ayerst, B.I.; Merry, C.L.R.; Day, A.J. The Good the Bad and the Ugly of Glycosaminoglycans in Tissue Engineering Applications. *Pharmaceuticals* **2017**, *10*, 54. [CrossRef] [PubMed]

19. Mizumoto, S.; Kosho, T.; Yamada, S.; Sugahara, K. Pathophysiological Significance of Dermatan Sulfate Proteoglycans Revealed by Human Genetic Disorders. *Pharmaceuticals* **2017**, *10*, 34. [CrossRef] [PubMed]

20. Wodicka, J.R.; Chambers, A.M.; Sangha, G.S.; Goergen, C.J.; Panitch, A. Development of a Glycosaminoglycan Derived, Selectin Targeting Anti-Adhesive Coating to Treat Endothelial Cell Dysfunction. *Pharmaceuticals* **2017**, *10*, 36. [CrossRef] [PubMed]

21. Takechi-Haraya, Y.; Aki, K.; Tohyama, Y.; Harano, Y.; Kawakami, T.; Saito, H.; Okamura, E. Glycosaminoglycan Binding and Non-Endocytic Membrane Translocation of Cell-Permeable Octaarginine Monitored by Real-Time In-Cell NMR Spectroscopy. *Pharmaceuticals* **2017**, *10*, 42. [CrossRef] [PubMed]

22. Tovar, A.M.; Santos, G.R.; Capille, N.V.; Piquet, A.A.; Glauser, B.F.; Pereira, M.S.; Vilanova, E.; Mourao, P.A. Structural and haemostatic features of pharmaceutical heparins from different animal sources: Challenges to define thresholds separating distinct drugs. *Sci. Rep.* **2016**, *6*, 35619. [CrossRef] [PubMed]

23. Pomin, V.H.; Mulloy, B. Current structural biology of the heparin interactome. *Curr. Opin. Struct. Biol.* **2015**, *34*, 17–25. [CrossRef] [PubMed]

24. Gresele, P.; Busti, C.; Paganelli, G. Heparin in the prophylaxis and treatment of venous thromboembolism and other thrombotic diseases. *Handb. Exp. Pharmacol.* **2012**, *207*, 179–209.

25. Hirsh, J.; Anand, S.S.; Halperin, J.L.; Fuster, V. Guide to anticoagulant therapy: Heparin: A statement for healthcare professionals from the American Heart Association. *Circulation* **2001**, *103*, 2994–3018. [CrossRef] [PubMed]

26. Hogwood, J.; Mulloy, B.; Gray, E. Precipitation and Neutralization of Heparin from Different Sources by Protamine Sulfate. *Pharmaceuticals* **2017**, *10*, 59. [CrossRef] [PubMed]

27. Mohamed, S.; Coombe, D.R. Heparin Mimetics: Their Therapeutic Potential. *Pharmaceuticals* **2017**, *10*, 78. [CrossRef] [PubMed]

28. Valachova, K.; Volpi, N.; Stern, R.; Soltes, L. Hyaluronan in Medical Practice. *Curr. Med. Chem.* **2016**, *23*, 3607–3617. [CrossRef] [PubMed]

29. Bishnoi, M.; Jain, A.; Hurkat, P.; Jain, S.K. Chondroitin sulphate: A focus on osteoarthritis. *Glycoconj. J.* **2016**, *33*, 693–705. [CrossRef] [PubMed]

30. Bruyere, O.; Cooper, C.; Pelletier, J.P.; Maheu, E.; Rannou, F.; Branco, J.; Luisa Brandi, M.; Kanis, J.A.; Altman, R.D.; Hochberg, M.C.; et al. A consensus statement on the European Society for Clinical and Economic Aspects of Osteoporosis and Osteoarthritis (ESCEO) algorithm for the management of knee osteoarthritis-From evidence-based medicine to the real-life setting. *Semin. Arthritis Rheum.* **2016**, *45*, S3–S11. [CrossRef] [PubMed]

31. McAlindon, T.E.; LaValley, M.P.; Gulin, J.P.; Felson, D.T. Glucosamine and chondroitin for treatment of osteoarthritis: A systematic quality assessment and meta-analysis. *JAMA* **2000**, *283*, 1469–1475. [CrossRef] [PubMed]

32. Santos, G.R.; Piquet, A.A.; Glauser, B.F.; Tovar, A.M.; Pereira, M.S.; Vilanova, E.; Mourao, P.A. Systematic Analysis of Pharmaceutical Preparations of Chondroitin Sulfate Combined with Glucosamine. *Pharmaceuticals* **2017**, *10*, 38. [CrossRef] [PubMed]

33. Burdick, J.A.; Prestwich, G.D. Hyaluronic acid hydrogels for biomedical applications. *Adv. Mater.* **2011**, *23*, H41–H56. [CrossRef] [PubMed]

34. Highley, C.B.; Prestwich, G.D.; Burdick, J.A. Recent advances in hyaluronic acid hydrogels for biomedical applications. *Curr. Opin. Biotechnol.* **2016**, *40*, 35–40. [CrossRef] [PubMed]

35. Juhlin, L. Hyaluronan in skin. *J. Intern. Med.* **1997**, *242*, 61–66. [CrossRef] [PubMed]

36. Anderegg, U.; Simon, J.C.; Averbeck, M. More than just a filler—The role of hyaluronan for skin homeostasis. *Exp. Dermatol.* **2014**, *23*, 295–303. [CrossRef] [PubMed]

37. Iozzo, R.V.; Schaefer, L. Proteoglycan form and function: A comprehensive nomenclature of proteoglycans. *Matrix Biol.* **2015**, *42*, 11–55. [CrossRef] [PubMed]

38. Lindahl, U. A personal voyage through the proteoglycan field. *Matrix Biol.* **2014**, *35*, 3–7. [CrossRef] [PubMed]

39. Lindahl, U.; Couchman, J.R.; Kimata, K.; Esko, J.D. Proteoglycans and Sulfated Glycosaminoglycans. In *Essentials of Glycobiology*, 3rd ed.; Varki, A., Cummings, R.D., Esko, J.D., Stanley, P., Hart, G.W., Aebi, M., Darvill, A.G., Kinoshita, T., Packer, N.H., Prestegard, J.H., et al., Eds.; Cold Spring Harbor Press: Cold Spring Harbor, NY, USA, 2015–2017.

40. Varki, A.; Kornfeld, S. Historical Background and Overview. In *Essentials of Glycobiology*, 3rd ed.; Varki, A., Cummings, R.D., Esko, J.D., Stanley, P., Hart, G.W., Aebi, M., Darvill, A.G., Kinoshita, T., Packer, N.H., Prestegard, J.H., et al., Eds.; Cold Spring Harbor Press: Cold Spring Harbor, NY, USA, 2015–2017.

41. Kolset, S.O.; Tveit, H. Serglycin–structure and biology. *Cell Mol. Life Sci.* **2008**, *65*, 1073–1085. [CrossRef] [PubMed]

42. Mulloy, B.; Lever, R.; Page, C.P. Mast cell glycosaminoglycans. *Glycoconj. J.* **2017**, *34*, 351–361. [CrossRef] [PubMed]

43. Mulloy, B.; Heath, A.; Shriver, Z.; Jameison, F.; Al-Hakim, A.; Morris, T.S.; Szajek, A.Y. USP compendial methods for analysis of heparin: Chromatographic determination of molecular weight distributions for heparin sodium. *Anal. Bioanal. Chem.* **2014**, *406*, 4815–4823. [CrossRef] [PubMed]

44. Fico, A.; Maina, F.; Dono, R. Fine-tuning of cell signaling by glypicans. *Cell. Mol. Life Sci.* **2011**, *68*, 923–929. [CrossRef] [PubMed]

45. Yoneda, A.; Lendorf, M.E.; Couchman, J.R.; Multhaupt, H.A.B. Breast and Ovarian Cancers: A survey and possible roles for the cell surface heparan sulfate proteoglycans. *J. Histochem. Cytochem.* **2012**, *60*, 9–21. [CrossRef] [PubMed]

46. Svensson, G.; Awad, W.; Hakansson, M.; Mani, K.; Logan, D.T. Crystal structure of N-glycosylated human glypican-1 core protein: Structure of two loops evolutionarily conserved in vertebrate glypican-1. *J. Biol. Chem.* **2012**, *287*, 14040–14051. [CrossRef] [PubMed]

47. Afratis, N.A.; Nikitovic, D.; Multhaupt, H.A.; Theocharis, A.D.; Couchman, J.R.; Karamanos, N.K. Syndecans - key regulators of cell signaling and biological functions. *FEBS J.* **2017**, *284*, 27–41. [CrossRef] [PubMed]

48. Ng, L.; Grodzinsky, A.J.; Patwari, P.; Sandy, J.; Plaas, A.; Ortiz, C. Individual cartilage aggrecan macromolecules and their constituent glycosaminoglycans visualized via atomic force microscopy. *J. Struct. Biol.* **2003**, *143*, 242–257. [CrossRef] [PubMed]

49. Whitelock, J.M.; Melrose, J.; Iozzo, R.V. Diverse cell signaling events modulated by perlecan. *Biochemistry* **2008**, *47*, 11174–11183. [CrossRef] [PubMed]

50. Watanabe, T.; Kametani, K.; Koyama, Y.I.; Suzuki, D.; Imamura, Y.; Takehana, K.; Hiramatsu, K. Ring-Mesh Model of Proteoglycan Glycosaminoglycan Chains in Tendon based on Three-dimensional Reconstruction by Focused Ion Beam Scanning Electron Microscopy. *J. Biol. Chem.* **2016**, *291*, 23704–23708. [CrossRef] [PubMed]

51. Dunlevy, J.R.; Neame, P.J.; Vergnes, J.P.; Hassell, J.R. Identification of the N-linked oligosaccharide sites in chick corneal lumican and keratocan that receive keratan sulfate. *J. Biol. Chem.* **1998**, *273*, 9615–9621. [CrossRef] [PubMed]

52. Amjadi, S.; Mai, K.; McCluskey, P.; Wakefield, D. The role of lumican in ocular disease. *ISRN Ophthalmol.* **2013**, *2013*, 632302. [CrossRef] [PubMed]

pharmaceuticals

MDPI

Review

Pathophysiological Significance of Dermatan Sulfate Proteoglycans Revealed by Human Genetic Disorders

Shuji Mizumoto [1,*], Tomoki Kosho [2], Shuhei Yamada [1] and Kazuyuki Sugahara [1,*]

[1] Department of Pathobiochemistry, Faculty of Pharmacy, Meijo University, 150 Yagotoyama, Tempaku-ku, Nagoya 468-8503, Japan; shuheiy@meijo-u.ac.jp
[2] Center for Medical Genetics, Shinshu University Hospital, 3-1-1 Asahi, Matsumoto, Nagano 390-8621, Japan; ktomoki@shinshu-u.ac.jp
* Correspondence: mizumoto@meijo-u.ac.jp (S.M.); k-sugar@sci.hokudai.ac.jp (K.S.); Tel.: +81-52-839-2652

Academic Editor: Barbara Mulloy
Received: 22 February 2017; Accepted: 24 March 2017; Published: 27 March 2017

Abstract: The indispensable roles of dermatan sulfate-proteoglycans (DS-PGs) have been demonstrated in various biological events including construction of the extracellular matrix and cell signaling through interactions with collagen and transforming growth factor-β, respectively. Defects in the core proteins of DS-PGs such as decorin and biglycan cause congenital stromal dystrophy of the cornea, spondyloepimetaphyseal dysplasia, and Meester-Loeys syndrome. Furthermore, mutations in human genes encoding the glycosyltransferases, epimerases, and sulfotransferases responsible for the biosynthesis of DS chains cause connective tissue disorders including Ehlers-Danlos syndrome and spondyloepimetaphyseal dysplasia with joint laxity characterized by skin hyperextensibility, joint hypermobility, and tissue fragility, and by severe skeletal disorders such as kyphoscoliosis, short trunk, dislocation, and joint laxity. Glycobiological approaches revealed that mutations in DS-biosynthetic enzymes cause reductions in enzymatic activities and in the amount of synthesized DS and also disrupt the formation of collagen bundles. This review focused on the growing number of glycobiological studies on recently reported genetic diseases caused by defects in the biosynthesis of DS and DS-PGs.

Keywords: biglycan; carbohydrate sulfotransferase 14; decorin; chondroitin sulfate; dermatan sulfate; dermatan sulfate epimerase; dermatan 4-*O*-sulfotransferase; Ehlers-Danlos syndrome; glycosaminoglycan; proteoglycan; spondyloepimetaphyseal dysplasia

---

1. Introduction

Dermatan sulfate (DS) is a linear polysaccharide that has been classified as a sulfated glycosaminoglycan, which is covalently attached to the core proteins of proteoglycans (PGs) [1–4]. PGs are widely distributed in extracellular matrices and at cell surfaces [1–4]. DS-PGs exist abundantly in skin, cartilage, and the aorta. Furthermore, they are ubiquitously expressed in various tissues such as brain, liver, lung, kidney and heart. DS chains consist of alternating disaccharide units comprising L-iduronic acid (IdoUA) and *N*-acetyl-D-galactosamine (GalNAc) residues with 50–200 repeats (Figure 1). DS chains are modified by sulfation at the C-2 and C-4 positions on IdoUA and GalNAc residues, respectively, which is a structural fundament to a wide range of biological events involving DS such as the assembly of extracellular matrices, signal transduction through binding to growth factors, wound healing, and anti-coagulation [2,3]. Chondroitin sulfate (CS) is composed of D-glucuronic acid (GlcUA) and GalNAc. After the synthesis of the chondroitin backbone, the GlcUA residue is epimerized to IdoUA by DS-epimerase (DSE). Thus, the content of IdoUA or DS is varied in each organ or developmental stage. CS-DS hybrid chains are also formed in specific cells and/or tissues.

Dermatan sulfate

Chondroitin sulfate

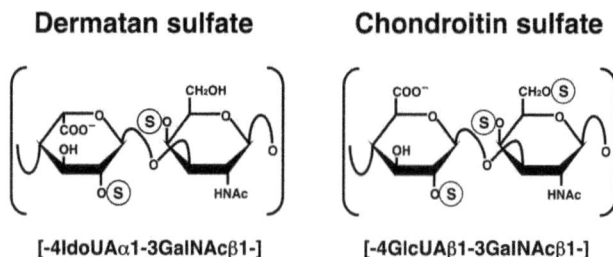

[-4IdoUAα1-3GalNAcβ1-]   [-4GlcUAβ1-3GalNAcβ1-]

Figure 1. Typical repeating disaccharide units in dermatan sulfate (DS) and chondroitin sulfate (CS), and their potential sulfation sites. The DS backbone consists of L-iduronic acid (IdoUA) and *N*-acetyl-D-galactosamine (GalNAc), whereas CS is a stereoisomer of DS that includes D-glucuronic acid (GlcUA) instead of IdoUA. These sugar moieties may be esterified by sulfate at various positions indicated by the circled 'S'.

The small leucine-rich DS-PGs, decorin, biglycan, and fibromodulin, contain leucine-rich regions and small protein cores [1]. The knockout mice of these PGs exhibit skin fragility, and osteoporosis in addition to collagen fibrils with irregular and rough outlines of the Achilles tendon, suggesting that DS-PGs play roles in the formation of skin and bone through the regulation of collagen [5–8]. Decorin core protein regulates the fibrogenesis of collagen [1]. The knockout mouse of decorin exhibited irregular collagen morphology and similar phenotypes of the human Ehlers-Danlos syndrome (EDS) [5]. In addition, the phenotypes of double-knockout mice of decorin and biglycan directly mimic the rare progeroid variant of the human EDS-like manifestation [9].

EDS is a heterogenous group of heritable connective tissue disorders characterized by skin hyperextensibility, joint hypermobility, and tissue fragility. EDS has been classified into six major types: The classical type (MIM#130000), hypermobility type (MIM#130020), vascular type (MIM#130050), kyphoscoliosis type (MIM#225400), arthrochalasia type (MIM#130060), and dermatospraxis type (MIM#225410) [10,11]. The dominant negative effects of a haploinsufficiency in the genes for the mutant procollagen α-chain or a deficiency in collagen-processing enzymes have been identified as the basis for these types of EDS [10]. Additional forms of EDS have also been reported in association with abnormalities in extracellular matrix proteins and DS [11,12].

This review focuses on DS-defective EDS, which was recently characterized from a glycobiological point of view in terms of disturbances in the biosynthesis of functional DS chains.

2. Biosynthesis of DS Chains

2.1. Glycosaminoglycan–Protein Linker Region

The repeating disaccharide regions of DS chains are attached to serine residues in core proteins through the common glycosaminoglycan–protein linker region tetrasaccharide, -O-xylose-galactose-galactose-GlcUA- (-O-Xyl-Gal-Gal-GlcUA-) (Figure 2) [1]. β-Xylosyltransferases (XylT), which is encoded by *XYLT1* or *XYLT2*, catalyze the transfer of a Xyl residue from uridine diphosphate (UDP)-Xyl to specific serine residues in the core proteins of PGs newly synthesized in the endoplasmic reticulum and cis-Golgi compartments, which initiates the biosynthesis of DS, CS, and heparan sulfate glycosaminoglycan chains (Figure 2) [13,14]. Two Gal residues are added to serine-O-Xyl in the core proteins from UDP-Gal by β1,4-galactosyltransferase-I (GalT-I) and β1,3-galactosyltransferase-II (GalT-II), which are encoded by *B4GALT7* and *B3GALT6*, respectively [15–17]. β1,3-Glucuronosyltransferase-I (GlcAT-I), which is encoded by *B3GAT3*, then transfers a GlcUA residue from UDP-GlcUA to serine-O-Xyl-Gal-Gal (Figure 2) [18].

2.2. Repeating Disaccharide Region of DS

The repeating disaccharide region in the chondroitin precursor chain, [-4GlcUAβ1-3GalNAcβ1-]$_n$, is constructed by chondroitin synthase family members (Figure 2) [19–24]. DSE, which is encoded by *DSE* or *DSE2*, subsequently converts GlcUA into IdoUA by epimerizing the C-5 OH group of GlcUA residues during or after the construction of a chondroitin backbone [25,26]. Dermatan chains are matured by sulfation reactions catalyzed by dermatan 4-*O*-sulfotransferase-1 (D4ST1) and uronosyl 2-*O*-sulfotransferase (UST), which are encoded by *CHST14* and *UST*, respectively. D4ST1 and UST transfer the sulfate group from the sulfate donor 3'-phosphoadenosine 5'-phosphosulfate to the C-4 position of GalNAc and C-2 position of IdoUA residues in dermatan, respectively [27–29].

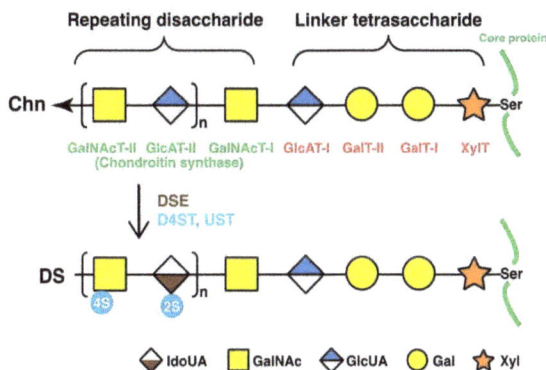

Figure 2. Biosynthetic assembly of DS chains by various glycosyltransferases, epimerases, and sulfotransferases. After specific core proteins are synthesized, the common glycosaminoglycan–protein linker region, GlcUAβ1-3Galβ1-3Galβ1-4Xylβ1-, is built up by XylT, GalT-I, GalT-II, and GlcAT-I on the specific serine (Ser) residue(s) of core proteins. These four groups of enzymes are common to the biosynthesis of glycosaminoglycans including DS, CS, and heparan sulfate. After the formation of the linker region, chondroitin synthases assemble the chondroitin backbone. Thereafter, the epimerization of some GlcUA residues and sulfation of each sugar residue are catalyzed by DSE and D4ST as well as UST, respectively. XylT, β-xylosyltransferase; GalT-I, β1,4-galactosyltransferase-I; GalT-II, β1,3-galactosyltransferase-II; GlcAT-I, β1,3-glucuronosyltransferase-I; GalNAcT-I, β1,4-*N*-acetylgalactosaminyltransferase-I; GlcAT-II, β1,3-glucuronosyltransferase-II; GalNAcT-II, β1,4-*N*-acetylgalactosaminyltransferase-II; DSE, dermatan sulfate epimerase; D4ST, dermatan 4-*O*-sulfotransferase; UST, uronosyl 2-*O*-sulfotransferase; Xyl, D-xylose; Gal, D-galactose; GlcUA, D-glucuronic acid; IdoUA, L-iduronic acid.

3. Human Disorders Affecting the Skeleton and Skin Caused by Disturbances in DS Biosynthetic Enzymes and DS-Proteoglycans

3.1. B4GALT7 (GalT-I) Deficiency

Mutations in *B4GALT7*, which encodes GalT-I, cause EDS-progeroid type 1 (Table 1, MIM#130070) [30–35]. The characteristics of EDS-progeroid type 1 include an aged appearance, developmental delays, a short stature, craniofacial dysmorphism, generalized osteopenia, defective wound healing, hypermobile joints, hypotonic muscles, and loose yet elastic skin [30–33]. GalT-I encoded by *B4GALT6* is responsible for the synthesis of the linkage region tetrasaccharide, -Xyl-Gal-Gal-GlcUA-, which is common to both CS/DS and heparan sulfate chains (Figure 2). Fibroblasts from patients with the compound heterozygous mutations of p.Ala186Asp/p.Leu206Pro in GalT-I showed weaker galactosyltransferase activity than that of control subjects, and synthesized de-glycanated decorin and biglycan core proteins in addition to their PG forms with shorter DS chains [33]. Furthermore, a homozygous mutation in *B4GALT7*, p.Arg270Cys, causes the same type of EDS, with patient fibroblasts exhibiting marked reductions in GalT-I activity in vitro and the lack of the DS side chain in 50% of decorin [33]. Fibroblasts with the mutation of p.Arg270Cys show reductions in the sulfation of heparan sulfate chains and the retardation of wound closure in vitro [35]. Thus, various clinical manifestations in EDS-progeroid type 1 may be partially caused by a lack of heparan sulfate as well as DS.

A variant of Larsen syndrome in Reunion Island in France is caused by a homozygous mutation in *B4GALT7* (p.Arg270Cys), and is characterized by multiple dislocations, dwarfism, distinctive facial features, and hyperlaxity [36]. The clinical manifestations of Larsen syndrome are congenital large-joint dislocations and characteristic craniofacial abnormalities including dislocations of the hip, elbow, and knee as well as foot deformities [37]. Therefore, EDS-progeroid type 1 and Larsen syndrome in Reunion Island may share clinical spectra including joint dislocations. However, the reason why these two disorders are caused by the same mutation in *B4GALT7* currently remains unclear. Further analyses are needed in order to elucidate the underlying pathogenic mechanisms.

3.2. B3GALT6 (GalT-II) Deficiency

Compound heterozygous mutations (p.Arg6Trp, p.Asp118Alafs*160, p.Met139Ala141del, p.Arg197Alafs*81, or p.Ser309Thr) in *B3GALT6* encoding GalT-II cause EDS-progeroid type 2 (Table 1, MIM#615349) [38]. The recombinant GalT-II mutant enzyme (p.Ser309Thr) exhibits significantly weaker GalT-II activity than that of the wild-type enzyme [38]. Furthermore, compound heterozygous or homozygous mutations (p.Met1?, p.Ser65Gly, p.Pro67Leu, p.Asp156Asn, p.Arg232Cys, and p.Cys300Ser) in *B3GALT6* cause an autosomal-recessive disorder, spondyloepimetaphyseal dysplasia with joint laxity type 1, which is characterized by kyphoscoliosis, clubfeet, hip dislocation, elbow contracture, platyspondyly, and craniofacial dysmorphisms including a small mandible with a cleft palate, prominent eyes, and a long upper lip (Table 1, MIM#271640) [38–40]. The skeletal and connective manifestations of EDS-progeroid type 2 and spondyloepimetaphyseal dysplasia with joint laxity type 1 largely overlap, whereas there are no common mutations in *B3GALT6* in these patients [38]. These findings suggest that the levels (amount) or length of glycosaminoglycan chains in patients with EDS-progeroid type 2 or spondyloepimetaphyseal dysplasia with joint laxity type 1 may differ, which gives rise to the number of clinical manifestations in these patients. The recombinant enzymes, p.Ser65Gly-, p.Pro67Leu-, p.Asp156Asn-, p.Arg232Cys-, and p.Cys300Ser-GalT-II exhibit significantly weaker galactosyltransferase activities than that of wild-type GalT-II [38]. Although wild-type GalT-II is expressed in the Golgi, mutant enzymes (p.Met1?, p.Ser65Gly, p.Pro67Leu, and p.Arg232Cys) are located in the cytoplasm and nucleus [38], indicating that the intracellular mislocalization of GalT-II may be partially or fully defective in glycosaminoglycan biosynthesis. Cultured lymphoblastoid cells from patients showed the reduced biosynthesis of heparan sulfate [38].

Malfait et al. identified homozygous missense mutations (p.Asp207His and p.Gly217Ser) and compound heterozygous mutations (p.Ala108Glyfs*163 and p.Asp207His) in *B3GALT6* in patients exhibiting various symptoms similar to those of EDS and spondyloepimetaphyseal dysplasia with joint hyperlaxity [39]. Cultured fibroblasts from the affected individuals synthesized markedly less DS and heparan sulfate. Beighton et al. reported that six patients with spondyloepimetaphyseal dysplasia with joint laxity from South African families had a homozygous missense mutation (p.Thr79Ala) and compound heterozygous mutations (p.Arg6Trp, p.Pro67Leu, or p.Thr79Ala) in *B3GALT6* [40]. Moreover, Alazami et al. detected a homozygous missense mutations (p.Phe186Lue and p.Arg179_Arg180dup) in patients with profound joint laxity, severe kyphoscoliosis, spondyloepimetaphyseal dysplasia, arthrogryposis, and joint dislocation [41].

These findings indicate that partial defects in DS, CS, and heparan sulfate due to mutations in *B3GALT6* affect the development of not only the skeleton, but also the skin with different or a wide range of symptoms in each patient.

4

Table 1. Human genetic disorders caused by defects in DS chains and core proteins of DS-PGs. B4GALT7, beta1,4-galactosyltransferase 7; B3GALT6, beta1,3-galactosyltransferase 6; DSE, dermatan sulfate epimerase; CHST14, carbohydrate sulfotransferase 14; UST, uronyl 2-sulfotransferase.

Enzymes and DS-PG Core Proteins	Coding Genes	MIM Number	Human Genetic Disorders	Clinical Features	Refs.
β4Galactosyltransferase-I (GalT-I)	B4GALT7	130070	Ehlers-Danlos syndrome progeroid type 1	Developmental delays, aged appearance, a short stature, craniofacial dysmorphism, and generalized osteopenia.	[30–36]
		604327	Larsen of Reunion Island syndrome	Multiple dislocations, hyperlaxity, dwarfism, and distinctive facial features.	
β3Galactosyltransferase-II (GalT-II)	B3GALT6	615349 615291	Ehlers-Danlos syndrome progeroid type 2	Sparse hair, wrinkled skin, defective wound healing with atrophic scars, osteopenia, and radial head dislocation.	[38–41]
		271640	Spondyloepimetaphyseal dysplasia with joint laxity type 1	Spatulate fingers with short nails, hip dislocation, elbow contracture, clubfeet, and mild craniofacial dysmorphism including prominent eyes, blue sclera, a long upper lip, and small mandible with a cleft palate.	
Dermatan sulfate epimerase	DSE	615539 605942	Ehlers-Danlos syndrome musculocontractural type 2	Characteristic facial features, congenital contracture of the thumbs and feet, hypermobility of the finger, elbow, and knee joints, atrophic scarring of the skin, and myopathy.	[42,43]
Dermatan 4-O-sulfotransferase	CHST14	601776 608429	Ehlers-Danlos syndrome musculocontractural type 1; EDS Kosho type; Adducted thumb-clubfoot syndrome	Craniofacial dysmorphism, multiple congenital contractures including adduction-flexion contracture of the thumbs and clubfeet, malformations of the heart, kidney, intestine, and eye; skin hyperextensibility, bruisability, and fragility with atrophic scars; recurrent joint dislocations, progressive foot or spinal deformities, pneumothorax, large subcutaneous hematomas, and diverticular perforation.	[41,43–58]
Uronosyl 2-O-sulfotransferase	UST	610752	Multiple congenital anomalies of the heart and central nervous system	Growth failure, congenital heart defect, underdeveloped cerebellar vermis, abnormal cutaneous elasticity, and joint laxity.	[59]
Decorin	DCN	610048 125255	Congenital stromal corneal dystrophy	Diffuse bilateral corneal clouding, corneal opacities, strabismus, nystagmus, photophobia, and esotropia.	[60–64]
		300106 301870	Spondyloepimetaphyseal dysplasia, X-linked	A short stature and osteoarthritic changes in joints; anomalies of the spine, and epiphyses and metaphyses of the long bones.	
Biglycan	BGN	300989	Meester-Loeys syndrome	Aortic aneurysm and dissection, hypertelorism, proptosis, downslanting palpebral fissures, frontal bossing, malar hypoplasia, pectus deformities, joint hypermobility or contracture, skin striae, a bifid uvula, cervical spine instability, ventricular dilation, hip dislocation, platyspondyly, phalangeal dysplasia, and dysplastic epiphyses of the long bones.	[65,66]

5

3.3. DSE Deficiency

A homozygous missense mutation in DSE (p.Ser268Leu) causes EDS musculocontractural type 2 (Table 1, MIM#615539) [42]. Clinical features including hypermobility of the finger, elbow, and knee joints, characteristic facial features, contracture of the thumbs and feet, and myopathy have been observed in a patient [42]. A marked reduction in the epimerase activity of the recombinant mutant DSE (p.Ser268Leu) as well as in the cell lysate from the patient has been demonstrated. Furthermore, a decrease in the biosynthesis of DS is accompanied by an increase in that of CS in the fibroblasts of patient [42]. Although the complete loss of DS from the fibroblasts of patients with *CHST14* mutations has been reported (see 3.4 *CHST14* deficiency) [46], a small amount of DS has been detected in fibroblasts from the DSE-deficient patient [42]. This finding suggests that the mutant enzyme, p.Ser268Leu-DSE, slightly residual enzymatic activity, or DSE2, which is a homologous protein to DSE in humans, partially synthesizes DS in the fibroblasts of patient.

Syx et al. reported another family with a homozygous DSE missense variant (p.Arg267Gly) [43]. The clinical manifestations of the two affected adult sisters showed craniofacial dysmorphic features, congenital clubfeet, long and slender fingers with contracture, muscle weakness, smooth, hyperextensible, and translucent skin, and the formation of large hematomas. No obvious alteration in the architecture of collagen fibrils was detected in DSE-deficient patients [43]. In contrast, CHST14-deficient patients show collagen bundles with collagen fibrils of various diameters, the intermittent presence of small flower-like fibrils, and irregular spaces filled with granulofilamentous deposits [43]. Thus, DSE-deficient patients may have a milder form of the EDS musculocontractural type than CHST14-deficient patients. However, difficulties are associated with describing the characterization due to the limited number of patients with mutations in DSE. Thus, the further characterization of DSE-deficient patients is needed in order to obtain a better understanding of this disorder.

The deficiencies associated with DSE affect the biosynthesis of DS, which implies that DSE and DS-PGs are both essential to the development of skin and bone as well as the maintenance of extracellular matrices in humans. $Dse^{-/-}$ mutant mice had fewer IdoUA residues in the skin and affected collagen fibrils [67]. Moreover, DSE appears to be more efficient at forming IdoUA blocks, which are characteristic of DS, than CS-DS hybrid structures, whereas DSE2 is more efficient at forming a CS-DS hybrid structure than IdoUA blocks [26]. These findings indicate that each function of DSE and DSE2 differs, and also that DSE2 may not be able to fully compensate for the loss-of-function observed in DSE.

3.4. CHST14 (D4ST1) Deficiency

Kosho et al. reported six unrelated Japanese patients with very similar features. They showed multiple congenital malformations, including craniofacial features such as a large fontanelle, hypertelorism, short and downslanting palpebral fissures, blue sclerae, a short nose with a hypoplastic columella, low-set and rotated ears, a high palate, long philtrum, thin upper lip vermilion, small mouth, and micro-retrognathia; multiple congenital contractures including adduction-flexion contracture and talipes equinovarus as well as other visceral or ophthalmological malformations. They also showed progressive multisystem fragility-related complications, including skin hyperextensibility, bruisability, and fragility with atrophic scars; recurrent dislocations; progressive talipes or spinal deformities; pneumothorax or pneumohemothorax; large subcutaneous hematomas; and diverticular perforation (Figure 3). These features are partially similar to those of EDS-kyphoscoliosis type VIA caused by a deficiency in lysyl hydroxylase (Table 1, MIM#601776) [44,45]. Homozygosity mapping of two independent consanguineous families revealed compound heterozygous mutations (p.Lys69*, p.Pro281Leu, p.Cys289Ser, or p.Tyr293Cys) or a homozygous mutation (p.Pro281Leu) in *CHST14*, which encodes D4ST1 [46]. Not only recombinant mutant D4ST1, but also fibroblasts from patients showed a marked reduction in D4ST activity [46]. CS chains, but not non-sulfated DS, have been produced on the decorin of fibroblasts from patients [46]. 4-O-Sulfation in CS and DS chains functions as an inhibitor of DSE [68]. Therefore, the defect in D4ST1 allows for a back-epimerization reaction converting IdoUA back to GlcUA to form chondroitin by DSE, followed by the 4-*O*-sulfation of GalNAc residues in chondroitin by C4ST. An aberrant reversed shift from the synthesis of DS to CS may affect the formation or maintenance of adequate collagen bundles in patients [46].

According to Dünder et al., mutations in *CHST14* cause an autosomal recessive disorder, adducted thumb-clubfoot syndrome (Table 1, MIM#601776) [47]. Three homozygous mutations, a 1-bp deletion (p.Val49*), two missense mutations (p.Arg213Pro and p.Tyr293Cys), and a compound heterozygous mutation (p.Arg135Gly and p.Leu137Gln), were found in *CHST14* in the three original adducted thumb-clubfoot syndrome families from Austria and Turkey as well as a consanguineous family from Japan [47]. The adducted thumb-clubfoot syndrome is characterized by adducted thumbs, clubfeet, craniofacial dysmorphism, arachnodactyly cryptorchidism, atrial septal defects, kidney defects, cranial ventricular enlargement, psychomotor retardation, thin and translucent skin, joint instability, and osteopenia from birth to early childhood [48,49]. Five out of eleven patients with the adducted thumb-clubfoot syndrome died in early infancy or childhood, suggesting that adducted thumb-clubfoot syndrome patients may have more severe manifestations than patients with the EDS-Kosho type. Malfait et al. previously reported that a homozygous deletion (p.Val49*) and homozygous 20-bp duplication (p.Glu334Glyfs*107) in *CHST14* from two Turkish siblings and an Indian patient, respectively, caused EDS-musculocontractural type 1 [50].

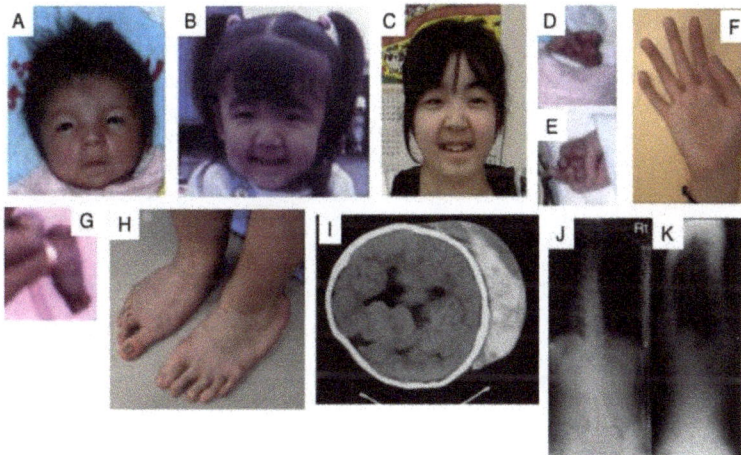

Figure 3. Clinical photographs of a patient with EDS caused by a carbohydrate sulfotransferase 14/dermatan 4-*O*-sulfotransferase-1 (CHST14/D4ST1) deficiency. Craniofacial features at the age of 23 days (**A**); three years (**B**); and 16 years (**C**) indicate hypertelorism; short and downslanting palpebral fissures, blue sclerae, a short nose with a hypoplastic columella, long philtrum, thin upper lip vermilion, small mouth, and micro-retrognathia at birth to early childhood. A slender and asymmetrical facial shape with a protruding jaw from adolescence is also observed. Congenital contracture of the fingers include adducted thumbs at 23 days (**D,E**); slender and cylindrical fingers and wrinkling palmar creases at 16 years (**F**); talipes equinovarus at birth (**G**); progressive foot deformities with talipes planus and valgus at 16 years (**H**); large subcutaneous hemtomas in a patient at the age of six years (**I**) and in another patient at the age of 16 years (**J**); kyphoscoliosis in a patient at the age of 16 years (**J, K**) (Figure (**I**) was reproduced from [44]; Figures (**A,B,D,E,G,J,K**) were reproduced from [45], with permission from Wiley-Liss, Inc., Hoboken, NJ, USA).

These disorders are currently considered to be a single clinical entity, with the proposed names 'D4ST1-deficient EDS' [51], 'EDS caused by a CHST14/D4ST1 deficiency' [12], or 'EDS, musculocontractural type 1' [50]. Forty patients from 27 families have been reported to date, including other mutations in *CHST14* (p.Arg29Glyfs*113, p.Gln133Argfs:14, p.Cys152Leufs*10, p.Phe209Ser, p.Arg218Ser, p.Gly228Leufs*13, p.Glu262Lys, p.Arg274Pro, p.Met280Leu, and pTrp327Cysfs*29) [11,12,41,43–58]. *CHST14* mutations cause a defect in DS side chains on the core protein, decorin, and affect the formation of collagen fibrils. Furthermore, DS side chains on other PGs such as biglycan, versican, epiphycan, endocan, and thrombomodulin may be affected by these mutations, which contribute to the wide range of the clinical manifestations of D4ST1-deficient EDS. Further analyses of the underlying molecular mechanisms may provide a clearer understanding of severe connective tissue disorders, and lead to the development of therapeutic approaches and agents.

$Chst14^{-/-}$ mice showed smaller body weights, kinked tails, more fragile skin, and lower fertility than wild-type mice [69]. Furthermore, the impaired proliferation of neural stem cells, reduced neurogenesis, and altered subpopulations of radial glial cells were observed in $Chst14^{-/-}$ mice [70]. These phenotypes are partially consistent with those of patients with D4ST1-deficient EDS. However, biochemical analyses such as the quantification of DS, characterization of DS-PGs, measurement of sulfotransferase activities, and pathological analyses of connective tissues including the skeleton and skin using $Chst14^{-/-}$ mice have yet be performed. Thus, pharmacotherapeutics for D4ST1-deficient EDS may be accelerated by further analyses using $Chst14^{-/-}$ mice.

3.5. UST Deficiency

A de novo 0.63 Mb deletion on chromosome 6q25.1 causes multiple congenital anomalies such as developmental delay, mild dysmorphic facial features, abnormally elastic and redundant skin, hyperextensible small joints, ventricular septal defect, and underdeveloped cerebellar vermis [59]. This region contains eight genes including *UST*, *TAB2*, and *LATS1*. TAB2 and LATS1 demonstrated to be essential for cardiac development and normal growth, respectively [71,72]. Thus, the patient with ventricular septal defect and developmental delay may be caused by defects in *TAB2* and *LATS1*, respectively. The characteristic joint and skin abnormalities were found in the patient, which are similar to the spectrum of those of the EDS. UST catalyzes the transfer a sulfate group from 3'-phosphoadenosine 5'-phosphosulfate to the C-2 position of IdoUA residues in DS chains [29]. Thus, the loss of *UST* gene may cause EDS-like symptoms.

3.6. DCN Deficiecny

Knockout mice of decorin exhibit the EDS-like phenotype [5]. Unexpectedly, mutations found to date in *DCN*, which encodes the decorin core protein, do not cause EDS. All mutations of *DCN* in human cause the truncated form of decorin core protein, resulting in the partial defects in functions of decorin. In fact, a congenital stromal dystrophy of the cornea (MIM#610048) is caused by heterozygous mutations (p.Pro314fs*14, p.Gly316Aspfs*12, p.Lys321Argfs*7, or p.Ser323fs*5,) in *DCN* [60–63]. Decorin, a prototype small leucine-rich proteoglycan, carries a DS side chain and plays roles in a number of cellular processes including collagen fibrillogenesis, wound repair, angiostasis, tumor growth, and autophagy [1–3,73]. This functional diversity may depend on interactions with various extracellular matrix components and growth factors through not only the core protein, but also the DS side chain of decorin. Congenital stromal corneal dystrophy is an autosomal dominant eye disease characterized by corneal clouding with fine opacities observed as small flakes and spots [60,61,64]. Furthermore, affected individuals show refractive errors, amblyopia, strabismus, nystagmus, and esotropia. Although the corneal epithelium and thin basement membrane are normal, not only normal, but also abnormal collagen fibrils have been detected in the stroma lamellae of patients [60–64,73]. The C-terminal truncation associated with mutations in the decorin of patients may affect the interaction with collagen in stroma, which is supported by structural informatics on decorin binding to collagen fibrils [63]. A mouse model of congenital stromal corneal dystrophy has been developed with a frameshift mutation in *DCN*, resulting in a C-terminal truncation lacking 33 amino acids [74]. Mutant mice show corneal opacities, abnormal fibril organization, and greater interfibrillar spaces and fibril diameters. Thus, truncated decorin may affect matrix assembly in the corneal stroma in a dominant-negative manner. Mellgren et al. have reported that that the knock-in mice with the truncated form of DCN exhibited a very low level in cornea, due to accumulation in the endoplasmic reticulum, whereas wild-type DCN was localized in Golgi [75]. Thus, it remains to be elucidated these differences of the phenotypes in both knock-in mice, and why only the corneal stroma is influenced by truncated decorin. The molecular composition of the corneal stroma is mainly type I collagen, which plays an important role in the maintenance of corneal transparency [76]. Therefore, the C-terminal domain of decorin may play roles in organ specific manner or function during the fibrillar organization of cornea.

$Dcn^{-/-}$ mice show skin fragility and an abnormal collagen morphology [5], which are similar to the symptoms of EDS. Thus, although defects in *DCN* may cause EDS, an EDS patient with a mutation in *DCN* has not been reported to date. Electron microscopic analyses revealed an abnormal morphology and organization of collagen fibrils in the periodontal ligament [77]. The number of periodontal ligament fibroblasts in $Dcn^{-/-}$ mice was reported to be higher than that in wild-type mice [77], suggesting that decorin regulates cell proliferation. Dcn/Bgn double knockout mice show severe skin fragility and marked osteopenia, which directly mimics the EDS-progeroid type [9], indicating the potential of this mouse to become a model for the EDS-progeroid type caused by mutations in *B4GALT7* and/or *B3GALT6*.

3.7. BGN Deficiency

Two missense mutations (p.Lys147Glu and p.Gly259Val) in *BGN*, which encodes biglycan, cause the X-linked form of spondyloepimetaphyseal dysplasia in Korean, Indian, and Italian families, and are characterized by anomalies of the spine as well as the epiphyses and metaphyses of the long bones, resulting in a short stature and osteoarthritic changes in joints [65] (Table 1, MIM#300106). A member of the small leucine-rich PGs, biglycan, is expressed in bones, and is essential to the assembly of the extracellular matrix and for cell signaling through interactions with type I collagen, transforming growth factor-β (TGFβ), bone morphogenetic protein 4, and Wnt [78–81]. Mutant proteins do not interact with TGFβ, as shown by an analysis of a molecular dynamics simulation [65]. In addition, the biglycan of fibroblasts from patients is degraded more rapidly than that from unaffected individuals [65]. These findings indicate that the identified variants, Lys147 and Gly259, are located in the leucine-rich region and their substitutions, p.Lys147Glu and p.Gly259Val, may affect decreases in biglycan stability and binding ability with TGFβ.

Meester et al. recently reported that thoracic aortic aneurysms and dissections are caused by mutations (p.Trp2* and p.Gln303Pro) or 21-kb and 28-kb deletions in *BGN* [66] (Table 1, MIM#300989). The clinical manifestation is characterized by the early-onset of aortic aneurysm and dissection, which involves the aortic root or more distal ascending aorta in all patients [66]. In addition, connective tissue features include joint hypermobility and contractures, deformities of skin striae and pectus, craniofacial dysmorphisms including dolichocephaly, hypertelorism, down-slanting eyes, a high-arched plate, proptosis, malar hypoplasia, and frontal bossing as well as the features of Loeys-Dietz syndrome (MIM#609192) such as a bifid uvula and cervical spine instability. Biglycan is not expressed in the aortic walls in affected individuals (p.Gly80Ser and 21-kb deletion). The disorder has been designated as Meester-Loeys syndrome (MIM#300989). The collagen content and elastin fibers in the aortic wall are lower in patients than in healthy controls. Furthermore, increased TGFβ signaling is observed in patients [66], which is similar to affected individuals with Loeys-Dietz syndrome caused by mutations in TGFβ signaling-related proteins such as TGFβ, the TGFβ receptor, and SMAD [82]. Biglycan has also been identified as a regulator of TGFβ signaling [79]. Thus, the clinical phenotypes of individuals with *BGN* mutations are similar to those with mutations in TGFβ-related genes.

BGN-deficient mice show a reduced growth rate and decreased bone mass [6]. A BGN deficiency promotes myofibroblast differentiation and proliferation, and this appears to be due to increased responses to TGFβ and SMAD2 signaling [83]. In addition, the aortas of *BGN*-deficient mice show structural abnormalities in collagen fibrils and reduced tensile strength [84], which indicate that biglycan, similar to decorin, is essential to the structural and functional integrity of the aortic wall through the regulation of collagen. These knockout mice may become models for spondyloepimetaphyseal dysplasia and Meester-Loeys syndrome in human *BGN* deficiencies, and may be helpful for developing therapeutic agents for these disorders.

4. Conclusions

Recent advances in genetic and glycobiological studies on connective tissue disorders have clarified the biological significance of DS side chains and the core proteins of DS-PGs. Thus, defects in the biosynthesis of DS and DS-PGs may affect the assembly of matrix proteins such as collagen and cell signaling through TGFβ during skeletal and skin formations; however, the underlying pathogenic mechanisms remain unclear. Furthermore, the clinical symptoms of DS-defective genetic disorders are not always similar to the different mutations in DS-biosynthetic enzymes. This number of phenotypes may be partially due to distinct residual functions including the enzymatic activities, cellular mislocalization, or partial compensation by other homologue(s) of each enzyme. A clearer understanding of molecular pathogeneses involving DS chains is essential for facilitating the development of therapeutics for these diseases.

Acknowledgments: This work was supported in part by a Grant-in-Aid for Young Scientists (B) 25860037 (to S.M.) and for Scientific Research (C) 16K08251 (to S.M.) from the Japan Society for the Promotion of Science, Japan; by a Grant-in-Aid for Challenging Scientific Research from the Research Institute of Meijo University (to S.M.); by the Nakatomi Foundation (to S.M.); and by the Practical Research Project for Rare/Intratable Diseases #105 from the Japan Agency for Medical Research and Development (AMED; 16ek0109105h0002) (to T.K., S.M., and S.Y.).

Author Contributions: S.M. wrote the manuscript. T.K., S.Y. and K.S. edited and elaborated on the manuscript.

Conflicts of Interest: The authors declare no conflict of interest.

References

1. Iozzo, R.V. Matrix proteoglycans: From molecular design to cellular function. *Annu. Rev. Biochem.* **1998**, *67*, 609–652. [CrossRef] [PubMed]
2. Neill, T.; Schaefer, L.; Iozzo, R.V. Decoding the matrix: Instructive roles of proteoglycan receptors. *Biochemistry* **2015**, *54*, 4583–4598. [CrossRef] [PubMed]
3. Trowbridge, J.M.; Gallo, R.L. Dermatan sulfate: New functions from an old glycosaminoglycan. *Glycobiology* **2002**, *12*, 117R–125R. [CrossRef] [PubMed]
4. Mizumoto, S.; Yamada, S.; Sugahara, K. Molecular interactions between chondroitin-dermatan sulfate and growth factors/receptors/matrix proteins. *Curr. Opin. Struct. Biol.* **2015**, *34*, 35–42. [CrossRef] [PubMed]
5. Danielson, K.G.; Baribault, H.; Holmes, D.F.; Graham, H.; Kadler, K.E.; Iozzo, R.V. Targeted disruption of decorin leads to abnormal collagen fibril morphology and skin fragility. *J. Cell Biol.* **1997**, *136*, 729–743. [CrossRef] [PubMed]
6. Xu, T.; Bianco, P.; Fisher, L.W.; Longenecker, G.; Smith, E.; Goldstein, S.; Bonadio, J.; Boskey, A.; Heegaard, A.M.; Sommer, B.; et al. Targeted disruption of the biglycan gene leads to an osteoporosis-like phenotype in mice. *Nat. Genet.* **1998**, *20*, 78–82. [CrossRef] [PubMed]
7. Svensson, L.; Aszódi, A.; Reinholt, F.P.; Fässler, R.; Heinegård, D.; Oldberg, A. Fibromodulin-null mice have abnormal collagen fibrils, tissue organization, and altered lumican deposition in tendon. *J. Biol. Chem.* **1999**, *274*, 9636–9647. [CrossRef] [PubMed]
8. Ameye, L.; Young, M.F. Mice deficient in small leucine-rich proteoglycans: novel in vivo models for osteoporosis, osteoarthritis, Ehlers-Danlos syndrome, muscular dystrophy, and corneal diseases. *Glycobiology* **2002**, *12*, 107R–116R. [CrossRef] [PubMed]
9. Corsi, A.; Xu, T.; Chen, X.D.; Boyde, A.; Liang, J.; Mankani, M.; Sommer, B.; Iozzo, R.V.; Eichstetter, I.; Robey, P.G.; et al. Phenotypic effects of biglycan deficiency are linked to collagen fibril abnormalities, are synergized by decorin deficiency, and mimic Ehlers-Danlos-like changes in bone and other connective tissues. *J. Bone Miner. Res.* **2002**, *17*, 1180–1189. [CrossRef] [PubMed]

10. Mao, J.R.; Bristow, J. The Ehlers-Danlos syndrome: On beyond collagens. *J. Clin. Investig.* **2001**, *107*, 1063–1069. [CrossRef] [PubMed]
11. Kosho, T. Discovery and delineation of dermatan 4-*O*-sulfotransferase-1 (D4ST1)-deficient Ehlers-Danlos syndrome. In *Current Genetics in Dermatology*; Oiso, N., Kawada, A., Eds.; InTech: Rijeka, Croatia, 2013; pp. 73–86.
12. Kosho, T. CHST14/D4ST1 deficiency: new form of Ehlers-Danlos syndrome. *Pediatr. Int.* **2016**, *58*, 88–99. [CrossRef] [PubMed]
13. Götting, C.; Kuhn, J.; Zahn, R.; Brinkmann, T.; Kleesiek, K. Molecular cloning and expression of Human UDP-D-xylose: Proteoglycan core protein β-D-xylosyltransferase and its first isoform XT-II. *J. Mol. Biol.* **2000**, *304*, 517–528. [CrossRef] [PubMed]
14. Pönighaus, C.; Ambrosius, M.; Casanova, J.C.; Prante, C.; Kuhn, J.; Esko, J.D.; Kleesiek, K.; Götting, C. Human xylosyltransferase II is involved in the biosynthesis of the uniform tetrasaccharide linkage region in chondroitin sulfate and heparan sulfate proteoglycans. *J. Biol. Chem.* **2007**, *282*, 5201–5206. [CrossRef] [PubMed]
15. Almeida, R.; Levery, S.B.; Mandel, U.; Kresse, H.; Schwientek, T.; Bennett, E.P.; Clausen, H. Cloning and expression of a proteoglycan UDP-galactose: β-xylose β1,4-galactosyltransferase I: A seventh member of the human β4-galactosyltransferase gene family. *J. Biol. Chem.* **1999**, *274*, 26165–26171. [CrossRef] [PubMed]
16. Okajima, T.; Yoshida, K.; Kondo, T.; Furukawa, K. Human homolog of *Caenorhabditis elegans sqv-3* gene is galactosyltransferase I involved in the biosynthesis of the glycosaminoglycan-protein linkage region of proteoglycans. *J. Biol. Chem.* **1999**, *274*, 22915–22918. [CrossRef] [PubMed]
17. Bai, X.; Zhou, D.; Brown, J.R.; Crawford, B.E.; Hennet, T.; Esko, J.D. Biosynthesis of the linkage region of glycosaminoglycans: Cloning and activity of galactosyltransferase II, the sixth member of the β1,3-galactosyltransferase family (β3GalT6). *J. Biol. Chem.* **2001**, *276*, 48189–48195. [PubMed]
18. Kitagawa, H.; Tone, Y.; Tamura, J.; Neumann, K.W.; Ogawa, T.; Oka, S.; Kawasaki, T.; Sugahara, K. Molecular cloning and expression of glucuronyltransferase I involved in the biosynthesis of the glycosaminoglycan-protein linkage region of proteoglycans. *J. Biol. Chem.* **1998**, *273*, 6615–6618. [CrossRef] [PubMed]
19. Kitagawa, H.; Uyama, T.; Sugahara, K. Molecular cloning and expression of a human chondroitin synthase. *J. Biol. Chem.* **2001**, *276*, 38721–38726. [CrossRef] [PubMed]
20. Kitagawa, H.; Izumikawa, T.; Uyama, T.; Sugahara, K. Molecular cloning of a chondroitin polymerizing factor that cooperates with chondroitin synthase for chondroitin polymerization. *J. Biol. Chem.* **2003**, *278*, 23666–23671. [CrossRef] [PubMed]
21. Izumikawa, T.; Uyama, T.; Okuura, Y.; Sugahara, K.; Kitagawa, H. Involvement of chondroitin sulfate synthase-3 (chondroitin synthase-2) in chondroitin polymerization through its interaction with chondroitin synthase-1 or chondroitin polymerizing factor. *Biochem. J.* **2007**, *403*, 545–552. [CrossRef] [PubMed]
22. Izumikawa, T.; Koike, T.; Shiozawa, S.; Sugahara, K.; Tamura, J.; Kitagawa, H. Identification of chondroitin sulfate glucuronyltransferase as chondroitin synthase-3 involved in chondroitin polymerization: Chondroitin polymerization is achieved by multiple enzyme complexes consisting of chondroitin synthase family members. *J. Biol. Chem.* **2008**, *283*, 11396–11406. [CrossRef] [PubMed]
23. Uyama, T.; Kitagawa, H.; Tamura, J.; Sugahara, K. Molecular cloning and expression of human chondroitin N-acetylgalactosaminyltransferase: The key enzyme for chain initiation and elongation of chondroitin/dermatan sulfate on the protein linkage region tetrasaccharide shared by heparin/heparan sulfate. *J. Biol. Chem.* **2002**, *277*, 8841–8846. [CrossRef] [PubMed]
24. Uyama, T.; Kitagawa, H.; Tanaka, J.; Tamura, J.; Ogawa, T.; Sugahara, K. Molecular cloning and expression of a second chondroitin N-acetylgalactosaminyltransferase involved in the initiation and elongation of chondroitin/dermatan sulfate. *J. Biol. Chem.* **2003**, *278*, 3072–3078. [CrossRef] [PubMed]
25. Maccarana, M.; Olander, B.; Malmström, J.; Tiedemann, K.; Aebersold, R.; Lindahl, U.; Li, J.P.; Malmström, A. Biosynthesis of dermatan sulfate: Chondroitin-glucuronate C5-epimerase is identical to SART2. *J. Biol. Chem.* **2006**, *281*, 11560–11568. [CrossRef] [PubMed]
26. Pacheco, B.; Malmström, A.; Maccarana, M. Two dermatan sulfate epimerases form iduronic acid domains in dermatan sulfate. *J. Biol. Chem.* **2009**, *284*, 9788–9795. [CrossRef] [PubMed]

27. Evers, M.R.; Xia, G.; Kang, H.G.; Schachner, M.; Baenziger, J.U. Molecular cloning and characterization of a dermatan-specific N-acetylgalactosamine 4-O-sulfotransferase. *J. Biol. Chem.* **2001**, *276*, 36344–36353. [CrossRef] [PubMed]
28. Mikami, T.; Mizumoto, S.; Kago, N.; Kitagawa, H.; Sugahara, K. Specificities of three distinct human chondroitin/dermatan N-acetylgalactosamine 4-O-sulfotransferases demonstrated using partially desulfated dermatan sulfate as an acceptor: Implication of differential roles in dermatan sulfate biosynthesis. *J. Biol. Chem.* **2003**, *278*, 36115–36127. [CrossRef] [PubMed]
29. Kobayashi, M.; Sugumaran, G.; Liu, J.; Shworak, N.W.; Silbert, J.E.; Rosenberg, R.D. Molecular cloning and characterization of a human uronyl 2-sulfotransferase that sulfates iduronyl and glucuronyl residues in dermatan/chondroitin sulfate. *J. Biol. Chem.* **1999**, *274*, 10474–10480. [CrossRef] [PubMed]
30. Quentin, E.; Gladen, A.; Rodén, L.; Kresse, H. A genetic defect in the biosynthesis of dermatan sulfate proteoglycan: Galactosyltransferase I deficiency in fibroblasts from a patient with a progeroid syndrome. *Proc. Natl. Acad. Sci. USA* **1990**, *87*, 1342–1346. [CrossRef] [PubMed]
31. Okajima, T.; Fukumoto, S.; Furukawa, K.; Urano, T.; Furukawa, K. Molecular basis for the progeroid variant of Ehlers-Danlos syndrome: Identification and characterization of two mutations in galactosyltransferase I gene. *J. Biol. Chem.* **1999**, *274*, 28841–28844. [CrossRef] [PubMed]
32. Faiyaz-Ul-Haque, M.; Zaidi, S.H.E.; Al-Ali, M.; Al-Mureikhi, M.S.; Kennedy, S.; Al-Thani, G.; Tsui, L.C.; Teebi, A.S. A novel missense mutation in the galactosyltransferase-I (B4GALT7) gene in a family exhibiting facioskeletal anomalies and Ehlers-Danlos syndrome resembling the progeroid type. *Am. J. Med. Genet. Part A* **2004**, *128*, 39–45. [CrossRef] [PubMed]
33. Seidler, D.G.; Faiyaz-Ul-Haque, M.; Hansen, U.; Yip, G.W.; Zaidi, S.H.; Teebi, A.S.; Kiesel, L.; Götte, M. Defective glycosylation of decorin and biglycan, altered collagen structure, and abnormal phenotype of the skin fibroblasts of an Ehlers-Danlos syndrome patient carrying the novel Arg270Cys substitution in galactosyltransferase I (β4GalT-7). *J. Mol. Med. (Berl.)* **2006**, *84*, 583–594. [CrossRef] [PubMed]
34. Götte, M.; Kresse, H. Defective glycosaminoglycan substitution of decorin in a patient with progeroid syndrome is a direct consequence of two point mutations in the galactosyltransferase I (β4GalT-7) gene. *Biochem. Genet.* **2005**, *43*, 65–77. [CrossRef] [PubMed]
35. Götte, M.; Spillmann, D.; Yip, G.W.; Versteeg, E.; Echtermeyer, F.G.; van Kuppevelt, T.H.; Kiesel, L. Changes in heparan sulfate are associated with delayed wound repair, altered cell migration, adhesion and contractility in the galactosyltransferase I (β4GalT-7) deficient form of Ehlers-Danlos syndrome. *Hum. Mol. Genet.* **2008**, *17*, 996–1009. [CrossRef] [PubMed]
36. Cartault, F.; Munier, P.; Jacquemont, M.L.; Vellayoudom, J.; Doray, B.; Payet, C.; Randrianaivo, H.; Laville, J.M.; Munnich, A.; Cormier-Daire, V. Expanding the clinical spectrum of B4GALT7 deficiency: Homozygous p.R270C mutation with founder effect causes Larsen of Reunion Island syndrome. *Eur. J. Hum. Genet.* **2015**, *23*, 49–53. [CrossRef] [PubMed]
37. Larsen, L.J.; Schottstaedt, E.R.; Bost, F.C. Multiple congenital dislocations associated with characteristic facial abnormality. *J. Pediatr.* **1950**, *37*, 574–581. [CrossRef]
38. Nakajima, M.; Mizumoto, S.; Miyake, N.; Kogawa, R.; Iida, A.; Ito, H.; Kitoh, H.; Hirayama, A.; Mitsubuchi, H.; Miyazaki, O.; et al. Mutations in *B3GALT6*, which encodes a glycosaminoglycan linker region enzyme, cause a spectrum of skeletal and connective tissue disorders. *Am. J. Hum. Genet.* **2013**, *92*, 927–934. [CrossRef] [PubMed]
39. Malfait, F.; Kariminejad, A.; Van Damme, T.; Gauche, C.; Syx, D.; Merhi-Soussi, F.; Gulberti, S.; Symoens, S.; Vanhauwaert, S.; Willaert, A.; et al. A. Defective initiation of glycosaminoglycan synthesis due to *B3GALT6* mutations causes a pleiotropic Ehlers-Danlos-syndrome-like connective tissue disorder. *Am. J. Hum. Genet.* **2013**, *92*, 935–945. [CrossRef] [PubMed]
40. Vorster, A.A.; Beighton, P.; Ramesar, R.S. Spondyloepimetaphyseal dysplasia with joint laxity (Beighton type): Mutation analysis in 8 affected South African families. *Clin. Genet.* **2015**, *87*, 492–495. [CrossRef] [PubMed]
41. Alazami, A.M.; Al-Qattan, S.M.; Faqeih, E.; Alhashem, A.; Alshammari, M.; Alzahrani, F.; Al-Dosari, M.S.; Patel, N.; Alsagheir, A.; Binabbas, B.; et al. Expanding the clinical and genetic heterogeneity of hereditary disorders of connective tissue. *Hum. Genet.* **2016**, *135*, 525–540. [CrossRef] [PubMed]
42. Müller, T.; Mizumoto, S.; Suresh, I.; Komatsu, Y.; Vodopiutz, J.; Dundar, M.; Straub, V.; Lingenhel, A.; Melmer, A.; Lechner, S.; et al. Loss of dermatan sulfate epimerase (DSE) function results in musculocontractural Ehlers-Danlos syndrome. *Hum. Mol. Genet.* **2013**, *22*, 3761–3772. [CrossRef] [PubMed]

43. Syx, D.; Van Damme, T.; Symoens, S.; Maiburg, M.C.; van de Laar, I.; Morton, J.; Suri, M.; Del Campo, M.; Hausser, I.; Hermanns-Lê, T.; et al. Genetic heterogeneity and clinical variability in musculocontractural Ehlers-Danlos syndrome caused by impaired dermatan sulfate biosynthesis. *Hum. Mutat.* **2015**, *36*, 535–547. [CrossRef] [PubMed]

44. Kosho, T.; Takahashi, J.; Ohashi, H.; Nishimura, G.; Kato, H.; Fukushima, Y. Ehlers-Danlos syndrome type VIB with characteristic facies, decreased curvatures of the spinal column, and joint contractures in two unrelated girls. *Am. J. Med. Genet. Part A* **2005**, *138*, 282–287. [CrossRef] [PubMed]

45. Kosho, T.; Miyake, N.; Hatamochi, A.; Takahashi, J.; Kato, H.; Miyahara, T.; Igawa, Y.; Yasui, H.; Ishida, T.; Ono, K.; et al. A new Ehlers-Danlos syndrome with craniofacial characteristics, multiple congenital contractures, progressive joint and skin laxity, and multisystem fragility-related manifestations. *Am. J. Med. Genet. Part A* **2010**, *152*, 1333–1346. [CrossRef] [PubMed]

46. Miyake, N.; Kosho, T.; Mizumoto, S.; Furuichi, T.; Hatamochi, A.; Nagashima, Y.; Arai, E.; Takahashi, K.; Kawamura, R.; Wakui, K.; et al. Loss-of-function mutations of *CHST14* in a new type of Ehlers-Danlos syndrome. *Hum. Mutat.* **2010**, *31*, 966–974. [CrossRef] [PubMed]

47. Dündar, M.; Müller, T.; Zhang, Q.; Pan, J.; Steinmann, B.; Vodopiutz, J.; Gruber, R.; Sonoda, T.; Krabichler, B.; Utermann, G.; et al. Loss of dermatan-4-sulfotransferase 1 function results in adducted thumb-clubfoot syndrome. *Am. J. Hum. Genet.* **2009**, *85*, 873–882. [CrossRef] [PubMed]

48. Dundar, M.; Demiryilmaz, F.; Demiryilmaz, I.; Kumandas, S.; Erkilic, K.; Kendirci, M.; Tuncel, M.; Ozyazgan, I.; Tolmie, J.L. An autosomal recessive adducted thumb-club foot syndrome observed in Turkish cousins. *Clin. Genet.* **1997**, *51*, 61–64. [CrossRef] [PubMed]

49. Sonoda, T.; Kouno, K. Two brothers with distal arthrogryposis, peculiar facial appearance, cleft palate, short stature, hydronephrosis, retentio testis, and normal intelligence: A new type of distal arthrogryposis? *Am. J. Med. Genet.* **2000**, *91*, 280–285. [CrossRef]

50. Malfait, F.; Syx, D.; Vlummens, P.; Symoens, S.; Nampoothiri, S.; Hermanns-Lê, T.; Van Laer, L.; De Paepe, A. Musculocontractural Ehlers-Danlos Syndrome (former EDS type VIB) and adducted thumb clubfoot syndrome (ATCS) represent a single clinical entity caused by mutations in the dermatan-4-sulfotransferase 1 encoding *CHST14* gene. *Hum. Mutat.* **2010**, *31*, 1233–1239. [CrossRef] [PubMed]

51. Kosho, T.; Miyake, N.; Mizumoto, S.; Hatamochi, A.; Fukushima, Y.; Yamada, S.; Sugahara, K.; Matsumoto, N. A response to: loss of dermatan-4-sulfotransferase 1 (D4ST1/CHST14) function represents the first dermatan sulfate biosynthesis defect, "dermatan sulfate-deficient Adducted Thumb-Clubfoot Syndrome". Which name is appropriate, "Adducted Thumb-Clubfoot Syndrome" or "Ehlers-Danlos syndrome?". *Hum. Mutat.* **2011**, *32*, 1507–1509. [PubMed]

52. Shimizu, K.; Okamoto, N.; Miyake, N.; Taira, K.; Sato, Y.; Matsuda, K.; Akimaru, N.; Ohashi, H.; Wakui, K.; Fukushima, Y.; et al. Delineation of dermatan 4-O-sulfotransferase 1 deficient Ehlers-Danlos syndrome: observation of two additional patients and comprehensive review of 20 reported patients. *Am. J. Med. Genet. Part A* **2011**, *155*, 1949–1958. [CrossRef] [PubMed]

53. Mendoza-Londono, R.; Chitayat, D.; Kahr, W.H.; Hinek, A.; Blaser, S.; Dupuis, L.; Goh, E.; Badilla-Porras, R.; Howard, A.; Mittaz, L.; et al. Extracellular matrix and platelet function in patients with musculocontractural Ehlers-Danlos syndrome caused by mutations in the CHST14 gene. *Am. J. Med. Genet. Part A* **2012**, *158*, 1344–1354. [CrossRef] [PubMed]

54. Voermans, N.C.; Kempers, M.; Lammens, M.; van Alfen, N.; Janssen, M.C.; Bönnemann, C.; van Engelen, B.G.; Hamel, B.C. Myopathy in a 20-year-old female patient with D4ST-1 deficient Ehlers-Danlos syndrome due to a homozygous CHST14 mutation. *Am. J. Med. Genet. Part A* **2012**, *158*, 850–855. [CrossRef] [PubMed]

55. Winters, K.A.; Jiang, Z.; Xu, W.; Li, S.; Ammous, Z.; Jayakar, P.; Wierenga, K.J. Re-assigned diagnosis of D4ST1-deficient Ehlers-Danlos syndrome (adducted thumb-clubfoot syndrome) after initial diagnosis of Marden-Walker syndrome. *Am. J. Med. Genet. Part A* **2012**, *158*, 2935–2940. [CrossRef] [PubMed]

56. Janecke, A.R.; Li, B.; Boehm, M.; Krabichler, B.; Rohrbach, M.; Müller, T.; Fuchs, I.; Golas, G.; Katagiri, Y.; Ziegler, S.G.; et al. The phenotype of the musculocontractural type of Ehlers-Danlos syndrome due to CHST14 mutations. *Am. J. Med. Genet. Part A* **2016**, *170*, 103–115. [CrossRef] [PubMed]

57. Kono, M.; Hasegawa-Murakami, Y.; Sugiura, K.; Ono, M.; Toriyama, K.; Miyake, N.; Hatamochi, A.; Kamei, Y.; Kosho, T.; Akiyama, M. A 45-year-old woman with Ehlers-Danlos syndrome caused by dermatan 4-O-sulfotransferase-1 deficiency: Implications for early ageing. *Acta Derm. Venereol.* **2016**, *96*, 830–831. [CrossRef] [PubMed]

58. Mochida, K.; Amano, M.; Miyake, N.; Matsumoto, N.; Hatamochi, A.; Kosho, T. Dermatan 4-O-sulfotransferase 1-deficient Ehlers-Danlos syndrome complicated by a large subcutaneous hematoma on the back. *J. Dermatol.* **2016**, *43*, 832–833. [CrossRef] [PubMed]

59. Salpietro, V.; Ruggieri, M.; Mankad, K.; Di Rosa, G.; Granata, F.; Loddo, I.; Moschella, E.; Calabro, M.P.; Capalbo, A.; Bernardini, L.; et al. A de novo 0.63 Mb 6q25.1 deletion associated with growth failure, congenital heart defect, underdeveloped cerebellar vermis, abnormal cutaneous elasticity and joint laxity. *Am. J. Med. Genet. Part A* **2015**, *167*, 2042–2051. [CrossRef] [PubMed]

60. Bredrup, C.; Knappskog, P.M.; Majewski, J.; Rodahl, E.; Boman, H. Congenital stromal dystrophy of the cornea caused by a mutation in the decorin gene. *Investig. Ophthalmol. Vis. Sci.* **2005**, *46*, 420–426. [CrossRef] [PubMed]

61. Rodahl, E.; Van Ginderdeuren, R.; Knappskog, P.M.; Bredrup, C.; Boman, H. A second decorin frame shift mutation in a family with congenital stromal corneal dystrophy. *Am. J. Ophthalmol.* **2006**, *142*, 520–521. [CrossRef] [PubMed]

62. Kim, J.; Ko, J.M.; Lee, I.; Kim, J.Y.; Kim, M.J.; Tchah, H. A novel mutation of the decorin gene identified in a Korean family with congenital hereditary stromal dystrophy. *Cornea* **2011**, *30*, 1473–1477. [CrossRef] [PubMed]

63. Jing, Y.; Kumar, P.R.; Zhu, L.; Edward, D.P.; Tao, S.; Wang, L.; Chuck, R.; Zhang, C. Novel decorin mutation in a Chinese family with congenital stromal corneal dystrophy. *Cornea* **2014**, *33*, 288–293. [CrossRef] [PubMed]

64. Van Ginderdeuren, R.; De Vos, R.; Casteels, I.; Foets, B. Report of a new family with dominant congenital heredity stromal dystrophy of the cornea. *Cornea* **2002**, *21*, 118–120. [CrossRef] [PubMed]

65. Cho, S.Y.; Bae, J.S.; Kim, N.K.; Forzano, F.; Girisha, K.M.; Baldo, C.; Faravelli, F.; Cho, T.J.; Kim, D.; Lee, K.Y.; et al. BGN mutations in X-linked spondyloepimetaphyseal dysplasia. *Am. J. Hum. Genet.* **2016**, *98*, 1243–1248. [CrossRef] [PubMed]

66. Meester, J.A.; Vandeweyer, G.; Pintelon, I.; Lammens, M.; Van Hoorick, L.; De Belder, S.; Waitzman, K.; Young, L.; Markham, L.W.; Vogt, J.; et al. Loss-of-function mutations in the X-linked biglycan gene cause a severe syndromic form of thoracic aortic aneurysms and dissections. *Genet. Med.* **2016**. [CrossRef] [PubMed]

67. Maccarana, M.; Kalamajski, S.; Kongsgaard, M.; Magnusson, S.P.; Oldberg, A.; Malmström, A. Dermatan sulfate epimerase 1-deficient mice have reduced content and changed distribution of iduronic acids in dermatan sulfate and an altered collagen structure in skin. *Mol. Cell. Biol.* **2009**, *29*, 5517–5528. [CrossRef] [PubMed]

68. Malmström, A. Biosynthesis of dermatan sulfate. II. Substrate specificity of the C-5 uronosyl epimerase. *J. Biol. Chem.* **1984**, *259*, 161–165. [PubMed]

69. Akyüz, N.; Rost, S.; Mehanna, A.; Bian, S.; Loers, G.; Oezen, I.; Mishra, B.; Hoffmann, K.; Guseva, D.; Laczynska, E.; et al. Dermatan 4-O-sulfotransferase1 ablation accelerates peripheral nerve regeneration. *Exp. Neurol.* **2013**, *247*, 517–530. [CrossRef] [PubMed]

70. Bian, S.; Akyüz, N.; Bernreuther, C.; Loers, G.; Laczynska, E.; Jakovcevski, I.; Schachner, M. Dermatan sulfotransferase Chst14/d4st1, but not chondroitin sulfotransferase Chst11/C4st1, regulates proliferation and neurogenesis of neural progenitor cells. *J. Cell Sci.* **2011**, *124*, 4051–4063. [CrossRef] [PubMed]

71. Thienpont, B.; Zhang, L.; Postma, A.V.; Breckpot, J.; Tranchevent, L.C.; Van Loo, P.; Møllgård, K.; Tommerup, N.; Bache, I.; Tümer, Z.; et al. Haploinsufficiency of TAB2 causes congenital heart defects in humans. *Am. J. Hum. Genet.* **2010**, *86*, 839–849. [CrossRef] [PubMed]

72. St John, M.A.; Tao, W.; Fei, X.; Fukumoto, R.; Carcangiu, M.L.; Brownstein, D.G.; Parlow, A.F.; McGrath, J.; Xu, T. Mice deficient of Lats1 develop soft-tissue sarcomas, ovarian tumours and pituitary dysfunction. *Nat. Genet.* **1999**, *21*, 182–186. [PubMed]

73. Gubbiotti, M.A.; Vallet, S.D.; Ricard-Blum, S.; Iozzo, R.V. Decorin interacting network: A comprehensive analysis of decorin-binding partners and their versatile functions. *Matrix Biol.* **2016**, *55*, 7–21. [CrossRef] [PubMed]

74. Chen, S.; Sun, M.; Meng, X.; Iozzo, R.V.; Kao, W.W.; Birk, D.E. Pathophysiological mechanisms of autosomal dominant congenital stromal corneal dystrophy: C-terminal-truncated decorin results in abnormal matrix assembly and altered expression of small leucine-rich proteoglycans. *Am. J. Pathol.* **2011**, *179*, 2409–2419. [CrossRef] [PubMed]

75. Mellgren, A.E.; Bruland, O.; Vedeler, A.; Saraste, J.; Schönheit, J.; Bredrup, C.; Knappskog, P.M.; Rødahl, E. Development of congenital stromal corneal dystrophy is dependent on export and extracellular deposition of truncated decorin. *Investig. Ophthalmol. Vis. Sci.* **2015**, *56*, 2909–2915. [CrossRef] [PubMed]
76. Massoudi, D.; Malecaze, F.; Galiacy, S.D. Collagens and proteoglycans of the cornea: importance in transparency and visual disorders. *Cell Tissue Res.* **2016**, *363*, 337–349. [CrossRef] [PubMed]
77. Häkkinen, L.; Strassburger, S.; Kähäri, V.M.; Scott, P.G.; Eichstetter, I.; Lozzo, R.V.; Larjava, H. A role for decorin in the structural organization of periodontal ligament. *Lab. Investig.* **2000**, *80*, 1869–1880. [CrossRef] [PubMed]
78. Schönherr, E.; Witsch-Prehm, P.; Harrach, B.; Robenek, H.; Rauterberg, J.; Kresse, H. Interaction of biglycan with type I collagen. *J. Biol. Chem.* **1995**, *270*, 2776–2783. [CrossRef] [PubMed]
79. Hildebrand, A.; Romarís, M.; Rasmussen, L.M.; Heinegård, D.; Twardzik, D.R.; Border, W.A.; Ruoslahti, E. Interaction of the small interstitial proteoglycans biglycan, decorin and fibromodulin with transforming growth factor beta. *Biochem. J.* **1994**, *302*, 527–534. [CrossRef] [PubMed]
80. Chen, X.D.; Fisher, L.W.; Robey, P.G.; Young, M.F. The small leucine-rich proteoglycan biglycan modulates BMP-4-induced osteoblast differentiation. *FASEB J.* **2004**, *18*, 948–958. [CrossRef] [PubMed]
81. Berendsen, A.D.; Fisher, L.W.; Kilts, T.M.; Owens, R.T.; Robey, P.G.; Gutkind, J.S.; Young, M.F. Modulation of canonical Wnt signaling by the extracellular matrix component biglycan. *Proc. Natl. Acad. Sci. USA* **2011**, *108*, 17022–17027. [CrossRef] [PubMed]
82. Van Laer, L.; Dietz, H.; Loeys, B. Loeys-Dietz syndrome. *Adv. Exp. Med. Biol.* **2014**, *802*, 95–105. [PubMed]
83. Melchior-Becker, A.; Dai, G.; Ding, Z.; Schäfer, L.; Schrader, J.; Young, M.F.; Fischer, J.W. Deficiency of biglycan causes cardiac fibroblasts to differentiate into a myofibroblast phenotype. *J. Biol. Chem.* **2011**, *286*, 17365–17375. [CrossRef] [PubMed]
84. Heegaard, A.M.; Corsi, A.; Danielsen, C.C.; Nielsen, K.L.; Jorgensen, H.L.; Riminucci, M.; Young, M.F.; Bianco, P. Biglycan deficiency causes spontaneous aortic dissection and rupture in mice. *Circulation* **2007**, *115*, 2731–2738. [CrossRef] [PubMed]

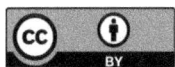

pharmaceuticals

MDPI

Review

Pathogenesis and Inhibition of Flaviviruses from a Carbohydrate Perspective

So Young Kim [1], Bing Li [2,3,*] and Robert J. Linhardt [1,4,5,6,7,*]

[1] Biochemistry and Biophysics Graduate Program, Center for Biotechnology and Interdisciplinary Studies, Rensselaer Polytechnic Institute, Troy, NY 12180, USA; pinkes2@rpi.edu

[2] Guangdong Province Key Laboratory for Green Processing of Natural Products and Product Safety, Guangzhou 510640, China

[3] School of Food Science and Technology, South China University of Technology, Guangzhou 510640, China

[4] Department of Chemistry and Chemical Biology, Center for Biotechnology and Interdisciplinary Studies, Rensselaer Polytechnic Institute, Troy, NY 12180, USA

[5] Department of Biological Science, Center for Biotechnology and Interdisciplinary Studies, Rensselaer Polytechnic Institute, Troy, NY 12180, USA

[6] Department of Chemical and Biological Engineering, Center for Biotechnology and Interdisciplinary Studies, Rensselaer Polytechnic Institute, Troy, NY 12180, USA

[7] Biomedical Engineering, Center for Biotechnology and Interdisciplinary Studies, Rensselaer Polytechnic Institute, Troy, NY 12180, USA

* Correspondence: lcbingli@scut.edu.cn (B.L.); linhar@rpi.edu (R.J.L.);
Tel.: +1-518-276-3404 (R.J.L.); Fax: +1-518-276-3405 (R.J.L.)

Academic Editor: Barbara Mulloy
Received: 3 March 2017; Accepted: 26 April 2017; Published: 4 May 2017

Abstract: Flaviviruses are enveloped, positive single stranded ribonucleic acid (RNA) viruses with various routes of transmission. While the type and severity of symptoms caused by pathogenic flaviviruses vary from hemorrhagic fever to fetal abnormalities, their general mechanism of host cell entry is similar. All pathogenic flaviviruses, such as dengue virus, yellow fever virus, West Nile virus, Japanese encephalitis virus, and Zika virus, bind to glycosaminglycans (GAGs) through the putative GAG binding sites within their envelope proteins to gain access to the surface of host cells. GAGs are long, linear, anionic polysaccharides with a repeating disaccharide unit and are involved in many biological processes, such as cellular signaling, cell adhesion, and pathogenesis. Flavivirus envelope proteins are *N*-glycosylated surface proteins, which interact with C-type lectins, dendritic cell-specific intercellular adhesion molecule-3-grabbing non-integrin (DC-SIGN) through their glycans. In this review, we discuss both host and viral surface receptors that have the carbohydrate components, focusing on the surface interactions in the early stage of flavivirus entry. GAG-flavivirus envelope protein interactions as well as interactions between flavivirus envelope proteins and DC-SIGN are discussed in detail. This review also examines natural and synthetic inhibitors of flaviviruses that are carbohydrate-based or carbohydrate-targeting. Both advantages and drawbacks of these inhibitors are explored, as are potential strategies to improve their efficacy to ultimately help eradicate flavivirus infections.

Keywords: dengue virus; DC-SIGN; envelope protein; flavivirus; flavivirus inhibitors; glycosaminoglycans; Japanese encephalitis virus; proteoglycans; viral infection; West Nile virus; yellow fever virus; Zika virus

1. Introduction

Each year, 13.4 million deaths worldwide are caused by various parasitic, bacterial, and viral infectious diseases [1]. Mosquito-borne infectious diseases annually cause several million deaths and hundreds of millions of cases [2]. Dengue virus (DENV), the world's most dangerous mosquito-borne flavivirus (FLV) disease, places 2.5 billion at risk of infection and results in 20 million cases each year in 100 countries and to date there is no completely effective vaccine [3]. Although more than 105 million people have been vaccinated for yellow fever virus (YFV) in West Africa, 84 to 170 thousand severe cases and 29 to 60 thousand deaths were estimated in Africa during 2013 [2]. While of less risk, West Nile virus (WNV) has no approved human vaccine and outbreaks in the U.S. from 1999–2010 reminds us that pandemic of vector-borne pathogens is still accessible due to frequent importation through global travel [2]. Recently, Zika virus (ZIKV) joined the list of FLVs of concern due to its ability to cross the placental barrier and cause serious birth defects with 2500 reported congenital syndromes worldwide and nearly 4000 ZIKV infection in pregnant women in the U.S. and its territories [4,5]. DENV, YFV, WNV, ZIKV, Japanese encephalitis virus (JEV), and tick-borne encephalitis virus (TBEV) belong to the *Flaviviridae* family. FLVs are enveloped, positive single stranded RNA viruses with varying symptoms from hemorrhagic fever and fatal neurological diseases to fetal defects. There are currently no approved antivirals for treating FLVs.

There are many similarities in pathogenesis of FLV in host cells. Glycosaminoglycans (GAGs), for example, are the initial co-receptors that all pathogenic FLVs utilize for the infection of host cell [6–13]. GAGs are anionic, unbranched polysaccharides comprised of repeating disaccharide units located on the surface of eukaryotic cells and in their extracellular matrix (ECM; Figure 1). GAGs are involved in many biological processes, including cell adhesion, cell migration, tissue repair, ECM assembly, inflammation, and pathogenesis [14]. After successfully making contact with the host cell surface through their binding to GAGs, FLV next interact with protein-based receptors [15–32]. Finally, FLVs infiltrate into the host cell through clathrin-mediated endocytosis, accompanied by a conformation change of envelope protein and membrane fusion and release of the viral genome (Figure 2) [33,34].

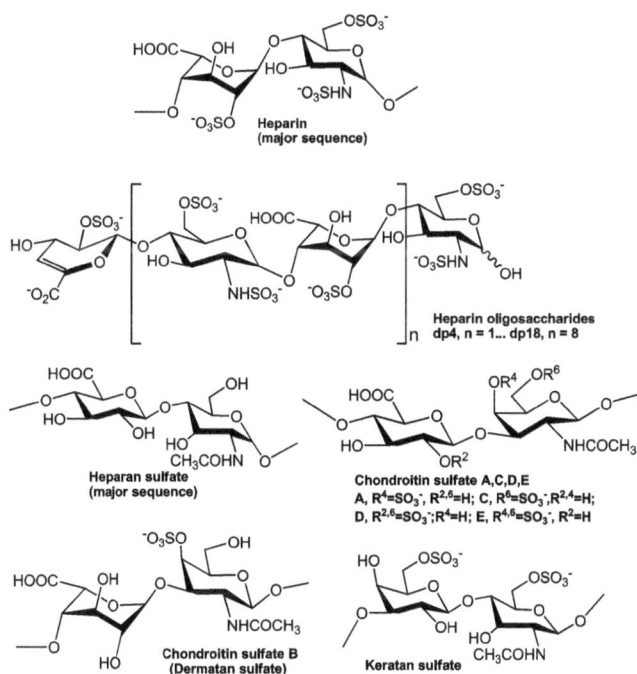

Figure 1. Chemical structures of glycosaminoglycans and heparin oligosaccharides.

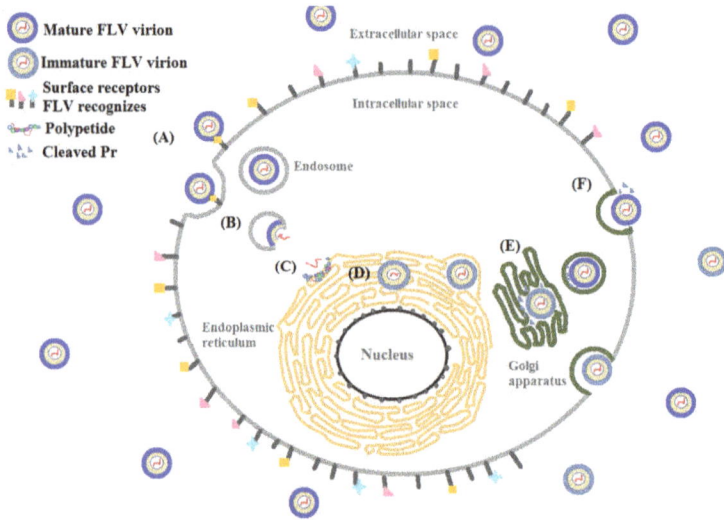

Figure 2. Host cell entry of flavivirus (FLV) (**A**) adsorption and (**B**) internalization confirmation change of envelope protein triggers membrane fusion and viral genome release; (**C**) replication and (**D**) translation beginning of *N*-linked glycosylation and viral assembly in the endoplasmic reticulum; (**E**) completed glycosylation and pre-membrane (prM) protein is cleaved to become a mature virion in the Golgi apparatus; (**F**) exocytosis of a mature virion.

This review examines the role of carbohydrates in the mechanism of FLV infection and the potential of carbohydrates in combating FLV pathogenesis. The roles of both host and viral glycans, including host cell GAGs and FLV envelope protein (FLVE) *N*-glycosylation, in FLV pathogenesis and the interactions of GAGs-FLVE and FLV envelope protein-dendritic cell-specific intercellular adhesion molecule-3-grabbing non-integrin (FLVE-DC-SIGN) will be addressed. This review will particularly focus on the viral and host surface interactions in the early stage of FLV entry. FLV inhibitors that are either glycan-based or target host or viral glycans are described. The pitfalls of currently investigated inhibitors and strategies that may improve them are discussed.

2. Glycan-Mediated Flavivirus Entry

From the perspective of not only pathogenesis but also therapy, understanding of FLVs entry into host cells with greater precision and resolution is of great importance. FLVs enter host cells through a receptor-mediated mechanism [35]. Multiple host cell receptors have been identified to facilitate FLV entry, including GAG [6,36], heat-shock proteins (heat-shock protein 70, 90, R67, R80) [15,25,37], a 45 kD mosquito glycoprotein [38], neolactotetraosylceramide [16], CD14 [17], GRP78/BiP [18], phosphatidylserine (PS) receptors such as T-cell immunoglobulin and mucin domain receptor (TIM) [39], Tyrosine-protein kinase receptor (TYRO3) [40], and AXL [41], and proto-oncogene tyrosine-protein kinase (MERTK) [42]. C-type lectins implicated in FLV entry include DC-SIGN [22,43], and the mannose receptor [23], C-type lectin domain family 5 member A (CLEC5A) [44]. Prohibitin was the first discovered receptor involved in pathogenesis of DENV in insect cells [45]. Among these receptors, GAGs, a 45 kD mosquito glycoprotein, and neolactotetraosylceramide are some of the carbohydrate-based host cell receptors. C-type lectins also involve carbohydrates as they function through their binding to glycans. Moreover, the structural glycoproteins, the envelope proteins in particular, are ligands that interact with cell surface receptors [46]. In this section, glycan-protein interactions that mediates the FLV entry into host cells on surface level, including FLVE, GAGs and C-type lectin are discussed (Figure 3).

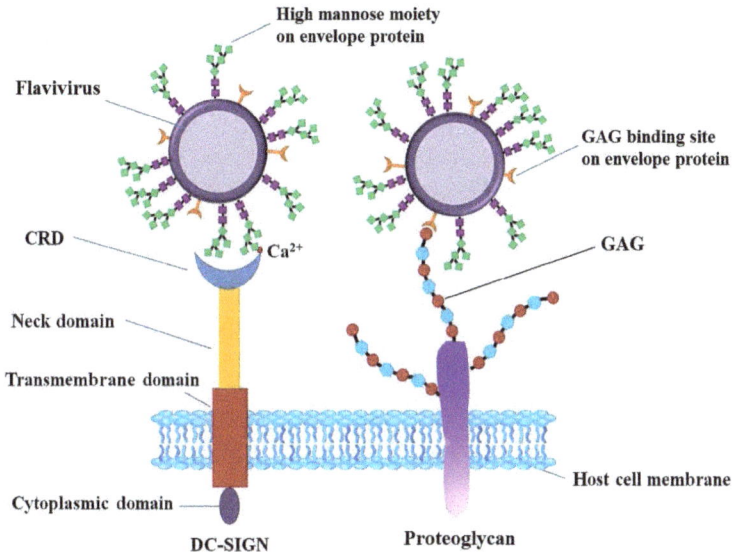

Figure 3. E protein binding to DC-SIGN or GAG. Carbohydrate recognition domain (CRD) of DC-SIGN with four domains (a cytoplasmic domain, a transmembrane domain, an extracellular neck domain, and a carbohydrate recognition domain) in molecular structure in the presence of Ca^{2+} recognizes the high mannose moiety on glycosylated E protein. Flavivirus binds to glycosaminoglycans (e.g., heparan sulfate or chondroitin sulfate depending on the virus) through their envelope proteins. DC-SIGN: dendritic cell-specific intercellular adhesion molecule-3-grabbing non-integrin; GAG: glycosaminoglycan.

2.1. The Flavivirus Envelope Proteins and Their Glycosylation

The FLV genome encodes for a single polypeptide that ultimately gets processed into the capsid (C), the membrane (prM/M), the envelope (E) protein, and seven nonstructural (NS) proteins, NS1, 2a, 2b, 3, 4a, 4b, and 5 [47,48]. The E protein mediate important processes in viral infection, such as viral attachment, fusion, penetration, hemagglutination; thus, it determines host range, cell tropism, virus virulence and attenuation [49,50]. The structures of the recombinant E proteins of TBEV [51], DENV [52], WNV [53,54], JEV [55] and ZIKV [56] have been solved by X-ray crystallography, and they exhibit great structural similarities. These E proteins consist of 500 amino acids and can be divided into three functional domains. Domain I is a central, stranded β-barrel, which contains a single *N*-linked glycan and is interspersed with domain II. Domain II is a long, finger-like protrusion from domain I, which contains the most of residues involved in dimeric interactions and houses the hydrophobic fusion peptide mediating post-entry endosomal fusion [57–61]. Domain III is an immunoglobulin-like fold, linked to the central domain I through a flexible stretch of amino acids, and characteristic of many cell receptors [62–66]. Domain III of FLVEs also contains GAG binding sites comprised of many surface basic and acidic residues that are contribute to hydrogen bonding [51,52,54–56]. Although the overall FLVE protein architecture is conserved, there are still significant differences within FLV family. In contrast to DENV E and TBEV E, WNV E does not form dimers in the crystal and contains more hydrogen bonds or buried surface area at the domain I-II interface [53]. An extra β strand (β5a) is formed in DENV-2 domain III, which is not found in DENV-3, DENV-4 [50]. The central domain I of JEV is composed of a nine stranded β-barrel [56], while domain I of DENV is an eight stranded β-barrel [57,59,61].

Glycosylation of FLVEs is an important determinant in the interaction of FLVs with host cells. Glycosylated variants of WNV were more virulent and had higher viremic levels in young chicks than the non-glycosylated variants [67]. The highly pathogenic WNV emerging in the late 1990s was attributed to glycosylation in WNV E. Viral replication in birds is enhanced by the glycosylation of E protein and may result in increased transmissibility among bird population and higher pathogenicity in birds [68]. Glycosylation of FLVEs takes place in the host cells that provide most or all of enzymes and saccharide substrates, since the FLVs themselves do not encode these enzymes [69,70]. During glycosylation, a pre-assembled oligosaccharide $Glc_3Man_9GlcNAc_2$ (Glc (glucose), Man (mannose), and GlcNAc (*N*-acetylglucosamine)) is trimmed stepwise by glucosidases and mannosidases and then elaborated through the action of *N*-acetylglucosaminyltransferase, galactosyltransferases, fucosyl-transferases, and sialyltransferases [71]. FLVs derived from different vectors may have structurally different *N*-linked glycans since the enzymes involved in glycosylation produced by different vectors, such as insect and mammalian cells, are different. For example, the structures of the *N*-linked glycans on the viral glycoproteins produced by insect cells are much less complex than those produced by mammalian cells [71]. Hacker et al. [43] analyzed mosquito-derived DENV glycoproteins using endoglycosidase, PNGaseF or EndoH, and lectins, *Galanthus nivalis* agglutinin (GNA) and *Datura stramonium* agglutinin (DSA), and found they have a mix of high-Man and paucimannose glycans. Further, using both lectin microarray and matrix assisted laser desorption ionization-time of flight mass spectrometry (MALDI-TOF-MS), Lei et al. proved that *N*-glycan structure on the surface of mature DENV-2 derived from mosquito cells was highly heterogeneous [72]. Five types of *N*-linked glycans were identified comprised of Man, *N*-acetylgalactosamine (GalNAc), GlcNAc, fucose (Fuc) and sialic acid (SA). High Man-type *N*-linked oligosaccharides and galactose (Gal)-containing of *N*-linked glycans were the major structures. In viruses derived from mammalian cells, the *N*-linked glycans were a mix of high-mannose and complex type glycans [43]. The number and location of glycosylation motifs in the E vary considerably both between and within FLV species [73]. It is well known that DENV E has two potential *N*-linked glycosylation sites at Asn-67 and Asn-153 [43]. The Asn-67 site is unique to DENV E whereas Asn-153 (or nearby Asn-154) is common to other FLVs, with the exception of Kunjin virus [51,74,75]. Interestingly, DENV2 E and DENV4 E proteins are glycosylated only at the Asn-67 site while DENV1 and DENV3 E proteins are glycosylated at both Asn-67 and Asn-153 sites [74]. *N*-linked glycosylation at Asn-67 (or nearby Asn-64) is critical for the survival of the virus in either mammalian or insect cell culture [76]. The high-mannose *N*-linked glycan at Asn-154 of JEV E was shown to be crucial for JEV binding to DC-SIGN [77]. The glycosylation site in WNV E was also confirmed at Asn-154 [49].

2.2. Glycans on Host Cells Mediating Flavivirus Entry

2.2.1. Flavivirus Binding to Glycosaminoglycans

GAGs are linear and negatively charged polysaccharides that have molecular weights of 10–100 kDa; and they contain repeating disaccharide units of uronic acid (D-glucuronic (GlcA) acid or L-iduronic acid (IdoA)) and hexosamine (D-GalN or D-GlcN) (Figure 1). Hence, GAGs differ according to the type of hexosamine, hexose or hexuronic acid unit that they contain, as well as the chirality and position of the glycosidic linkage between their saccharide units [78]. Heparan sulfate proteoglycans (HSPGs) are sulfated GAGs that represent a major GAGs component of the cell surface of eukaryotes [8]. HSPGs have the common characteristic of containing one or more covalently attached heparan sulfate (HS) chain [79]. The HS GAG has the major repeating unit of monosulfated →4)GlcNAc(1→4)GlcA/IdoA(1→ per disaccharide [80,81]. HS contains a considerable number of negatively charged sulfo and carboxyl groups that can interact with numerous proteins that carry positive charges including growth factors, morphogens, ECM proteins and pathogen surface proteins [6,82–86]. HS on host cell surface plays a very important role in the process of many virus infections, and the affinity of the viral surface for HS may be a crucial determinant of tissue tropism, virus spread, or the establishment of latent infection. In most cases, the binding of the virus to HS seems to be relatively low-affinity, thus, HS may serve the purpose of concentrating the virus on the cell surface to facilitate the interaction with one or more high-affinity receptors, which induce endocytosis and subsequent cell membrane fusion [8,87–89].

HS also serves as an attachment factor in the host cell entry of many FLVs, including DENV, JEV, YFV, and TBEV. The efficiency of HS binding is virus-dependent. In multiple studies, HS has been shown to serve as a receptor or co-receptor for DENV infection of host cells [6,8,36,90]. Clinical strains of DENV1 can specifically interact with HS and heparin (HP). HP is the most negatively charged occurring natural polymer with an excellent anticoagulant activity. DENV2 binding to the two mutant cell lines of Chinese hamster ovary (CHO) cells defective in GAG expression was reduced by more than 75% compared to binding to wild-type CHO K1 [7]. Human endothelial cells express HSPGs that DENV4 specifically and efficiently interacts with in vitro. This was demonstrated by >60% reduction in DENV4 infection when human endothelial cells were pretreated with HP or HS [91]. The level of sulfation in GAGs on cell surfaces was found to be an important factor in success of in vitro JEV infection in both neurovirulent (RP-9) and attenuated (RP-2ms) strains [92]. In a separate study, both wild type (T1P1, CC27 and CJN) and laboratory-adapted strains (T1P1-L4, T1P1-S1, CJN-L1, CJN-S1, CC27-L1, CC27-L3, CC27-S6 and CC27-S8) of JEV infected BHK-21 and C6/36 cells by binding to surface HS [93]. An evident difference in attachment efficiency for JEV infection between CHO-K1 cells and its mutant with defects in GAG biosynthesis proved the importance of HS during JEV infection [94]. Recombinant TBEV with mutations in a defined genetic backbone showed HS-dependent phenotypes, resulting in an increased specific infectivity and binding affinity for BHK-21 cells and significant attenuation of neuro-invasiveness in adult mice [12]. Mutants of TBEV attached to HS-expressing cell lines with a 10-fold to 13-fold higher affinity than wild-type TBEV [95]. Although it was reported that mutations in the WNV E protein that enhanced binding to GAG molecules in vitro led to attenuation of virulence in a mouse model, the role of GAG in attachment of WNV is not clear [96]. A study conducted in our laboratory showed that ZIKV might also utilize GAGs to mediate host cell entry [13]. Surface plasmon resonance (SPR) kinetic measurements revealed that ZIKV E binds commercial HP strongly (K_D = 443 nM). Screening ability of ZIKV E binding to various natural GAGs with different disaccharide units, and varying length of HP oligosaccharides revealed that ZIKV E exhibits structural specificity of binding in addition to being electrostatically driven. The chondroitin sulfate (CS) GAG, isolated from human placenta tissues, showed comparable binding to ZIKV E (K_D = 658 nM) and it may be one of the candidate receptors for ZIKV. Main driving force of FLV-GAG interaction is electrostatically driven between surface basic and acidic residues on the FLVE and concentrated negative charge density on the sulfated polysaccharide chain [13,86,97]. Along the HS chain, relatively rigid, highly *N*-sulfo group rich domains (NS domains) of approximately 12–20 residues are adjacent to relatively flexible *N*-acetyl group rich domains (NA domains). This domain organization influences the orientation of the sulfate residues in space, and facilitates protein interactions with the sulfate residue [86]. Degree of sulfation in GAGs influences binding avidity and infection rate of FLVs shown in cell based studies. Treatment of BHK-21 target cells by a potent sulfation inhibitor, sodium chlorate, greatly reduced JEV binding avidity and infection [92]. When TBEV mutants with high HS affinity were incubated with sulfate-depleted BHK-21 cells, the growth was significantly delayed by the inhibition of sulfation [12]. HP and highly sulfated HS substantially inhibit DENV infection on Vero cells, with 99% and 87% inhibition respectively at the highest doses used, whereas the low-sulfate form of HS had no significant effect [6].

Both basic and acidic surface residues that contribute to hydrogen bonding play an important role in GAG-protein interactions in terms of both binding avidity and specificity [68]. Positively charged amino acids such Arg, Lys and His confer the envelope E protein to bind with negative-charged GAG. The GAG binding sites within FLVEs can be tentatively identified the crystal structures of FLVs [51,52,54–56]. Three basic residues, K305, K307, and K310, at a lateral ridge of domain III were speculated to form a potential GAG binding motif within DENV2 E [6]. Using an enzyme-linked immunosorbent assay (ELISA)-based GAG-binding assay, cell-based binding analysis and antiviral-activity assays, two critical residues, K291 and K295, in domain III were identified in GAG interaction with DENV E [61]. The highly DENV- and JEV-serogroup conserved K or R basic residues at positions 282, 284, and/or 288 in the domain I-HS-binding cluster are essential for virus function in both C6/36 and Vero cells [98]. Point mutations at E-138 and E-306 on the envelope protein of JEV may alter its ability to bind to HS on the cell surface and consequently change JEV infectivity, indicating these two sites are rather likely to be involved in determining efficiencies of JEV attachment, penetration, and eventual infection [94].

2.2.2. Glycan-Mediated Dendritic Cell-Specific Intercellular Adhesion Molecule-Grabbing Non-Integrin Binding to Flavivirus

DC-SIGN, a carbohydrate binding, C-type, lectin-like molecule, is abundant in immature dendritic cells and is involved in the interaction with viruses, being an ancillary receptor [27,99]. DC-SIGN is composed of four domains, including a cytoplasmic domain, a transmembrane domain, an extracellular neck domain, and a carbohydrate recognition domain (CRD) [27,100].

Like other C-type lectins, DC-SIGN can recognize the glycosylation sites on the envelope FLVEs, including DENV E and WNV E (Table 1), thus facilitating the virus infection to host cells. DC-SIGN is a very important receptor for DENV E. Although Man receptor expressed on macrophages is another carbohydrate-binding receptor for DENV DC-SIGN is abundant in dendritic cells (DC) on human skin which is the first target for DENV once the infected mosquitos bite [21,101]. All four DENV serotypes derived from mosquito and mammalian cells infected DC-SIGN-expressing human monocytic cell line U937 cells with similar efficiency [44]. DC-SIGN transfected THP-1 monocytic cells also render these cells permissive to infection with all DENV serotypes [22]. DENV cannot bind nor infect the human B-cell line Raji, whereas DENV productively infects DC-SIGN transfected Raji cells [102]. Glycosylated WNV strains L1 infected DC-SIGN expressing THP-1 monocytic cell lines more efficiently than DC-SIGN negative cells [103]. Comparison of DC-SIGN and DC-SIGNR (a DC-SIGN related molecule, expressed on microvascular endothelial cells) in viral infection has been reported for WNV and JEV. DC-SIGNR promoted WNV infection much more efficiently than did DC-SIGN, particularly when the virus was grown in human cell types [28]. Growth of JEV derived from pig in DC-SIGNR expressing Daudi cells was greater than in DC-SIGN expressing Daudi cells [104]. ZIKV was also reported to infect DC-SIGN expressing HEK293T cells [40]. In contrast to DENV, WNV, and JEV, YF17D can infect immature and mature human DCs, but is independent of DC-SIGN [105]. It seems that YF17D interacts with DCs via different mechanism rather than DC-SIGN binding.

Table 1. Dendritic cell-specific intercellular adhesion molecule-grabbing nonintegrin (DC-SIGN) are involved in receptor mediated host cell entry of many pathogenic flaviviruses.

Receptor	Virus	Cell	Reference
DC-SIGN	DENV-1, DENV-2, DENV-3, DENV-4	human monocytic cell line (U937)	[43]
DC-SIGN	DENV-2	Raji	[102]
DC-SIGN	DENV-1, DENV-2, DENV-3, DENV-4	HEK-293T, HeLa, Raji, monocyte-derived dendritic cell (MDDC)	[20]
DC-SIGN	DENV-1, DENV-2, DENV-3, DENV-4	THP-1	[22]
DC-SIGN	WNV	THP-1	[103]
DC-SIGN, DC-SIGNR	WNV	K562, MDDC	[28]
DC-SIGN, DC-SIGNR	JEV	Daudi	[104]
DC-SIGN	ZIKV	HEK293T	[40]

DENV: dengue virus; WNV: West Nile virus; JEV: Japanese encephalitis virus; ZIKV: Zika virus.

The interaction between DC-SIGN and the glycans of E protein on virus surface are essential for virus infection. The CRD domain in DC-SIGN C-terminal is responsible for responsible for recognition of high-Man glycans in the presence of Ca^{2+} (Figure 3) [46,104,106,107]. Molecular docking analysis between carbohydrates on DENV-2 virions and DC-SIGN revealed that hydrogen bonding and hydrophobic interactions are two of the forces that exist between glycan receptors and DC-SIGN, and most of the persistent H-bonds were formed from hydroxyl groups on Asn36, Glu366, Ser363 and Man [72]. The structural organization of *N*-linked glycans on the surface of E protein can favor the engagement of multiple E proteins dimers by each tetrameric lectin, enhancing the interaction between oligomeric DC-SIGN and virus [20]. The affinity of CRD to *N*-linked glycans on viral E proteins is dependent on the glycosylation level, increasing with the number of Man residues in the glycan [107,108]. Treatment of JEV particles with endoglycosidase H, which removes only *N*-linked sugars containing more than three terminal Man residues [109], or use of de-glycosylated JEV mutants reduced JEV infection of DC-SIGN-expressing cells [77]. DC-SIGN preferentially recognizes mannosylated E protein, rather than E protein with complex glycosylation [20]. DENV infection inhibited by Concanavalin A supported that α-Man carbohydrate residues participate in the attachment of DENV to DC-SIGN [21]. The involvement of Man during the interaction between JEV and DC-SIGN is further supported by the fact that JEV infection is significantly reduced in DC-SIGN expressing Raji cells in the presence of mannan, a competitor of insect-derived glycans [77].

3. Combating Flaviviruses with Carbohydrate-Based Or -Targeting Compounds

Extensive research has been performed to eliminate FLV entry at every step of host cell invasion including adsorption, membrane fusion, polypeptide processing, and viral assembly (Figure 2). The majority of the FLV inhibitors tested are comprised of carbohydrates, proteins, peptides, and small molecules, which are described in some excellent reviews [110–113]. The current review focuses on the inhibitors that are carbohydrate-based or carbohydrate-targeting (both viral and host cell glycan targeting). First, we examine the compounds that block the interactions between the host glycan, GAGs, and the viral envelope protein either by mimicking structure and activity of GAGs or binding to GAGs. Next, we investigate the compounds that block the interactions between viral glycan (*N*-linked glycan on FLVEs) and host receptor DC-SIGN by mimicking, attaching to, or permanently modifying the viral glycan on its envelope protein. Finally, we revisit the obstacles that were encountered when these compounds were studied and explore prospective strategies to eradicate FLVs infections.

3.1. Glycan-Based Entry Inhibitors Targeting Host Cell Glycans by Mimicking Structures and Activity of GAGs

Anionic surface GAGs provide an excellent starting point for preventing the initial attachment of FLV to the surface of host cells. HS is a universal eukaryotic surface GAG that all pathogenic FLVs bind to and, thus, various natural and synthetic HS mimetics have tested for their ability to inhibit GAG-FLVE interactions (Table 2).

3.1.1. Natural and Synthetic GAGs

A previous study in our laboratory, we screened small polyanionic drugs, larger GAGs and their semisynthetic derivatives for their binding affinity to DENV2 E to investigate their structure-activity relationships [114]. Small polyanionic drugs (having two to six sugars), such as sucrose octasulfate, sulfated lactobionic acid, and sulfated β-cyclodextrin, failed to efficiently bind to DENV2 E despite their high level of charge density. This is presumably due to inability to efficiently occupy the entire putative GAG binding sites within DENV2 E. However, suramin, synthetic sulfonated aromatic, was able to bind to DENV2 E at comparable affinity, 40 nM, to that of HP, 15 nM. Next, we screened persulfated GAGs and HA (hyaluronan) oligosaccharides (decasaccharide to eicosisaccharide) where every hydroxyl group was sulfated. Binding affinity of persulfated GAGs, 4–15 nM, was similar or greater than that of HP whereas HA oligosaccharides showed size dependent binding, 57–100 nM. Using SPR, more rapid on-rate and off-rate were observed in HP and suramin than those of persulfated GAGs due to higher level of conformational flexibility HP and suramin possessed. Structure-activity relationships that promoted effective interactions between DENV2 E and polyanions were concluded:

(1) minimum size 39 Å; (2) high charge density; and (3) high level of structural flexibility. In a separate study, we also demonstrated inhibition of DENV2 infection using highly sulfated HS, HP, and suramin in vitro model involving Vero cells [6]. In our recent study, we concluded similar requirements for the structure-activity relationships between ZIKV E and natural GAGs and HP oligosaccharides, however HP bound ZIKV E with lower avidity, 443 nM, potentially due to less basic surface residue observed in GAG binding sites within ZIKV E [13]. Germi et al. reported that HP, but not CS-type B, inhibited binding of DENV2 and YFV in Vero cells [7]. Varying concentrations of HP (0.2 to 200 µg/mL) also inhibited YFV infection in Vero cells up to 97% with an ID_{50} of about 0.2 µg/mL. Despite having same degree of sulfation, CS-type E (CSE), but not CS-type D (CSD), was found to inhibit DENV infection in Vero cells [115]. Interestingly, CSE showed comparable inhibition of all serotypes of DENV and JEV infection to HP in Vero cells. The EC_{50} for the inhibition of DENV1-4 infection was 0.5–1.89 and 0.3–3.80 µg/mL for HP and CSE, respectively. EC_{50} of JEV infection inhibition by HP and CSE were 0.77 and 0.93 µg/mL, respectively. HS, CS-type A and B showed 50–70% inhibition activity against DENV4 in human endothelial cells at high concentrations (>10 µg/mL) whereas HP inhibited by >60% even at low concentration ($\geq$1 µg/mL) [91]. These concentrations of GAGs can be easily achieved in plasma without toxicity.

3.1.2. Fucoidan

Fucoidan, a natural polysaccharide from the marine algae, *Cladosiphon okamuranus*, is comprised of carbohydrate units containing glucuronic acid and sulfated Fuc residues [116]. Fucoidan was reported to selectively inhibit DENV2 infection, but not other serotypes, in BHK-21 cells. The IC_{50} against DENV2 by fucoidan was 4.7 µg/mL while those against DENV1, 3, and 4 ranged from 365 to greater than 1000 µg/mL. The inability of desulfated fucoidan, carboxyl-reduced fucoidan, and Fuc polymer (fucan) to inhibit DENV infection demonstrated that sulfation on the Fuc units and carboxyl group at the C6 of glucuronic acid were important for effective binding to DENV2 E. Structure analysis revealed that Arg 323 is also important for binding to DENV2 E. While fucoidans from many species of brown algae possess anticoagulant activity, those from *C. okamuranus* did not exhibit significant level of anticoagulant activity [117]. Thus, fucoidan from *C. okamuranus* makes an excellent natural polysaccharide candidate for selective inhibitor of DENV2 infection.

3.1.3. Carrageenans

Talarico et al. tested the anti-FLV activity of sulfated polysaccharides, k/ι/ν carrageenan G3d, from *Gymnogongrus griffithsiae* against all serotypes of DENV and reported these to be selective inhibitors of DENV2 infection in vitro models [118]. Carrageenans consist of linear chains of alternating (1→3)-β-D-Gal and (1→4)-α-D-Gal (or 3,6-anhydro-Gal). The IC_{50} of k/ι/ν carrageenan against DENV1, 2, 3, and 4 infections were >50, 0.9, 13.9, and >50 µg/mL in Vero cells, respectively. The IC_{50} of k/ι/ν carrageenan against DENV2 infection were 1.8 and 0.31 µg/mL in human hepatoma HepG2 and foreskin PH cells, respectively. In DENV3, IC_{50} was 10.4 and 9.5 µg/mL for HepG2 and PH cells, respectively. Surprisingly, neither k/ι/ν carrageenan, HP, nor dextran sulfate 8000 could inhibit DENV infection even at the maximum concentration tested, 50 µg/mL, in C6/36 HT cells that are derived from *Aedes albopictus* mosquitoes that are main vector of DENV. In a subsequent study, k/ι/ν carrageenans were used to test their inhibition against DENV2 infection in Vero and C6/36 HT cells [119,120]. All three carrageenans inhibited against DENV2 infection with ι-carrageenan being a most potent inhibitor (EC_{50} = 0.4 µg/mL) in Vero cells. However, only ι-carrageenan was able to inhibit DENV2 infection in C6/36 HT cells and at a 17.5-fold lower potency (EC_{50} = 7 µg/mL). The mode of action of ι-carrageenan differed in Vero and mosquito cells. Inhibition occurred at adsorption of DENV2 in Vero cells whereas it did not in mosquito cells. The order from the greatest degree of sulfation to the least per disaccharide unit follows: λ (3) > ι (2) > k (1). It is interesting that ι-carrageenan demonstrated greatest inhibition against DENV2 infection even though ι-carrageenan had the greatest degree of sulfation. This reinforces that polyanion-DENV E interaction possesses structural specificity and is not entirely dependent upon electrostatic forces as found in our previous studies [6,114]. Carrageenans also have been reported to have anticoagulant activity and effects to enhance their activity has been employed by oversulfation and regioselective sulfation modification [121–123].

3.1.4. Sulfated K5 Polysaccharides from *Escherichia coli*

K5 polysaccharides from *E. coli* and their chemically modified sulfated derivatives were evaluated for their anti-FLV activities against DENV2 [124]. K5 polysaccharides have the disaccharide unit of →4)-β-GlcA (1→4)-α-GlcNAc(1→, which is similar to de-sulfonated HS [125]. They were previously reported for their antiviral activity against human immunodeficiency virus (HIV), herpes simplex virus (HSV), human papillomavirus (HPV) and human cytomegalovirus (HCMV) [126–129]. Out of native form K5 and its sulfated derivatives (*N*-sulfo K5 (K5-NS), *O*-sulfo K5-OS (L) and *N,O*-sulfo K5-N,OS (L) with low degree of sulfation and K5 with high degree of sulfation K5-OS (H) and K5-N,OS (H)), K5-OS (H) and K5-N,OS (H) were most potent in inhibiting DENV2 infection in HMEC-1 and HMVEC-d. K5-OS (H) and K5-N,OS (H) inhibited DENV2 infection with EC_{50} of with an EC_{50} value of 113 and 111 nM in HMEC-1 cells, and 266 and 330 nM in HMVEC-d cells, respectively. HP, HS, CSA, and CSB were used as references and their EC_{50} against DENV2 infection in HMEC-1 cells were 77 nM (or 1 μg/mL), 6000 nM (60 μg/mL), 4200 nM (67 μg/mL), and 3300 nM (46 μg/mL), respectively. K5-OS (H) and K5-N,OS (H) present promising inhibitors against DENV2 because they not only have comparable level of inhibition of infection to HP, but K5 and its sulfated derivatives were evaluated to be devoid of anticoagulant activity [130].

3.1.5. Curdlan Sulfate (Sulfated Glucan)

A sulfated 1R3-β-D-glucan, curdlan sulfate, showed excellent inhibition against infection of all serotype DENV and selectively against DENV2 infection (selectivity index > 1428) in various types of cell lines, such as BHK-21, C6/36, LLC-MK2, HL-60, and THP-1 [131]. The order of EC_{50} values in LLC-MK2 cells were as follows: DENV1 (262 μg/mL) > DENV4 (69 μg/mL) > DENV3 (10 μg/mL) > DENV2 (7 μg/mL). Curdlan sulfate was also reported as effective inhibitors of HIV and to exhibit anticoagulant activity [132,133].

3.1.6. Sulfated Galactomannans

Chemically sulfated forms of galactomannans from seeds of *M. scabrella* (BRS) and *L. leucocephala* (LLS) demonstrated antiviral activity against DENV1 and YFV in vitro and in vivo models [134]. Galactomannans has a main chain of (1→4)-linked β-D-Man units substituted by α-D-Gal units with varying degree of D-Man units, which ranges from 60 to 80% [135,136]. Their structural analysis showed that galactomannans from BRS and LLS have Man to Gal ratio of 1:1 and 1:4, respectively. After sulfation, galactomannans from BRS and LLS had 0.62 and 0.5 degree of sulfation per unit and the average molecular weight of 620 kDa and 574 kDa. In C6/36 cells, concentration that reduced the YFV viral titer 100-fold in comparison to that of the positive control were 586 and 387 mg/L for BRS and LLS, respectively. In DENV1, these concentrations were 347 and 37 mg/L for BRS and LLS, respectively. At a dose of 49 mg/kg^{-1}, BRS and LLS gave protection against death caused by YFV infection in 87.7 and 96.5% of young mice, respectively. In a separate study, chemically sulfated forms of galactomannans from fenugreek gum, guargum, tara gum, and locust bean gum were reported to for their antiviral activity against HIV and DENV2 [137]. Sulfated galactomannans generally had higher anticoagulant activity, 13.4–36.6 unit/mg, compared to that of dextran and curdlan sulfates, 22.7 and 10.0 unit/mg. They also exhibited similar anti-HIV and anti-DENV2 activities, 0.04–0.8 and 0.2–1.1 μg/mL, to those curdlan sulfates, 0.1 μg/mL, respectively.

3.1.7. Sulfated Xylomannans

A diverse group of sulfated polysaccharides isolated from red, brown, and green seaweeds were tested for their anti-DENV activity [138]. Composition analysis revealed that the polysaccharides from *Grateloupia indica* (Gi) and *Gracilaria corticate* (Gc) were sulfated galactans, *Scinaia hatei* (Sh) gave sulfated xylomannans, *Stoechospermum marginatum* (Sm) and *Cystoseira indica* (Ci) sulfated fucans, and those from *Caulerpa racemose* (Cr) were heteropolysaccharides made up of Gal, Glc, arabinose (Ara) and xylose (Xyl). All sulfated polysaccharides most effectively inhibited against DENV2 in Vero cells with IC_{50} ranging from 0.12–20 μg/mL. Sulfated galactans (Gi), sulfated xylomannan (Sh), and sulfated fucan (Cr) had even greater anti-DENV2 activities with IC_{50} of 0.12–0.6 μg/mL compared to those of reference HP and dextran sulfate 8000 of 1.9 and 0.9 μg/mL. Sulfated polysaccharides from seaweeds have been generally reported to possess many biological activities including anticoagulant activity [139,140].

3.1.8. Methyl-α-3-*O*-Sulfated Glucuronic Acid

A series of monomer carbohydrate compounds with varying conformations at anomeric center (α/β) and degree and position of sulfation on 1-methyl glucose (MeGlc), glucuronic acid (MeGlcA), and galactose (MeGal) were synthesize to evaluate their anti-DENV2 activities in BHK-21 cells [141]. The 3-*O*-sulfated MeGlcA was the most anti-DENV2 compound, inhibiting DENV2 infection by 87.5%, which is comparable to that of a reference compound sucrose octasulfate, 92.4%, at 500 μM. The EC_{50} of 3-*O*-sulfated MeGlcA was 120 μM, which was lower than that of sucrose octasulfate. Although lower than sucrose octasulfate, 3-*O*-sulfated MeGlcA still may not be a potent inhibitor. The chain length of sucrose octasulfate is only a disaccharide, which was not long enough to occupy the GAG binding site of DENV E in our previous study [6,114]. Thus, 3-*O*-sulfated MeGlcA being as a monosaccharide surely cannot efficiently bind DENV E to inhibit DENV infection. All the other derivatives with higher degree of sulfation also did not successfully inhibit DENV2 infection as expected. However, this study provides a structural rationale for designing low molecular weight sulfated carbohydrate compounds as anti-DENV agents. Two negatively charged groups a 3-*O*-sulfo and carboxyl group at C6 of GlcA were found important for anti-DENV activity. Carboxyl group at C6 of GlcA was also important in fucoidan [116]. No anticoagulant activity is expected at the monosaccharide length due to the importance of chain length for HP's anticoagulant activity.

3.1.9. Phosphomannopentaose Sulfate, Pentosan Polysulfate, and Suramin

Lee et al. evaluated the in vitro and in vivo anti-FLV activity of compounds that are currently approved or in clinical trials for DENV2 and encephalitis FLV, including phosphomannopentaose sulfate (PI-88), pentosan polysulfate (PPS), and suramin [142]. In BHK-21 cells, the EC_{50} against DENV2 infection followed the order from the highest to the lowest: PI-88 (200 μg/mL) > suramin (60 μg/mL) > PPS (30 μg/mL). However, EC_{50} against JEV infection followed the order: suramin (50 μg/mL) > PI-88 (40 μg/mL) > PPS (7 μg/mL). In both DENV2 and JEV, PPS was the most potent inhibitor in vitro models. The EC_{50} of PI-88 against WNV and MVE infections was 50 μg/mL. Surprisingly, PI-88 was the only compound with potent antiviral activity in vivo experiments. PI-88 inhibited against JEV, DENV2, and MEV infection in C57B1/6 mice at an acceptable toxicity concentration (0.5 mg/injection). In interferon-α and -γ receptor knockout mice, PI-88 increased the survival time from 15 to 22 days. This study is an excellent example of additional factors, such as physiochemical and pharmacological properties, alter the in vitro potency in vivo and must be carefully monitored. PI-88, PPS, and suramin have been reported to exhibit anticoagulant activities [143–145].

3.1.10. Multivalent Lacto-*N*-Neotetraose Glycodendrimers

Aoki et al. identified that glycosphingolipid, neolactotetraosylceramide (nLc4Cer) was a host receptor for all serotypes of DENV in mammalian cells and that the non-reducing terminal disaccharide residue →4)Galβ(1→4)GlcNAcβ(1→ was critical for DENV2 binding [146]. Multivalent dendrimers containing lacto-N-neotetraose (nLc4, Galβ(1→4)GlcNAcβ(1→3)Gal β(1→4)Glcβ(1→) or lactose (Lac, Galβ(1→4)Glcβ(1→) in three different structures named Fan(0)3, Ball(0)4, and Dumbbell(1)6, were synthesized and tested for their anti-DENV2 activities in BHK-21 cells. At 500 μM concentration, the inhibition of DENV2 infection follows: Dumbbell(1)6-nLc4 (57%), Fan(0)3-nLc4 (44%), and Ball(0)4-nLc4 (32%). However, the same dendrimer structures synthesized with lactose did not show effective inhibition at this concentration. While this is not a HP/HS mimetic, it attempted to mimic the carbohydrate moiety of glycosphingolipid and amplify its binding to DENV by multivalency.

3.2. Non Glycan-Based GAG Binding Agents

Although these are not glycan based, peptides and proteins deserve attention for their anti-FLV activity resulting from specifically binding to cell surface GAGs.

3.2.1. Lactoferrin

An antimicrobial protein, bovine lactoferrin, demonstrated anti-JEV activity by binding to cell surface HS in vitro [93]. Lactoferrin showed concentration-dependent inhibition against infection from HS-adapted JEV (CJN-S1) with IC_{50} of 25 μg/mL in BHK-21 cells. The inhibition was lower against infection from non-HS adapted JEV, reaching only 40% inhibition even at 200 μg/mL. HS binding of lactoferrin was determined by reduced anti-JEV activity from its binding to HP-Sepharose as well as the co-incubation with soluble HS. However, another potential pathway was discovered by the reduced anti-JEV activity when co-incubated with each low-density lipoprotein receptor and its antibodies.

3.2.2. Basic Chemokine Derived Peptide

Basic peptides derived from antimicrobial chemokines, CXCL9 and CXCL12γ, with high affinity for GAGs have shown to inhibit DENV2 by its ability to bind to GAGs [147]. Using SPR, peptides derived from the carboxyl terminal regions of CXCL9 and CXCL12γ exhibited broad range of affinity to HP (K_D = 3.1–3559 nM). Inhibition of DENV2 infection in HMEC-1 cells by CXCL9 and CXCL12γ peptides ranged from EC_{50} of 11 to 48 μM with CXCL9 (74–103) being the most potent peptide. Using SPR competition assay, CXCL9 (74–103) blocked domain III of DENV2 envelope protein (DENV2 E) binding to immobilized HP even at 1:10 ratio for their concentrations in the sample.

3.3. Entry Inhibitors Targeting Viral Glycans

3.3.1. Multivalent Mannose Glycodendrimers Mimicking Viral Envelope Protein Glycans

FLVs bind to a C type receptor DC-SIGN through the high-Man on their envelope proteins. Varga et al. synthesized multivalent Man glycodendrimers with varying valency to better compete with the high mannose expressed on the viral envelope protein to inhibit its interactions with DC-SIGN [148]. Surface plasmon resonance competition assay showed that the hexavalent glycodendrimer bearing six copies of bisamide gave the lowest IC_{50} of 6 μM to inhibit DC-SIGN binding to immobilized mannosylated bovine serum albumin. Interestingly, this same hexavalent glycodendrimer most successfully inhibited HIV and DENV2 infection in B-THP-1/DC-SIGN and Raji cells over-expressing DC-SIGN, respectively. Hexavalent glycodendrimer comparably inhibited against HIV and DENV2 infection with IC_{50} of 1 and 5.9 μM. This is an interesting approach to mimic the viral glycans, rather than the host glycans to compete for the carbohydrate-binding region on the host cell receptor.

3.3.2. Lectin Based Inhibitors Targeting Viral Glycans

Rather than mimicking the viral glycans, several plant lectins were utilized to bind to the viral glycan on its envelope protein to block the viral envelope protein and DC-SIGN interactions. Three plant lectins, *Hippeastrum* hybrid agglutinin (HHA), *Galanthus nivalis* agglutinin (GNA) and *Urtica dioica* (UDA) isolated from the amaryllis, the snowdrop and the stinging nettle showed anti-DENV2 activities in vitro [149]. HHA specifically recognizes α1→3 and α1→6 Man residues, GNA recognizes α1→3 Man residues, and finally UDA recognizes GlcNAc residues. These lectins showed cell type dependent inhibition of DENV2 infection with EC_{50} of 0.1–2.2 and 4–56 μM in DC-SIGN transfected Raji cells and interleukin 4 (IL-4) treated monocytes, respectively. However, they did not exhibit any antiviral activities in Vero-B (DC-SIGN$^-$). Both Raji/DC-SIGN$^+$ and IL-4 treated monocytes express DC-SIGN on their cellular surface while Vero-B did not, which may explain the absence of anti-FLV activity in Vero-B cells.

Griffithsin (GRFT) is a lectin isolated from red algae *Griffithsia* and has been reported to exhibit antiviral activities against many enveloped viruses. It is 121 amino acid residues long, yet contains three distinctive carbohydrate-binding sites for Man and Glc [150]. GRFT successfully inhibited against JEV infection both in vitro and in vivo [151]. Pretreatment of GRFT in BHK-21 cells inhibited against JEV infection with IC$_{50}$ of 265 ng/mL. In vivo data showed that *intraperitoneal* administration of GRFT (5 mg/kg) into BALB/c mice completely prevented mortality of JEV infection with a lethal dose. In a separate study, it was postulated that GRFT inhibits against JEV infection by binding to the viral glycan on the envelope protein [152].

3.3.3. α-Glucosidase Inhibitors: Disrupting Proper N-Linked Glycosylation of Viral Glycoproteins

While 3.2.1 and 3.2.2 deal with competitive inhibitors to successfully interrupt viral glycan on the envelope protein and DC-SIGN in the extracellular space, glucosidase inhibitors permanently modify the "original" glycan structure of viral glycan in cytoplasm. Glucosidases first must properly trim the terminal glycans on the lumen of endoplasmic reticulum (ER) before sending the proteins over to Golgi apparatus for further processing. FLVs have three main glycoproteins: prM/M (premembrane/membrane protein), E (envelope protein), and NS1 (nonstructural protein 1). Improper N-glycosylation of viral glycoproteins can interrupt proper folding of prM, leading to destabilization of the prM/E complex, and improper viral particle assembly [153]. Iminosugar derivatives, such as castanospermine (CST), celgosivir (6-O-butanoyl-CST), and N-nonyldeoxynojirimycin (NN-DNJ), are some of the most well studied glucosidase inhibitors in FLV infection. The pathway of N-glycosylation and chemical structures of these inhibitors are shown in Figure 4.

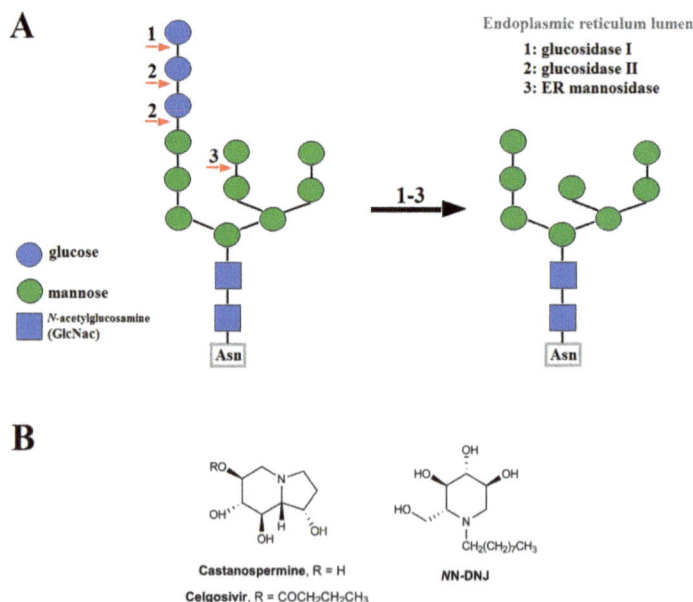

Figure 4. (**A**) Schematic of glucose- and mannose-removal by glucosidase I, II, and endoplasmic reticulum (ER) mannosidase during asparagine (Asn)-linked glycosylation in the ER lumen; (**B**) Chemical structures of α-glucosidase inhibitors, castanospermine, celgosivir, and N-nonyldeoxynojirimycin (NN-DNJ).

Table 2. Chemical and anti-flavivirus properties of heparin and heparan sulfate mimetics.

Compounds	Chemical Structures	Antiviral Activity				Anticoagulant Activity (Y/N)	References
		In Vitro (EC$_{50}$ or IC$_{50}$)	Flavivirus	Cell Type	In Vivo		
Heparin	→4)-N-sulfo 6-O-sulfo-α-D-glucosamine (1→4)-2-O-sulfo-α-L-iduronic acid(1→ per disaccharide unit	0.2 µg/mL; 0.5–1.89 µg/mL, 0.77 µg/mL; 1 µg/mL	YFV; DENV1-4, JEV; DENV2	Vero; Vero; HMEC-1		Y	[131]; [115]; [124]
CSE	β-D-glucuronic acid 1→3, N-acetyl, 4,6-di-O-sulfo β-D-galactosamine 1→4	0.3–3.8 µg/mL; 0.93 µg/mL	DENV1-4; JEV	Vero		Y	[115]
Fucoidan	α-(1→3) linked fucose with sulfate groups substituted at the C-4 position on some of the fucose residues	4.7 µg/mL; 0.9 µg/mL	DENV2	BHK-21; Vero.		Generally, Y	[116]
Carrageenans Kappa/iota/nu	Alternating (1→3)-β-D-galactopyranoses and (1→4)-α-D-galactopyranoses (or 3,6-anhydrogalactopyranoses)	1.8–10.4 µg/mL; 0.31–9.5 µg/mL; >50 µg/mL	DENV2; DENV1-4	HepG2; PH; C6/36 HT (Aedes albopictus mosquito cells)		Y	[118]
iota		0.4 µg/mL	DENV2	Vero			[119]
K5 K5-OS(H)		7 µg/mL		C6/36 HT			[120]
K5-N,OS(H)	4-β-glucuronyl-1,4-α-N-acetylglucosamine	113 µg/mL; 226 µg/mL; 111 µg/mL; 330 µg/mL	DENV2	HMEC-1; HMVEC-d; HMEC-1; HMVEC-d		N	[124]
Curdlan sulfate (sulfated glucan)	branched β-D-(1→3) glucan backbone with piperidine-N-sulfonic acid	262 µg/mL; 7 µg/mL; 10 µg/mL; 69 µg/mL	DENV1; DENV2; DENV3; DENV4	LLC-MK2		Y	[131]
Sulfated galactomannans	(1→4)-linked β-D-mannopyranosyl units substituted by α-D-galactopyranosyl units. M. scabrella (BRS): 1:1 mannose to galactose and L. leucocephala (LLS): 1:4	586 mg/L (BRS) 387 mg/L (LLS); 347 mg/L (BRS) 37 mg/L (LLS)	YFV; DENV1	C6/36	Swiss mice, 87.7 and 96.5% protection at 48 mg/kg of animal weight.	Y	[134]
Sulfated polysaccharides from red, green, and brown seaweeds	Sulfated galactans, xylomannans, fucans, and heteropolysaccharides	0.12–20 µg/mL	DENV2	Vero		Y	[138]
Methyl-α-3-O-sulfated glucuronic acid	Methyl-α-3-O-sulfated glucuronic acid	120 µM	DENV2	BHK-21		N	[141]
PI-88 (phosphomannopentaose sulfate)	A mixture of highly sulfated, monophosphorylated mannose oligosaccharides	200 µg/mL; 40 µg/mL	DENV2; JEV		Increased survival time from 15 to 22 days in C57BL/6 mice.	Y	
PPS (pentosan polysulfate)	(1→4)-β-Xylan 2,3-bis (hydrogen sulfate) with a 4 O-methyl-α-D-glucuronate), this for PPS	60 µg/mL; 7 µg/mL; 30 µg/mL	DENV2; JEV; DENV2	BHK-21		Y	[142]
Suramin	8,8'-[carbonylbis[imino-3,1-phenylenecarbonylimino(4-methyl-3,1-phenylene)carbonylimino]] bis-1,3,5-naphthalenetrisulfonic acid	50 µg/mL	DENV2			Y	

BHK-21: baby hamster kidney fibroblasts; BRS: Sulfated galactomannans from M. scabrella; CSE: chondroitin sulfate type E; DENV1-4: dengue virus serotypes 1-4; EC$_{50}$: half maximal effective concentration; HepG2: human liver cancer cell line; HMEC-1: immotalized human dermal microvascular endothelial cell line; IC$_{50}$: half maximal inhibitory concentration; JEV: Japanese encephalitis virus; LLS: Sulfated galactomannans from L. leucocephala; YFV: yellow fever virus.

3.3.4. Castanospermine

Whitby et al. tested antiviral activity of castanospermine (CST) against all four types of DENV, YFV, and WNV in vitro and in vivo [154]. CST showed comparable inhibition level against all serotypes of DENV in Huh-7 and BHK-21 cells, however this activity was cell type dependent. For example, the IC_{50} against DENV2 infection was 85.7 and 1 µM in Huh-7 and BHK-21 cells, respectively. CST also showed inhibition against YFV by 57 and 93% at 50 and 500 µM. However, CST did not show significant inhibition against WNV even at high concentration (500 µM). In C57BL/6 and A/J mice, CST promoted survival at 10, 50, and 250 mg/kg of body weight per day. However, no protective effect was shown against WNV. It was postulated that the mechanism of inhibition was due to ineffective secretion of virus with improper N-glycosylation.

3.3.5. Celgosivir (6-O-Butanoyl-CST)

Celgosivir is an oral prodrug of CST and inhibits α-glucosidase I and II, and its antiviral activities were tested in DENV [155–157]. Celgosivir effectively inhibited against DENV infections in BHK-21 cells with EC_{50} ranging from 0.16 to 0.68 µM depending on the serotype, which was partly due to accumulation of misfolded NS1 of DENV in the ER [156]. Interestingly, Celogosivir showed two-fold higher efficacy than that of CST when ADE mice were challenged with 50 mg/kg. However, a recent study demonstrated that celgosivir was not a potent inhibitor of ZIKV in Vero cells (EC_{50} was not determined even at 50 µM) [158]. Despite its great efficacy in vitro and in vivo, celgosivir did not succeed at treating DENV patients due to its rapid elimination [159].

3.3.6. N-Nonyldeoxynojirimycin (NN-DNJ)

N-Nonyldeoxynojirimycin (NN-DNJ), a 9-carbon alkyl iminosugar derivative, was found to inhibit against DENV, JEV, and WNV [160,161]. Wu et al. reported that NN-DNJ inhibited more successfully against DENV than JEV in BHK-21 cells although the IC_{50} values were not reported.

In Institute of Cancer Research (ICR) mice, NN-DNJ successfully increased the survival rate by 40% against JEV infection, compared to the control group, at 200 mg/kg/day. Secretion of the E and NS1 proteins was greatly reduced, indicating that the proper N-glycosylation steps must be followed for successful virus assembly. In a separate study, NN-DNJ showed anti-WNV activity with IC_{50} of 4 µM in BHK cells [161].

4. Future Directions and Conclusion

A number of strategies might be used to improve GAGs and other sulfated polysaccharides to more effectively inhibit against FLV infections. The first classes of compounds studied were natural GAGs and then GAG mimetics that inhibit GAG-FLVE interactions. Although these compounds have the required level of charge density and structural flexibility to successfully occupy the GAG binding sites of FLV and inhibit against FLV infections in vitro, the majority of these also possess anticoagulant activities. Anticoagulant activity is problematic because it will promote plasma leakage in the patients infected with DENV and YFV, diseases that cause haemorrhagic fever. This undesired characteristic might be attenuated by processing these polysaccharides into smaller oligosaccharides that reach the minimum size required for occupying the E protein GAG-binding site (a HP decasaccharide corresponding to 39 Å in the case of DENV). For example, HP is a very potent anticoagulant drug, however its anticoagulant activity was relatively low until it reaches a hexadecasaccharide [140,162,163]. Several different chain lengths of oligosaccharides must be prepared to retain anti-FLV activity while minimizing its anticoagulant activity. Sulfated polysaccharides can also go through chemical modifications to reduce their anticoagulant activity. In our laboratory, non-anticoagulant heparin (NACH) has been synthesized by periodate cleavage at the GlcA and IdoA residues located within and adjacent to the antithrombin III [164]. Upon chemical modification, NACH completely loses its anticoagulant activity. However, these structurally modified sulfated polysaccharides can also result in a reduced level of interactions to the GAG-binding sites of FLVE as shown in our interactions studies of DENV E and ZIKV E [6,13]. Multivalent glycopolymers or glycodendrimers can also be produced to amplify glycan-protein binding, as this is often how glycans and proteins are presented on the surface of cells in nature. Another potential pitfall of sulfated polysaccharides is their poor bioavailability. While exhibiting excellent in vitro antiviral activities, those activities of PPS and suramin did not translate well to in vivo experiments. The least potent inhibitor, PI-88, in vitro, showed the greatest efficacy, which was postulated to be caused by their interactions with other HP-binding proteins in vivo [142]. This drawback may be overcome by improved in vivo delivery approaches. The simplest approach would be to conjugate the sulfated polysaccharides to a molecule that has higher specificity towards the target such as envelope protein, or specific cell or organ types. There are antibodies against FLVE for research use, however no effective antibody is available for clinical treatment due to antibody dependent enhancement between different serotypes of DENV. DNA or RNA aptamers may be excellent alternatives to specifically target FLVE; they are cost efficient, nontoxic, non-immunogenic, and exhibit incredible specificity against their targets once the "hit" compound is found from a large library. Highly specific DNA based aptamers were discovered against FLVE in recent studies [165,166]. Conjugating sulfated polysaccharides with highly specific and synergistic compounds, such as DNA aptamers, may improve the potential hurdle of oral bioavailability. Lastly, an additional hurdle is presented in the treatment of pregnant women infected with ZIKV infection. Inhibitors against congenital ZIKV infection must be large enough and not readily metabolized in the blood stream so that they do not enter the cells and cross the placental barrier to avoid undesired additional harm to the fetus.

In conclusion, this review examined the role of carbohydrates in the pathogenesis of pathogenic FLVs and their antiviral inhibitors. First, we briefly introduced the general mechanism of host cell entry of FLVs. Then we described the glycosylation of FLV envelope protein, host surface GAGs, DC-SIGN, and interactions between them. FLV inhibitors that are both glycan-based and targeting were reviewed and strategies to improve carbohydrate-based inhibitors were discussed.

Acknowledgments: We acknowledge the National Institutes of Health (grant HL125371) for funding our work on glycosaminoglycans.

Author Contributions: S.Y.K. wrote the abstract, Section 1, Section 3, and Section 4 of the manuscript. B.L. wrote Section 2 of the manuscript. R.J.L. oversaw the writing and provided critical feedback on the manuscript. All authors participated in the revision process.

Conflicts of Interest: The authors declare no conflict of interest.

References

1. World Health Organization. Vector-Borne Diseases. Available online: http://www.who.int/mediacentre/factsheets/fs387/en/ (accessed on 2 February 2017).
2. World Health Organization. Mosquito-Borne Diseases. Available online: http://www.who.int/neglected_diseases/vector_ecology/mosquito-borne-diseases/en/ (accessed on 2 February 2017).
3. World Health Organization. Dengue and Severe Dengue. Available online: http://www.who.int/mediacentre/factsheets/fs117/en/ (accessed on 2 February 2017).
4. World Health Organization. WHO Director-General Summarizes the Outcome of the Emergency Committee Regarding Clusters of Microcephaly and Guillain-Barré Syndrome. Available online: http://www.who.int/mediacentre/news/statements/2016/emergency-committee-zika-microcephaly/en/ (accessed on 2 February 2017).
5. Centers for Disease Control and Prevention. Pregnant Women with Any Laboratory Evidence of Possible Zika Virus Infection in the United States and Territories. Available online: https://www.cdc.gov/zika/geo/pregwomen-uscases.html (accessed on 2 February 2017).
6. Chen, Y.; Maguire, T.; Hileman, R.E.; Fromm, J.R.; Esko, J.D.; Linhardt, R.J.; Marks, R.M. Dengue virus infectivity depends on envelope protein binding to target cell heparan sulfate. *Nat. Med.* **1997**, *3*, 866–871. [CrossRef] [PubMed]

7. Germi, R.; Crance, J.M.; Garin, D.; Guimet, J.; Lortat-Jacob, H.; Ruigrok, R.W.; Zarski, J.P.; Drouet, E. Heparan sulfate-mediated binding of infectious dengue virus type 2 and yellow fever virus. *Virology* **2002**, *292*, 162–168. [CrossRef] [PubMed]

8. Hilgard, P.; Stockert, R. Heparan sulfate proteoglycans initiate dengue virus infection of hepatocytes. *Hepatology* **2000**, *32*, 1069–1077. [CrossRef] [PubMed]

9. Chen, H.L.; Her, S.Y.; Huang, K.C.; Cheng, H.T.; Wu, C.W.; Wu, S.C.; Cheng, J.W. Identification of a heparin binding peptide from the Japanese encephalitis virus envelope protein. *Biopolymers* **2010**, *94*, 331–338. [CrossRef] [PubMed]

10. Kozlovskaya, L.I.; Osolodkin, D.I.; Shevtsova, A.S.; Romanova, L.I.; Rogova, Y.V.; Dzhivanian, T.I.; Lyapustin, V.N.; Pivanova, G.P.; Gmyl, A.P.; et al. GAG binding variants of tick-borne encephalitis virus. *Virology* **2010**, *398*, 262–272. [CrossRef] [PubMed]

11. Lee, E.; Lobigs, M. E protein domain III determinants of yellow fever virus 17D vaccine strain enhance binding to glycosaminoglycans, impede virus spread, and attenuate virulence. *J. Virol.* **2008**, *82*, 6024–6033. [CrossRef] [PubMed]

12. Mandl, C.W.; Kroschewski, H.; Allison, S.L.; Kofler, R.; Holzmann, H.; Meixner, T.; Heinz, F.X. Adaptation of tick-borne encephalitis virus to BHK-21 cells results in the formation of multiple heparan sulfate binding sites in the envelope protein and attenuation in vivo. *J. Virol.* **2001**, *75*, 5627–5637. [CrossRef] [PubMed]

13. Kim, S.Y.; Zhao, J.; Liu, X.; Fraser, K.; Lin, L.; Zhang, X.; Zhang, F.; Dordick, J.S.; Linhardt, R.J. Interaction of Zika Virus Envelope Protein with Glycosaminoglycans. *Biochemistry* **2017**, *56*, 1151–1162. [CrossRef] [PubMed]

14. Kamhi, E.; Joo, E.J.; Dordick, J.S.; Linhardt, R.J. Glycosaminoglycans in infectious disease. *Biol. Rev.* **2013**, *88*, 928–943. [CrossRef] [PubMed]

15. Reyes-del Valle, J.; Chavez-Salinas, S.; Medina, F.; del Angel, R.M. Heat Shock Protein 90 and Heat Shock Protein 70 Are Components of Dengue Virus Receptor Complex in Human Cells. *J. Virol.* **2005**, *79*, 4557–4567. [CrossRef] [PubMed]

16. Aoki, C.; Hidari, K.I.P.J.; Itonori, S.; Yamada, A.; Takahashi, N.; Kasama, T.; Hasebe, F.; Islam, M.A.; Hatano, K.; Matsuoka, K.; et al. Identification and characterization of carbohydrate molecules in mammalian cells recognized by dengue virus type 2. *J. Biochem.* **2006**, *139*, 607–614. [CrossRef] [PubMed]

17. Chen, Y.C.; Wang, S.Y.; King, C.C. Bacterial lipopolysaccharide inhibits dengue virus infection of primary human monocytes/macrophages by blockade of virus entry via a CD14-dependent mechanism. *J. Virol.* **1999**, *73*, 2650–2657. [PubMed]

18. Jindadamrongwech, S.; Thepparit, C.; Smith, D.R. Identification of GRP 78 (BiP) as a liver cell expressed receptor element for dengue virus serotype 2. *Arch. Virol.* **2004**, *149*, 915–927. [CrossRef] [PubMed]

19. Thepparit, C.; Smith, D.R. Serotype-specific entry of dengue virus into liver cells: identification of the 37-kilodalton/67-kilodalton high-affinity laminin receptor as a dengue virus serotype 1 receptor. *J. Virol.* **2004**, *78*, 12647–12656. [CrossRef] [PubMed]

20. Lozach, P.Y.; Burleigh, L.; Staropoli, I.; Navarro-Sanchez, E.; Harriague, J.; Virelizier, J.L.; Rey, F.A.; Desprès, P.; Arenzana-Seisdedos, F.; Amara, A. Dendritic cell-specific intercellular adhesion molecule 3-grabbing non-integrin (DC-SIGN)-mediated enhancement of dengue virus infection is independent of DC-SIGN internalization signals. *J. Biol. Chem.* **2005**, *280*, 23698–23708. [CrossRef] [PubMed]

21. Navarro-Sanchez, E.; Altmeyer, R.; Amara, A.; Schwartz, O.; Fieschi, F.; Virelizier, J.L.; Arenzana-Seisdedos, F.; Despres, P. Dendritic-cell-specific ICAM3-grabbing non-integrin is essential for the productive infection of human dendritic cells by mosquito-cell-derived dengue viruses. *EMBO Rep.* **2003**, *4*, 723–728. [CrossRef] [PubMed]

22. Tassaneetrithep, B.; Burgess, T. H.; Granelli-Piperno, A.; Trumpfheller, C.; Finke, J.; Sun, W.; Eller, M.A.; Pattanapanyasat, K.; Sarasombath, S.; Birx, D.L.; Steinman, R.M.; Schlesinger, S.; Marovich, M. A. DC-SIGN (CD209) mediates dengue virus infection of human dendritic cells. *J. Exp. Med.* **2003**, *197*, 823–829. [CrossRef] [PubMed]

23. Miller, J.L.; deWet, B.J.M.; Martinez-Pomares, L.; Radcliffe, C.M.; Dwek, R.A.; Rudd, P.M.; Gordon, S. The Mannose Receptor Mediates Dengue Virus Infection of Macrophages. *PLoS Pathog.* **2008**, *4*, 1–11. [CrossRef]

24. Chen, S.-T.; Lin, Y.-L.; Huang, M.-T.; Wu, M.-F.; Cheng, S.-C.; Lei, H.-Y.; Lee, C.-K.; Chiou, T.-W.; Wong, C.-H.; Hsieh, S.-L. CLEC5A is critical for dengue-virus-induced lethal disease. *Nature* **2008**, *453*, 672–676. [CrossRef] [PubMed]

25. Mercado-Curiel, R.F.; Esquinca-Avilés, H.A.; Tovar, R.; Díaz-Badillo, A.; Camacho-Nuez, M.; de Lourdes Muñoz, M. The four serotypes of dengue recognize the same putative receptors in *Aedes aegypti* midgut and *Ae. albopictus* cells. *BMC Microbiol.* **2006**, *6*, 1–10. [CrossRef] [PubMed]

26. Mendoza, M.Y.; Salas-Benito, J.S.; Lanz-Mendoza, H.; Hernández-Martinez, S.; Del Angel, R.M. A putative receptor for dengue virus in mosquito tissues: Localization of a 45-kDa glycoprotein. *Am. J. Trop. Med. Hyg.* **2002**, *67*, 76–84.

27. Pokidysheva, E.; Zhang, Y.; Battisti, A.J.; Bator-Kelly, C.M.; Chipman, P.R.; Xiao, C.; Gregorio, G. G.; Hendrickson, W.A.; Kuhn, R.J.; Rossmann, M.G. Cryo-EM reconstruction of dengue virus in complex with the carbohydrate recognition domain of DC-SIGN. *Cell* **2006**, *124*, 485–493. [CrossRef] [PubMed]

28. Davis, C.W.; Nguyen, H.-Y.; Hanna, S.L.; Sánchez, M.D.; Doms, R.W.; Pierson, T.C. West Nile virus discriminates between DC-SIGN and DC-SIGNR for cellular attachment and infection. *J. Virol.* **2006**, *80*, 1290–1301. [CrossRef] [PubMed]

29. Davis, C.W.; Mattei, L.M.; Nguyen, H.Y.; Ansarah-Sobrinho, C.; Doms, R.W.; Pierson, T.C. The location of asparagine-linked glycans on West Nile virions controls their interactions with CD209 (dendritic cell-specific ICAM-3 grabbing nonintegrin). *J. Biol. Chem.* **2006**, *281*, 37183–37194. [CrossRef] [PubMed]

30. Chu, J.J.H.; Ng, M.L. Interaction of West Nile virus with $\alpha V\beta 3$ integrin mediates virus entry into cells. *J. Biol. Chem.* **2004**, *279*, 54533–54541. [CrossRef] [PubMed]

31. Lee, J.W.-M.; Chu, J.J.-H.; Ng, M.-L. Quantifying the specific binding between West Nile virus envelope domain III protein and the cellular receptor $\alpha V\beta 3$ integrin. *J. Biol. Chem.* **2006**, *281*, 1352–1360. [CrossRef] [PubMed]

32. Medigeshi, G.R.; Hirsch, A.J.; Streblow, D.N.; Nikolich-Zugich, J.; Nelson, J.A. West Nile virus entry requires cholesterol-rich membrane microdomains and is independent of $\alpha v\beta 3$ integrin. *J. Virol.* **2008**, *82*, 5212–5219. [CrossRef] [PubMed]

33. Van der Schaar, H.M.; Rust, M. J.; Chen, C.; van der Ende-Metselaar, H.; Wilschut, J.; Zhuang, X.; Smit, J.M. Dissecting the cell entry pathway of dengue virus by single-particle tracking in living cells. *PLoS Pathog.* **2008**, *4*, 1–9. [CrossRef] [PubMed]

34. Ishak, R.; Tovey, D.G.; Howard, C.R. Morphogenesis of yellow fever virus 17D in infected cell cultures. *J. Gen. Virol.* **1988**, *69*, 325–335. [CrossRef] [PubMed]

35. Pierson, T.C.; Kielian, M. Flaviviruses: braking the entering. *Curr. Opin. Virol.* **2013**, *3*, 3–12. [CrossRef] [PubMed]

36. Martinez-Barragan, J.J.; del Angel, R.M. Identification of a putative coreceptor on Vero cells that participates in dengue 4 virus infection. *J. Virol.* **2001**, *75*, 7818–7827. [CrossRef] [PubMed]

37. Das, S.; Laxminarayana, S.V.; Chandra, N.; Ravi, V.; Desai, A. Heat shock protein 70 on Neuro2a cells is a putative receptor for Japanese encephalitis virus. *Virology* **2009**, *385*, 47–57. [CrossRef] [PubMed]

38. Salas-Benito, J.; Reyes-Del Valle, J.; Salas-Benito, M.; Ceballos-Olvera, I.; Mosso, C.; del Angel, R.M. Evidence that the 45 kD glycoprotein, part of a putative dengue virus receptor complex in the mosquito cell line C6/36, is a heat-shock related protein. *Am. J. Trop. Med. Hyg.* **2007**, *77*, 283–290. [PubMed]

39. Jemielity, S.; Wang, J.J.; Chan, Y.K.; Ahmed, A.A.; Li, W.; Monahan, S.; Bu, X.; Farza, M.; Freeman, J.J.; Umetsu, D.T.; et al. TIM-family proteins promote infection of multiple enveloped viruses through virion-associated phosphatidylserine. *PLoS Pathog* **2013**, *9*, e1003232. [CrossRef] [PubMed]

40. Hamel, R.; Dejarnac, O.; Wichit, S.; Ekchariyawat, P.; Neyret, A.; Luplertlop, N.; Perera-Lecoin, M.; Surasombatpattana, P.; Talignani, L.; Thomas, F.; et al. Biology of Zika virus infection in human skin cells. *J. Virol.* **2015**, *89*, 8880–8896. [CrossRef] [PubMed]

41. Richard, A.S.; Shim, B.S.; Kwon, Y.C.; Zhang, R.; Otsuka, Y.; Schmitt, K.; Berri, F.; Diamond, M.S.; Choe, H. AXL-dependent infection of human fetal endothelial cells distinguishes Zika virus from other pathogenic flaviviruses. *Proc. Natl. Acad. Sci. USA* **2017**, *114*, 2024–2029. [CrossRef] [PubMed]

42. Miner, J.J.; Daniels, B.P.; Shrestha, B.; Proenca-Modena, J.L.; Lew, E.D.; Lazear, H.M.; Gorman, M.J.; Lemke, G.; Klein, R.S.; Diamond, M.S. The Tam Receptor Mertk Protects Against Neuroinvasive Viral Infection by Maintaining Blood-brain Barrier Integrity. *Nat. Med.* **2015**, *21*, 1464–1472. [CrossRef] [PubMed]

43. Hacker, K.; White, L.; de Silva, A.M. N-linked glycans on dengue viruses grown in mammalian and insect cells. *J. Gen. Virol.* **2009**, *90*, 2097–2106. [CrossRef] [PubMed]

44. Chen, S.T.; Liu, R.S.; Wu, M.F.; Lin, Y.L.; Chen, S.Y.; Tan, D.T.; Chou, T.Y.; Tsai, I.S.; Li, L.; Hsieh, S.L. CLEC5A regulates Japanese encephalitisvirus-induced neuroinflammation and lethality. *PLoS Pathog.* **2012**, *8*, e1002655. [CrossRef] [PubMed]

45. Kuadkitkan, A.; Wikan, N.; Fongsaran, C.; Smith, D.R. Identification and characterization of prohibitin as a receptor protein mediating DENV-2 entry into insect cells. *Virology* **2010**, *406*, 149–161. [CrossRef] [PubMed]

46. Idris, F.; Muharram, S.H.; Diah, S. Glycosylation of dengue virus glycoproteins and their interactions with carbohydrate receptors: possible targets for antiviral therapy. *Arch. Virol.* **2016**, *161*, 1751–1760. [CrossRef] [PubMed]
47. Beesetti, H.; Khanna, N.; Swaminathan, S. Drugs for dengue: a patent review (2010–2014). *Exp. Opin. Ther. Pat.* **2014**, *24*, 1171–1184. [CrossRef] [PubMed]
48. Herrero, L.J.; Zakhary, A.; Gahan, M.E.; Nelson, M.A.; Herring, B.L.; Hapel, A.J.; Keller, P.A.; Obeyseker, M.; Chen, W.; Sheng, K.C.; et al. Dengue virus therapeutic intervention strategies based on viral, vector and host factors involved in disease pathogenesis. *Pharmacol. Ther.* **2013**, *137*, 266–282. [CrossRef] [PubMed]
49. Hanna, S.L.; Pierson, T.C.; Sanchez, M.D.; Ahmed, A.A.; Murtadha, M.M.; Doms, R.W. *N*-linked glycosylation of West Nile virus envelope proteins influences particle assembly and infectivity. *J. Virol.* **2005**, *79*, 13262–13274. [CrossRef] [PubMed]
50. Huang, K.C.; Lee, M.C.; Wu, C.W.; Huang, K.J.; Lei, H.Y.; Cheng, J.W. Solution structure and neutralizing antibody binding studies of domain III of the dengue-2 virus envelope protein. *Proteins* **2008**, *70*, 1116–1119. [CrossRef] [PubMed]
51. Rey, F.A.; Heinz, F.X.; Mandl, C.; Kunz, C.; Harrison, S.C. The envelope glycoprotein from tick-borne encephalitis virus at 2 angstrom resolution. *Nature* **1995**, *375*, 291–298. [CrossRef] [PubMed]
52. Ji, G.H.; Deng, Y.Q.; Yu, X.J.; Jiang, T.; Wang, H.J.; Shi, X.; Zhang, D.P.; Li, X.F.; Zhu, S.Y.; Zhao, H.; et al. Characterization of a Novel Dengue Serotype 4 Virus-Specific Neutralizing Epitope on the Envelope Protein Domain III. *PLoS ONE* **2015**, *10*, e0139741. [CrossRef] [PubMed]
53. Kanai, R.; Kar, K.; Anthony, K.; Gould, L.H.; Ledizet, M.; Fikrig, E.; Marasco, W.A.; Koski, R.A.; Modis, Y. Crystal structure of West Nile virus envelope glycoprotein reveals viral surface epitopes. *J. Virol.* **2006**, *80*, 11000–11008. [CrossRef] [PubMed]
54. Nybakken, G.E.; Nelson, C.A.; Chen, B.R.; Diamond, M.S.; Fremont, D.H. Crystal structure of the West Nile virus envelope glycoprotein. *J. Virol.* **2006**, *80*, 11467–11474. [CrossRef] [PubMed]
55. Luca, V.C.; AbiMansour, J.; Nelson, C.A.; Fremont, D.H. Crystal structure of the Japanese encephalitis virus envelope protein. *J. Virol.* **2012**, *86*, 2337–2346. [CrossRef] [PubMed]
56. Sirohi, D.; Chen, Z.; Sun, L.; Klose, T.; Pierson, T.C.; Rossmann, M.G.; Kuhn, R.J. The 3.8 Å resolution cryo-EM structure of Zika virus. *Science* **2016**, *352*, 467–470. [CrossRef] [PubMed]
57. Huang, C.Y.H.; Butrapet, S.; Moss, K.J.; Childers, T.; Erb, S.M.; Calvert, A.E.; Silengo, S.J.; Kinne, R.M.; Blair, C.D.; Roehrig, J.T. The dengue virus type 2 envelope protein fusion peptide is essential for membrane fusion. *Virology* **2010**, *396*, 305–315. [CrossRef] [PubMed]
58. Kuhn, R.J.; Zhang, W.; Rossmann, M.G.; Pletnev, S.V.; Corver, J.; Lenches, E.; Jones, C.T.; Mukhopadhyay, S.; Chipman, P.R.; Strauss, E.G. Structure of dengue virus: implications for flavivirus organization, maturation, and fusion. *Cell* **2002**, *108*, 717–725. [CrossRef]
59. Goncalvez, A.P.; Purcell, R.H.; Lai, C.J. Epitope determinants of a chimpanzee Fab antibody that efficiently cross-neutralizes dengue type 1 and type 2 viruses map to inside and in close proximity to fusion loop of the dengue type 2 virus envelope glycoprotein. *J. Virol.* **2004**, *78*, 12919–12928. [CrossRef] [PubMed]
60. Watterson, D.; Kobe, B.; Young, P.R. Residues in domain III of the dengue virus envelope glycoprotein involved in cell-surface glycosaminoglycan binding. *J. Gen. Virol.* **2012**, *93*, 72–82. [CrossRef] [PubMed]
61. Zhang, Y.; Zhang, W.; Ogata, S.; Clements, D.; Strauss, J.H.; Baker, T.S.; Kuhn, R.J.; Rossmann, M.G. Conformational changes of the flavivirus E glycoprotein. *Structure* **2004**, *12*, 1607–1618. [CrossRef] [PubMed]
62. Batra, G.; Raut, R.; Dahiya, S.; Kamran, N.; Swaminathan, S.; Khanna, N. *Pichia pastoris*-expressed dengue virus type 2 envelope domain III elicits virus-neutralizing antibodies. *J. Virol. Methods* **2010**, *67*, 10–16. [CrossRef] [PubMed]
63. Chin, J.F.; Chu, J.J.; Ng, M.L. The envelope glycoprotein domain III of dengue virus serotypes 1 and 2 inhibit virus entry. *Microbes Infect.* **2007**, *9*, 1–6. [CrossRef] [PubMed]
64. Modis, Y.; Ogata, S.; Clements, D.; Harrison, S.C. Structure of the dengue virus envelope protein after membrane fusion. *Nature* **2004**, *427*, 313–319. [CrossRef] [PubMed]
65. Modis, Y.; Ogata, S.; Clements, D.; Harrison, S.C. Variable surface epitopes in the crystal structure of dengue virus type 3 envelope glycoprotein. *J. Virol* **2005**, *79*, 1223–1231. [CrossRef] [PubMed]
66. Pitcher, T.J.; Sarathy, V.V.; Matsui, K.; Gromowski, G.D.; Huang, C.Y.H.; Barrett, A.D. Functional analysis of dengue virus (DENV) type 2 envelope protein domain 3 type-specific and DENV complex-reactive critical epitope residues. *J. Gen. Virol.* **2015**, *96*, 288–293. [CrossRef] [PubMed]

67. Murata, R.; Eshita, Y.; Maeda, A.; Maeda, J.; Akita, S.; Tanaka, T.; Yoshii, K.; Kariwa, H.; Umemura, T.; Takashima, I. Glycosylation of the West Nile Virus envelope protein increases in vivo and in vitro viral multiplication in birds. *Am. J. Trop. Med. Hyg.* **2010**, *82*, 696–704. [CrossRef] [PubMed]

68. Kariwa, H.; Murata, R.; Totani, M.; Yoshii, K.; Takashima, I. Increased pathogenicity of West Nile virus (WNV) by glycosylation of envelope protein and seroprevalence of WNV in wild birds in Far Eastern Russia. *Int. J. Environ. Res. Public Health* **2013**, *10*, 7144–7164. [CrossRef] [PubMed]

69. Hebert, D.N.; Foellmer, B.; Helenius, A. Glucose trimming and reglucosylation determine glycoprotein association with calnexin in the endoplasmic reticulum. *Cell* **1995**, *81*, 425–433. [CrossRef]

70. Ruddock, L.W.; Molinari, M. N-glycan processing in ER quality control. *J. Cell Sci.* **2006**, *119*, 4373–4380. [CrossRef] [PubMed]

71. Jarvis, D.L. Developing baculovirus-insect cell expression systems for humanized recombinant glycoprotein production. *Virology* **2003**, *310*, 1–7. [CrossRef]

72. Lei, Y.; Yu, H.; Dong, Y.; Yang, J.; Ye, W.; Wang, Y.; Chen, W.; Jia, Z.; Xu, Z.; Li, Z.; et al. Characterization of N-glycan structures on the surface of mature dengue 2 virus derived from insect cells. *PLoS ONE* **2015**, *10*, e0132122. [CrossRef] [PubMed]

73. Ishak, H.; Takegami, T.; Kamimura, K.; Funada, H. Comparative sequences of two type 1 dengue virus strains possessing different growth characteristics in vitro. *Microbiol. Immunol.* **2001**, *45*, 327–331. [CrossRef] [PubMed]

74. Johnson, A.J.; Guirakhoo, F.; Roehrig, J.T. The envelope glycoproteins of dengue 1 and dengue 2 viruses grown in mosquito cells differ in their utilization of potential glycosylation sites. *Virology* **1994**, *203*, 241–249. [CrossRef] [PubMed]

75. Scherret, J.H.; Mackenzie, J.S.; Khromykh, A.A.; Hall, R.A. Biological significance of glycosylation of the envelope protein of Kunjin virus. *Ann. N. Y. Acad. Sci.* **2001**, *951*, 361–363. [CrossRef] [PubMed]

76. Bryant, J.E.; Calvert, A.E.; Mesesan, K.; Crabtree, M.B.; Volpe, K.E.; Silengo, S.; Kinney, R.M.; Huang, C.Y.; Miller, B.R.; Roehrig, J.T. Glycosylation of the dengue 2 virus E protein at N67 is critical for virus growth in vitro but not for growth in intrathoracically inoculated *Aedes aegypti* mosquitoes. *Virology* **2007**, *366*, 415–423. [CrossRef] [PubMed]

77. Wang, P.; Hu, K.; Luo, S.; Zhang, M.; Deng, X.; Li, C.; Jin, W.; Hu, B.; He, S.; Li, M.; et al. DC-SIGN as an attachment factor mediates Japanese encephalitis virus infection of human dendritic cells via interaction with a single high-mannose residue of viral E glycoprotein. *Virology* **2016**, *488*, 108–119. [CrossRef] [PubMed]

78. Gandhi, N.S.; Mancera, R.L. The structure of glycosaminoglycans and their interactions with proteins. *Chem. Biol. Drug Des.* **2008**, *72*, 455–482. [CrossRef] [PubMed]

79. Sarrazin, S.; Lamanna, W.C.; Esko, J.D. Heparan sulfate proteoglycans. *Cold Spring Harb. Perspect. Biol.* **2011**, *3*, a004952. [CrossRef] [PubMed]

80. Lindahl, U.; Li, J. Interactions between heparan sulfate and proteins—design and functional implications. *Int. Rev. Cell Mol. Biol.* **2009**, *276*, 105–159. [PubMed]

81. Sasisekharan, R.; Raman, R.; Prabhakar, V. Glycomics approach to structure function relationships of glycosaminoglycans. *Annu. Rev. Biomed. Eng.* **2006**, *8*, 181–231. [CrossRef] [PubMed]

82. Cladera, J.; Martin, I.; O'Shea, P. The fusion domain of HIV gp41 interacts specifically with heparan sulfate on the T-lymphocyte cell surface. *EMBO J.* **2001**, *20*, 19–26. [CrossRef] [PubMed]

83. Shukla, D.; Liu, J.; Blaiklock, P.; Shworak, N.W.; Bai, X.; Esko, J.D.; Cohen, G.H.; Eisenberg, R.J.; Rosenberg, R.D.; Spear, P.G. A novel role for 3-O-sulfated heparan sulfate in herpes simplex virus 1 entry. *Cell* **1999**, *99*, 13–22. [CrossRef]

84. Shukla, D.; Spear, P.G. Herpesviruses and heparan sulfate: an intimate relationship in aid of viral entry. *J. Clin. Investig.* **2001**, *108*, 503–510. [CrossRef] [PubMed]

85. Wadstrom, T.; Ljungh, A. Glycosaminoglycan-binding microbial proteins in tissue adhesion and invasion: Key events in microbial pathogenicity. *J. Med. Microbiol.* **1999**, *48*, 223–233. [CrossRef] [PubMed]

86. Zhu, W.Y.; Li, J.J.; Liang, G.D. How does cellular heparan sulfate function in viral pathogenicity? *Biomed. Environ. Sci.* **2011**, *24*, 81–87. [PubMed]

87. Añez, G.; Men, R.; Eckels, K.H.; Lai, C.J. Passage of dengue virus type 4 vaccine candidates in fetal rhesus lung cells selects heparin-sensitive variants that result in loss of infectivity and immunogenicity in rhesus macaques. *J. Virol.* **2009**, *83*, 10384–10394. [CrossRef] [PubMed]

88. Gopal, S.; Bober, A.; Whiteford, J.R.; Multhaupt, H.A.; Yoneda, A.; Couchman, J.R. Heparan sulfate chain valency controls syndecan-4 function in cell adhesion. *J. Biol. Chem.* **2010**, *285*, 14247–14258. [CrossRef] [PubMed]

89. Putnak, J.R.; Niranjan, K.T.; Innis, B.L. A putative cellular receptor for dengue viruses. *Nat. Med.* **1997**, *3*, 828–829. [CrossRef] [PubMed]

90. Thepparit, C.; Phoolcharoen, W.; Suksanpaisan, L.; Smith, D.R. Internalization and propagation of the dengue virus in human hepatoma (HepG2) cells. *Intervirology* **2004**, *47*, 78–86. [CrossRef] [PubMed]

91. Dalrymple, N.; Mackow, E.R. Productive dengue virus infection of human endothelial cells is directed by heparan sulfate-containing proteoglycan receptors. *J. Virol.* **2011**, *85*, 9478–9485. [CrossRef] [PubMed]

92. Su, C.M.; Liao, C.L.; Lee, Y.L.; Lin, Y.L. Highly sulfated forms of heparin sulfate are involved in Japanese encephalitis virus infection. *Virology* **2001**, *286*, 206–215. [CrossRef] [PubMed]

93. Chien, Y.J.; Chen, W.J.; Hsu, W.L.; Chiou, S.S. Bovine lactoferrin inhibits Japanese encephalitis virus by binding to heparan sulfate and receptor for low density lipoprotein. *Virology* **2008**, *379*, 143–151. [CrossRef] [PubMed]

94. Liu, H.; Chiou, S.S.; Chen, W.J. Differential binding efficiency between the envelope protein of Japanese encephalitis virus variants and heparan sulfate on the cell surface. *J. Med. Virol.* **2004**, *72*, 618–624. [CrossRef] [PubMed]

95. Kroschewski, H.; Allison, S.L.; Heinz, F.X.; Mandl, C.W. Role of heparan sulfate for attachment and entry of tick-borne encephalitis virus. *Virology* **2003**, *308*, 92–100. [CrossRef]

96. Lee, E.; Hall, R.A.; Lobigs, M. Common E protein determinants for attenuation of glycosaminoglycan-binding variants of Japanese encephalitis and West Nile viruses. *J. Virol.* **2004**, *78*, 8271–8280. [CrossRef] [PubMed]

97. Hileman, R.E.; Fromm, J.R.; Weiler, J.M.; Linhardt, R.J. Glycosaminoglycan–protein interactions: definition of consensus sites in glycosaminoglycan binding proteins. *Bioessays* **1998**, *20*, 156–167. [CrossRef]

98. Roehrig, J.T.; Butrapet, S.; Liss, N.M.; Bennett, S.L.; Luy, B.E.; Childers, T.; Boroughs, K.L.; Stovall, J.L.; Calvert, A.E.; Blair, C.D.; et al. Mutation of the dengue virus type 2 envelope protein heparan sulfate binding sites or the domain III lateral ridge blocks replication in Vero cells prior to membrane fusion. *Virology* **2013**, *441*, 114–125. [CrossRef] [PubMed]

99. Cambi, A.; Figdor, C.G. Dual function of C-type lectin-like receptors in the immune system. *Curr. Opin. Cell Biol.* **2003**, *15*, 539–546. [CrossRef] [PubMed]

100. Van Kooyk, Y.; Unger, W.W.; Fehres, C.M.; Kalay, H.; Garcia-Vallejo, J.J. Glycan-based DC-SIGN targeting vaccines to enhance antigen cross-presentation. *Mol. Immunol.* **2013**, *55*, 143–145. [CrossRef] [PubMed]

101. Perera-Lecoin, M.; Meertens, L.; Carnec, X.; Amara, A. Flavivirus entry receptors: An update. *Viruses* **2013**, *6*, 69–88. [CrossRef] [PubMed]

102. Alen, M.M.; Kaptein, S.J.; De Burghgraeve, T.; Balzarini, J.; Neyts, J.; Schols, D. Antiviral activity of carbohydrate-binding agents and the role of DC-SIGN in dengue virus infection. *Virology* **2009**, *387*, 67–75. [CrossRef] [PubMed]

103. Martina, B.E.; Koraka, P.; van den Doel, P.; Rimmelzwaan, G.F.; Haagmans, B.L.; Osterhaus, A.D. DC-SIGN enhances infection of cells with glycosylated West Nile virus in vitro and virus replication in human dendritic cells induces production of IFN-α and TNF-α. *Virus Res.* **2008**, *135*, 64–71. [CrossRef] [PubMed]

104. Shimojima, M.; Takenouchi, A.; Shimoda, H.; Kimura, N.; Maeda, K. Distinct usage of three C-type lectins by Japanese encephalitis virus: DC-SIGN, DC-SIGNR, and LSECtin. *Arch. Virol.* **2014**, *159*, 2023–2031. [CrossRef] [PubMed]

105. Barba-Spaeth, G.; Longman, R.S.; Albert, M.L.; Rice, C.M. Live attenuated yellow fever 17D infects human DCs and allows for presentation of endogenous and recombinant T cell epitopes. *J. Exp. Med.* **2005**, *202*, 1179–1184. [CrossRef] [PubMed]

106. Guo, Y.; Feinberg, H.; Conroy, E.; Mitchell, D.A.; Alvarez, R.; Blixt, O.; Taylor, M.E.; Weis, W.I.; Drickamer, K. Structural basis for distinct ligand-binding and targeting properties of the receptors DC-SIGN and DC-SIGNR. *Nat. Struct. Mol. Biol.* **2004**, *11*, 591–598. [CrossRef] [PubMed]

107. Mitchell, D.A.; Fadden, A.J.; Drickamer, K. A novel mechanism of carbohydrate recognition by the C-type lectins DC-SIGN and DC-SIGNR. Subunit organization and binding to multivalent ligands. *J. Biol. Chem.* **2001**, *276*, 28939–28945. [CrossRef] [PubMed]

108. Lozach, P.Y.; Lortat-Jacob, H.; De Lacroix De Lavalette, A.; Staropoli, I.; Foung, S.; Amara, A.; Houles, C.; Fieschi, F.; Schwartz, O.; Virelizier, J.L.; et al. DC-SIGN and L-SIGN are high affinity binding receptors for hepatitis C virus glycoprotein E2. *J. Biol. Chem.* **2003**, *278*, 20358–20366. [CrossRef] [PubMed]

109. Maley, F.; Trimble, R.B.; Tarentino, A.L.; Plummer, T.H. Characterization of glycoproteins and their associated oligosaccharides through the use of endoglycosidases. *Anal. Biochem.* **1989**, *180*, 195–204. [CrossRef]

110. Wang, Q.Y.; Shi, P.Y. Flavivirus Entry Inhibitors. *ACS Infect. Dis.* **2015**, *1*, 428–434. [CrossRef] [PubMed]

111. Hidari, K.I.; Abe, T.; Suzuki, T. Carbohydrate-related inhibitors of dengue virus entry. *Viruses* **2013**, *5*, 605–618. [CrossRef] [PubMed]
112. Castilla, V.; Piccini, L.E.; Damonte, E.B. Dengue virus entry and trafficking: perspectives as antiviral target for prevention and therapy. *Future Virol.* **2015**, *10*, 625–645. [CrossRef]
113. Lim, S.P.; Shi, P.Y. West Nile virus drug discovery. *Viruses* **2013**, *5*, 2977–3006. [CrossRef] [PubMed]
114. Marks, R.M.; Lu, H.; Sundaresan, R.; Toida, T.; Suzuki, A.; Imanari, T.; Hernáiz, M.J.; Linhardt, R.J. Probing the interaction of dengue virus envelope protein with heparin: Assessment of glycosaminoglycan-derived inhibitors. *J. Med. Chem.* **2001**, *44*, 2178–2187. [CrossRef] [PubMed]
115. Kato, D.; Era, S.; Watanabe, I.; Arihara, M.; Sugiura, N.; Kimata, K.; Suzuki, Y.; Morita, K.; Hidari, K.I.; Suzuki, T. Antiviral activity of chondroitin sulphate E targeting dengue virus envelope protein. *Antivir. Res.* **2010**, *88*, 236–243. [CrossRef] [PubMed]
116. Hidari, K.I.; Takahashi, N.; Arihara, M.; Nagaoka, M.; Morita, K.; Suzuki, T. Structure and anti-dengue virus activity of sulfated polysaccharide from a marine alga. *Biochem. Biophys. Res. Commun.* **2008**, *376*, 91–95. [CrossRef] [PubMed]
117. Cumashi, A.; Ushakova, N.A.; Preobrazhenskaya, M.E.; D'incecco, A.; Piccoli, A.; Totani, L.; Tinari, N.; Morozevich, G.E.; Berman, A.E.; Bilan, M.I.; et al. A comparative study of the anti-inflammatory, anticoagulant, antiangiogenic, and antiadhesive activities of nine different fucoidans from brown seaweeds. *Glycobiology* **2007**, *17*, 541–552. [CrossRef] [PubMed]
118. Talarico, L.B.; Pujol, C.A.; Zibetti, R.G.M.; Faria, P.C.S.; Noseda, M.D.; Duarte, M.E.R.; Damonte, E.B. The antiviral activity of sulfated polysaccharides against dengue virus is dependent on virus serotype and host cell. *Antivir. Res.* **2005**, *66*, 103–110. [CrossRef] [PubMed]
119. Talarico, L.B.; Noseda, M.D.; Ducatti, D.R.; Duarte, M.E.; Damonte, E.B. Differential inhibition of dengue virus infection in mammalian and mosquito cells by iota-carrageenan. *J. Gen. Virol.* **2011**, *92*, 1332–1342. [CrossRef] [PubMed]
120. Talarico, L.B.; Damonte, E.B. Interference in dengue virus adsorption and uncoating by carrageenans. *Virology* **2007**, *363*, 473–485. [CrossRef] [PubMed]
121. Anderson, W.; Duncan, J.G.C.; Harthill, J.E. The anticoagulant activity of carrageenan. *J. Pharm. Pharmacol.* **1965**, 647–654. [CrossRef]
122. Opoku, G.; Qiu, X.; Doctor, V. Effect of oversulfation on the chemical and biological properties of kappa carrageenan. *Carbohydr. Polym.* **2006**, *65*, 134–138. [CrossRef]
123. De Araújo, C.A.; Noseda, M.D.; Cipriani, T.R.; Gonçalves, A.G.; Duarte, M.E.R.; Ducatti, D.R. Selective sulfation of carrageenans and the influence of sulfate regiochemistry on anticoagulant properties. *Carbohydr. Polym.* **2013**, *91*, 483–491. [CrossRef] [PubMed]
124. Vervaeke, P.; Alen, M.; Noppen, S.; Schols, D.; Oreste, P.; Liekens, S. Sulfated Escherichia coli K5 polysaccharide derivatives inhibit dengue virus infection of human microvascular endothelial cells by interacting with the viral envelope protein E domain III. *PLoS ONE* **2013**, *8*, e74035. [CrossRef] [PubMed]
125. Vann, W.F.; Schmidt, M.A.; JANN, B.; JANN, K. The Structure of the Capsular Polysaccharide (K5 Antigenn) of Urinary-Tract-Infective *Escherichia coli* 010:K5:H4. *Eur. J. Biochem.* **1981**, *116*, 359–364. [CrossRef] [PubMed]
126. Vicenzi, E.; Gatti, A.; Ghezzi, S.; Oreste, P.; Zoppetti, G.; Poli, G. Broad spectrum inhibition of HIV-1 infection by sulfated K5 *Escherichia coli* polysaccharide derivatives. *Aids* **2003**, *17*, 177–181. [CrossRef] [PubMed]
127. Pinna, D.; Oreste, P.; Coradin, T.; Kajaste-Rudnitski, A.; Ghezzi, S.; Zoppetti, G.; Rotola, A.; Argnani, R.; Poli, G.; Manservigi, R.; et al. Inhibition of herpes simplex virus types 1 and 2 in vitro infection by sulfated derivatives of Escherichia coli K5 polysaccharide. *Antimicrob. Agents Chemother.* **2008**, *52*, 3078–3084. [CrossRef] [PubMed]
128. Lembo, D.; Donalisio, M.; Rusnati, M.; Bugatti, A.; Cornaglia, M.; Cappello, P.; Giovarelli, M.; Oreste, P.; Landolfo, S. Sulfated K5 *Escherichia coli* polysaccharide derivatives as wide-range inhibitors of genital types of human papillomavirus. *Antimicrob. Agents Chemother.* **2008**, *52*, 1374–1381. [CrossRef] [PubMed]
129. Mercorelli, B.; Oreste, P.; Sinigalia, E.; Muratore, G.; Lembo, D.; Palù, G.; Loregian, A. Sulfated derivatives of Escherichia coli K5 capsular polysaccharide are potent inhibitors of human cytomegalovirus. *Antimicrob. Agents Chemother.* **2010**, *54*, 4561–4567. [CrossRef] [PubMed]
130. Rusnati, M.; Vicenzi, E.; Donalisio, M.; Oreste, P.; Landolfo, S.; Lembo, D. Sulfated K5 *Escherichia coli* polysaccharide derivatives: A novel class of candidate antiviral microbicides. *Clin. Pharmacol. Ther.* **2009**, *123*, 310–322. [CrossRef] [PubMed]

131. Ichiyama, K.; Reddy, S.B.G.; Zhang, L.F.; Chin, W.X.; Muschin, T.; Heinig, L.; Suzuki, Y.; Nanjundappa, H.; Yoshinaka, Y.; Ryo, A.; et al. Sulfated polysaccharide, curdlan sulfate, efficiently prevents entry/fusion and restricts antibody-dependent enhancement of dengue virus infection in vitro: a possible candidate for clinical application. *PLoS Negl. Trop. Dis.* **2013**, *7*, e2188. [CrossRef] [PubMed]

132. Yutaro, K.; Osamu, Y.; Ryusuke, N.; Takashi, Y.; Sadahiko, O.; Shigeru, S.; Yoshimasa, M.; Nobuya, N.; Yasuo, I.; Tohoru, M.; et al. Inhibition of HIV-1 infectivity with curdlan sulfate in vitro. *Biochem. Pharmacol.* **1990**, *39*, 793–797. [CrossRef]

133. Gordon, M.; Guralnik, M.; Kaneko, Y.; Mimura, T.; Baker, M.; Lang, W. A phase I study of curdlan sulfate—An HIV inhibitor. Tolerance, pharmacokinetics and effects on coagulation and on CD4 lymphocytes. *J. Med.* **1993**, *25*, 163–180.

134. Ono, L.; Wollinger, W.; Rocco, I.M.; Coimbra, T.L.; Gorin, P.A.; Sierakowski, M.R. In vitro and in vivo antiviral properties of sulfated galactomannans against yellow fever virus (BeH111 strain) and dengue 1 virus (Hawaii strain). *Antivir. Res.* **2003**, *60*, 201–208. [CrossRef]

135. Dey, P.M. Biochemistry of plant galactomannans. *Adv. Carbohydr. Chem. Biochem.* **1978**, *35*, 341–376.

136. Whistler, R.L.; Smart, C.L. *Polysaccharide Chemistry*; Academic Press: New York, NY, USA, 1953; pp. 292–301.

137. Muschin, T.; Budragchaa, D.; Kanamoto, T.; Nakashima, H.; Ichiyama, K.; Yamamoto, N.; Shuqin, H.; Yoshida, T. Chemically sulfated natural galactomannans with specific antiviral and anticoagulant activities. *Int. J. Biol. Macromol.* **2016**, *89*, 415–420. [CrossRef] [PubMed]

138. Pujol, C.A.; Ray, S.; Ray, B.; Damonte, E.B. Antiviral activity against dengue virus of diverse classes of algal sulfated polysaccharides. *Int. J. Biol. Macromol.* **2012**, *51*, 412–416. [CrossRef] [PubMed]

139. Pereira, M.G.; Benevides, N.M.; Melo, M.R.; Valente, A.P.; Melo, F.R.; Mourão, P.A. Structure and anticoagulant activity of a sulfated galactan from the red alga, *Gelidium crinale*. Is there a specific structural requirement for the anticoagulant action? *Carbohydr. Res.* **2005**, *340*, 2015–2023. [CrossRef] [PubMed]

140. Patel, S. Therapeutic importance of sulfated polysaccharides from seaweeds: Updating the recent findings. *3 Biotech.* **2012**, *2*, 171–185. [CrossRef]

141. Hidari, K.I.; Ikeda, K.; Watanabe, I.; Abe, T.; Sando, A.; Itoh, Y.; Tokiwa, H.; Morita, K.; Suzuki, T. 3-O-sulfated glucuronide derivative as a potential anti-dengue virus agent. *Biochem. Biophys. Res. Commun.* **2012**, *424*, 573–578. [CrossRef] [PubMed]

142. Lee, E.; Pavy, M.; Young, N.; Freeman, C.; Lobigs, M. Antiviral effect of the heparan sulfate mimetic, PI-88, against dengue and encephalitic flaviviruses. *Antivir. Res.* **2006**, *69*, 31–38. [CrossRef] [PubMed]

143. Khachigian, L.M.; Parish, C.R. Phosphomannopentaose Sulfate (PI-88): Heparan Sulfate Mimetic with Clinical Potential in Multiple Vascular Pathologies. *Cardiovasc. Drug Rev.* **2004**, *22*, 1–6. [CrossRef] [PubMed]

144. Barrowcliffe, T.W.; Gray, E.; Merton, R.E.; Dawes, J.; Jennings, C.A.; Hubbard, A.R.; Thomas, D.P. Anticoagulant activities of pentosan polysulphate (Hemoclar) due to release of hepatic triglyceride lipase (HTGL). *Thromb. Haemost.* **1986**, *56*, 202–206. [PubMed]

145. Olson, J.J.; Polk, D.M.; Reisner, A. The efficacy and distribution of suramin in the treatment of the 9L gliosarcoma. *Neurosurgery* **1994**, 297–308. [CrossRef] [PubMed]

146. Aoki, C.; Hidari, K.I.; Itonori, S.; Yamada, A.; Takahashi, N.; Kasama, T.; Hasebe, F.; Islam, M.A.; Hatano, K.; Matsuoka, K.; et al. Identification and characterization of carbohydrate molecules in Mammalian cells recognized by dengue virus type 2. *J. Biochem.* **2006**, *139*, 607–614. [CrossRef] [PubMed]

147. Vanheule, V.; Vervaeke, P.; Mortier, A.; Noppen, S.; Gouwy, M.; Snoeck, R.; Andrei, G.; Van Damme, J.; Liekens, S.; Proost, P. Basic chemokine-derived glycosaminoglycan binding peptides exert antiviral properties against dengue virus serotype 2, herpes simplex virus-1 and respiratory syncytial virus. *Biochem. Pharmacol.* **2016**, *100*, 73–85. [CrossRef] [PubMed]

148. Varga, N.; Sutkeviciute, I.; Ribeiro-Viana, R.; Berzi, A.; Ramdasi, R.; Daghetti, A.; Vettoretti, G.; Amara, A.; Clerici, M.; Rojo, J.; et al. A multivalent inhibitor of the DC-SIGN dependent uptake of HIV-1 and Dengue virus. *Biomaterials* **2014**, *35*, 4175–4184. [CrossRef] [PubMed]

149. Alen, M.M.; Burghgraeve, T.D.; Kaptein, S.J.; Balzarini, J.; Neyts, J.; Schols, D. Broad Antiviral Activity of Carbohydrate-Binding Agents against the Four Serotypes of Dengue Virus in Monocyte-Derived Dendritic Cells. *PLoS ONE* **2011**, *6*, e21658. [CrossRef]

150. O'Keefe, B.R.; Giomarelli, B.; Barnard, D.L.; Shenoy, S.R.; Chan, P.K.; McMahon, J.B.; Palmer, K.E.; Barnett, B.W.; Meyerholz, D.K.; Wohlford-Lenane, C.L.; et al. Broad-spectrum in vitro activity and in vivo efficacy of the antiviral protein griffithsin against emerging viruses of the family Coronaviridae. *J. Virol.* **2010**, *84*, 2511–2521. [CrossRef] [PubMed]

151. Ishag, H.Z.; Li, C.; Huang, L.; Sun, M.X.; Wang, F.; Ni, B.; Malik, T.; Chen, P.Y.; Mao, X. Griffithsin inhibits Japanese encephalitis virus infection in vitro and in vivo. *Arch. Virol.* **2013**, *158*, 349–358. [CrossRef] [PubMed]

152. Ishag, H.Z.; Li, C.; Wang, F.; Mao, X. Griffithsin binds to the glycosylated proteins (E and prM) of Japanese encephalitis virus and inhibit its infection. *Virus Res.* **2016**, *215*, 50–54. [CrossRef] [PubMed]

153. Courageot, M.P.; Frenkiel, M.P.; Dos Santos, C.D.; Deubel, V.; Desprès, P. α-Glucosidase inhibitors reduce dengue virus production by affecting the initial steps of virion morphogenesis in the endoplasmic reticulum. *J. Virol.* **2000**, *74*, 564–572. [CrossRef] [PubMed]

154. Whitby, K.; Pierson, T.C.; Geiss, B.; Lane, K.; Engle, M.; Zhou, Y.; Doms, R.W.; Diamond, M.S. Castanospermine, a potent inhibitor of dengue virus infection in vitro and in vivo. *J. Virol.* **2005**, *79*, 8698–8706. [CrossRef] [PubMed]

155. Watanabe, S.; Rathore, A.P.; Sung, C.; Lu, F.; Khoo, Y.M.; Connolly, J.; Low, J.; Ooi, E.E.; Lee, H.S.; Vasudevan, S.G. Dose-and schedule-dependent protective efficacy of celgosivir in a lethal mouse model for dengue virus infection informs dosing regimen for a proof of concept clinical trial. *Antivir. Res.* **2012**, *96*, 32–35. [CrossRef] [PubMed]

156. Rathore, A.P.; Paradkar, P.N.; Watanabe, S.; Tan, K.H.; Sung, C.; Connolly, J.E.; Low, J.; Ooi, E.E.; Vasudevan, S.G. Celgosivir treatment misfolds dengue virus NS1 protein, induces cellular pro-survival genes and protects against lethal challenge mouse model. *Antivir. Res.* **2011**, *92*, 453–460. [CrossRef] [PubMed]

157. Watanabe, S.; Rathore, A.P.; Sung, C.; Lu, F.; Khoo, Y.M.; Connolly, J.; Low, J.; Ooi, E.E.; Lee, H.S.; Vasudevan, S.G. Dose- and schedule-dependent protective efficacy of celgosivir in a lethal mouse model for dengue virus infection informs dosing regimen for a proof of concept clinical trial. *Antivir. Res.* **2012**, *96*, 32–35. [CrossRef] [PubMed]

158. Adcock, R.S.; Chu, Y.K.; Golden, J.E.; Chung, D.H. Evaluation of anti-Zika virus activities of broad-spectrum antivirals and NIH clinical collection compounds using a cell-based, high-throughput screen assay. *Antivir. Res.* **2017**, *138*, 47–56. [CrossRef] [PubMed]

159. Low, J.G.; Sung, C.; Wijaya, L.; Wei, Y.; Rathore, A.P.; Watanabe, S.; Tan, B.H.; Toh, L.; Chua, L.T.; Hou, Y.A.; et al. Efficacy and safety of celgosivir in patients with dengue fever (CELADEN): A phase 1b, randomised, double-blind, placebo-controlled, proof-of-concept trial. *Lancet Infect. Dis.* **2004**, *14*, 706–715. [CrossRef]

160. Wu, S.F.; Lee, C.J.; Liao, C.L.; Dwek, R.A.; Zitzmann, N.; Lin, Y.L. Antiviral effects of an iminosugar derivative on flavivirus infections. *J. Virol.* **2002**, *76*, 3596–3604. [CrossRef] [PubMed]

161. Gu, B.; Mason, P.; Wang, L.; Norton, P.; Bourne, N.; Moriarty, R.; Mehta, A.; Despande, M.; Shah, R.; Block, T. Antiviral profiles of novel iminocyclitol compounds against bovine viral diarrhea virus, West Nile virus, dengue virus and hepatitis B virus. *Antivir. Chem. Chemother.* **2007**, *18*, 49–59. [CrossRef] [PubMed]

162. Lane, D.A.; Denton, J.; Flynn, A.M.; Thunberg, L.; Lindahl, U. Anticoagulant activities of heparin oligosaccharides and their neutralization by platelet factor 4. *Biochem. J.* **1984**, *218*, 725–732. [CrossRef] [PubMed]

163. Linhardt, R.J.; Rice, K.G.; Kim, Y.S.; Engelken, J.D.; Weiler, J.M. Homogeneous, structurally defined heparin-oligosaccharides with low anticoagulant activity inhibit the generation of the amplification pathway C3 convertase in vitro. *J. Biol. Chem.* **1988**, *263*, 13090–13096. [PubMed]

164. Islam, T.; Butler, M.; Sikkander, S.A.; Toida, T.; Linhardt, R.J. Further evidence that periodate cleavage of heparin occurs primarily through the antithrombin binding site. *Carbohydr. Res.* **2002**, *337*, 2239–2243. [CrossRef]

165. Chen, H.L.; Hsiao, W.H.; Lee, H.C.; Wu, S.C.; Cheng, J.W. Selection and characterization of DNA aptamers targeting all four serotypes of dengue viruses. *PLoS ONE* **2015**, *10*, e0131240. [CrossRef] [PubMed]

166. Bruno, J.G.; Carrillo, M.P.; Richarte, A.M.; Phillips, T.; Andrews, C.; Lee, J.S. Development, screening, and analysis of DNA aptamer libraries potentially useful for diagnosis and passive immunity of arboviruses. *BMC Res. Notes* **2012**, *5*, 633. [CrossRef] [PubMed]

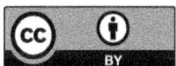

pharmaceuticals

MDPI

Review

Glycosaminoglycan Interactions with Chemokines Add Complexity to a Complex System

Amanda E. I. Proudfoot [1,*], Zoë Johnson [1], Pauline Bonvin [2] and Tracy M. Handel [3,*]

[1] Novimmune SA, 1228 Plan-les-Ouates, Switzerland; zjohnson@novimmune.com
[2] Novartis Pharma Schweiz A.G., Suurstoffi 14, 6343 Rotkreuz, Switzerland; pauline.bonvin@novartis.com
[3] Skaggs School of Pharmacy and Pharmaceutical Sciences, University of California, San Diego, La Jolla, CA 92093, USA
* Correspondence: amandapf@orange.fr (A.E.I.P.); thandel@ucsd.edu (T.M.H.);
  Tel.: +33-450-941-376 (A.E.I.P.); +1-858-822-6656 (T.M.H.)

Received: 1 July 2017; Accepted: 24 July 2017; Published: 9 August 2017

Abstract: Chemokines have two types of interactions that function cooperatively to control cell migration. Chemokine receptors on migrating cells integrate signals initiated upon chemokine binding to promote cell movement. Interactions with glycosaminoglycans (GAGs) localize chemokines on and near cell surfaces and the extracellular matrix to provide direction to the cell movement. The matrix of interacting chemokine–receptor partners has been known for some time, precise signaling and trafficking properties of many chemokine–receptor pairs have been characterized, and recent structural information has revealed atomic level detail on chemokine–receptor recognition and activation. However, precise knowledge of the interactions of chemokines with GAGs has lagged far behind such that a single paradigm of GAG presentation on surfaces is generally applied to all chemokines. This review summarizes accumulating evidence which suggests that there is a great deal of diversity and specificity in these interactions, that GAG interactions help fine-tune the function of chemokines, and that GAGs have other roles in chemokine biology beyond localization and surface presentation. This suggests that chemokine–GAG interactions add complexity to the already complex functions of the receptors and ligands.

Keywords: chemokines; glycosaminoglycans/GAGs; heparan sulfate; chemokine therapeutics; chemokine structure; chemokine oligomerization

1. Introduction

Chemokines have been known to interact with glycosaminoglycans (GAGs) for more than 40 years, since the discovery of Platelet Factor 4 (PF-4, now referred to as CXCL4). CXCL4 was best known for its role in neutralizing heparin in the context of coagulation [1] and this interaction ultimately enabled its isolation by heparin affinity chromatography [2]. When γ-interferon inducible cytokine (IP-10/CXCL10) was cloned in 1985 [3], a common pattern of four cysteine residues was noted in CXCL10, CXCL4, and the previously identified platelet-derived protein β-thromboglobulin/CXCL7 [4], and led to the suggestion that these proteins might belong to a common family of inflammatory mediators [3]. With the cloning and functional characterization of interleukin-8 (IL-8/CXCL8) as a neutrophil chemoattractant in the late 1980s, the role of this family of proteins in directing cell migration was firmly established, and led to their classification as chemokines (derived from *chemo*attractant cyto*kines*) [5,6]. The signature cysteine motif facilitated the identification of many additional members of the chemokine family, which is now the largest cytokine sub-class, with approximately 50 members [7,8].

Although it was initially thought that soluble chemokines promoted cell migration, this notion was challenged in 1992, and an alternative hypothesis was put forward suggesting that cell migration occurs along gradients of chemokines bound to substrates such as endothelial cells or the extracellular matrix (ECM) [9,10]. Support for a haptotactic mechanism came shortly thereafter with the identification of heparan sulfate (HS) as a plausible component of endothelial cells and the ECM that could facilitate the creation of solid phase gradients [11]. CXCL8 was subsequently shown to be associated with endothelial cell (EC) projections in vivo; moreover, the presence of an intact GAG binding domain at its C-terminus was required for EC presentation and transcytosis of the chemokine, and correspondingly, the induction of neutrophil migration [12]. In more recent studies, tissue bound gradients of CXCL8 have been observed in vivo in zebrafish, with neutrophil migration dependent on the ability of CXCL8 to bind HS [13]. HS-dependent gradients of the chemokine, CCL21, have also been directly visualized within lymphatic vessels in mouse skin, and shown to be required for guiding dendritic cells toward the vessels, thereby firmly establishing the concept of haptotaxis along GAG-immobilized sources of chemokine [14].

The above and other seminal studies support the paradigm illustrated in Figure 1, where GAGs and chemokine receptors both function as chemokine-interacting partners to promote cell migration [15–19]. According to this mechanism, chemokines are secreted from the blood vessel wall or underlying tissue in response to inflammatory signals (e.g., infection and damage), transported to the luminal surface of the endothelial cells, and immobilized on the GAG chains of endothelial proteoglycans. Bound to GAGs, the chemokines are concentrated at the source and form an immobilized gradient that provides directional signals to guide the migration of leukocytes towards the inflammatory site. In this scenario, infiltrating leukocytes first roll along the endothelial cell surface due to weak interactions with adhesion molecules such as selectins [20,21]. Once they encounter chemokines at or near the source, the chemokines engage their cognate chemokine receptors on the surface of leukocytes, resulting in leukocyte arrest via integrin activation, followed by diapedesis through the endothelium to resolve the physiological insult [20–22]. This glycosaminoglycan-mediated mechanism for spatially restricting the encounter between chemokine and receptor (at a surface near the source) is thought to prevent premature activation of leukocytes before reaching the inflammatory site [10,23].

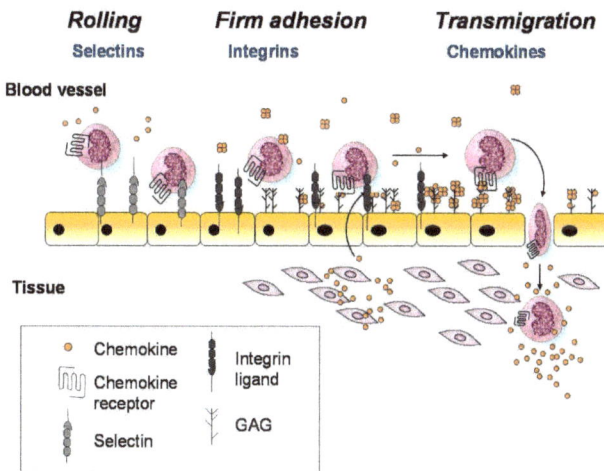

Figure 1. The role of GAGs in cell recruitment. Chemokines (yellow circles) produced by the underlying tissue are immobilized on cell surface GAGs. Circulating leukocytes first roll upon interaction with selectins (pale gray symbols), followed by firm adhesion to integrin ligands (dark gray symbols) following integrin activation on the leukocytes after which they transmigrate into the tissue. Although chemokines are depicted as a single species, many different chemokines may be involved.

The type of leukocyte recruited during an inflammatory response is determined in large part by the nature of the secreted chemokines and corresponding receptors expressed on the migrating cells [7,8,24]. Thus, a large number of molecular players make up the chemokine network (discussed below) to selectively control the migration of specific leukocyte subpopulations towards specific tissues and microenvironments. However, in addition to the chemokine–receptor interaction, chemokine–GAG interactions may impose another level of control, adding complexity to an already complex system [15–19]. In this review we summarize the structural diversity of chemokine–GAG interactions, which suggests chemokine-specific regulation by GAGs. These diverse interactions not only regulate the formation and location of the chemokine gradient, but also its physical properties (e.g., composition, steepness and duration [14,25–29]). We also highlight emerging evidence for the involvement of chemokine–GAG interactions in other aspects of chemokine function, such as chemokine stability, negative and positive regulation of receptor activation, and remodeling the cellular glycocalyx, potentially to facilitate cell–cell interactions and transcytosis [30–36]. Finally, we address the implications of chemokine–GAG interactions on the development of therapeutics, which may explain puzzling results observed with anti-chemokine antibodies [37].

2. Overview of the Chemokine–Receptor and Chemokine–GAG Interactome

Approximately 50 human chemokines have been identified [7,8], most of which promote cell migration. They share a characteristic pattern of cysteine residues that defines them as belonging to CC, CXC, CX3C or C subfamilies, and led to the modern chemokine/receptor nomenclature (e.g., CXCL8, previously called IL-8, is a CXC ligand; and CCL2, previously called MCP-1, is a CC chemokine). Twenty-three human receptors have also been discovered [7,8], 18 of which belong to the G protein-coupled receptor (GPCR) family of receptors (e.g., CXCR1 belongs to the CXC receptor family), while five are "atypical receptors" (ACKR1-4, CCRL2) that neither couple to G proteins nor induce cell migration, but have other functions such as chemokine scavenging and transport [38,39]. Many chemokines bind multiple receptors and similarly many receptors bind several chemokines, leading to a dense network of interacting partners. The system is further complicated by the fact that the interactions can be regulated by post-translational modifications (PTMs, such as tyrosine sulfation), alternative splicing of the receptors, proteolysis and other PTMs of the ligands, ligand and receptor dimerization, and many other mechanisms [8].

Much less is known about precise chemokine–GAG interacting partners because of the many challenges of studying carbohydrates at the biochemical and cellular level. This is largely due to the heterogeneous non-template nature of GAGs [17,19,40]. GAGs are long, linear, sulfated and highly charged heterogeneous polysaccharides that are expressed throughout the body. They consist of repeating disaccharide units, and form chains that range from one to over a hundred disaccharide units, thus representing incredible biological diversity. According to an estimate by Shriver and colleagues, a GAG containing six disaccharide units could theoretically encode for more than 12 billion different sequences, which is 100 times greater than that of a hexapeptide and two million times greater than DNA [41]. As a consequence, the composition and structures of relevant chemokine–GAG complexes are likely quite heterogeneous and large in number, even for a single chemokine.

GAGs are also difficult to produce synthetically and to characterize analytically [42–44]; thus even though heparan sulfate (HS) is biologically more relevant, heparin is often used for in vitro studies due to the availability of reagents including short GAGs that are size-defined and homogeneous in composition [45,46]. Demonstrating that specific chemokine–GAG complexes are relevant in vivo is even more challenging because antibodies to specific GAG sequences are not available and siRNA strategies against specific enzymes broadly affect GAG composition. Nevertheless two decades of mutagenesis, biophysical, structural and in vivo studies, have lead to a basic understanding of the structural principles of chemokine–GAG interactions, their functional consequences, and strategies to exploit or interfere with their interactions for therapeutic purposes [16,17,47].

3. Structural Biology of Chemokine–Glycosaminoglycan Interactions

3.1. Chemokine Tertiary Structure, Receptor-Binding Domains and Glycosaminoglycan-Binding Epitopes

The structure of CXCL8 [48] revealed what has proven to be the consensus fold of all chemokines known to date [7,8,49]. It consists of a disordered N-terminus, an irregular loop referred to as the "N-loop", a three stranded β-sheet connected by loops (the 30s-, 40s- and 50s-loop), and a C-terminal helix. The "core" globular domain of the chemokine (everything beyond the N-terminus) is stapled to the N-terminus via one, and usually two, disulfide bonds (Figure 2A). The N-terminus of the chemokine functions as a key signaling domain, and binds within the pocket of chemokine receptors where it interacts with receptor transmembrane helices (chemokine recognition site 2, CRS2) to promote activation, similar to small molecule activation of GPCRs [50–52]. The chemokine core domain interacts with the receptor N-termini and extracellular loops (CRS1 and CRS1.5) and functions primarily as a binding determinant (Figure 2B). However, it also serves as the binding site for GAGs [53–56] (Figure 2C).

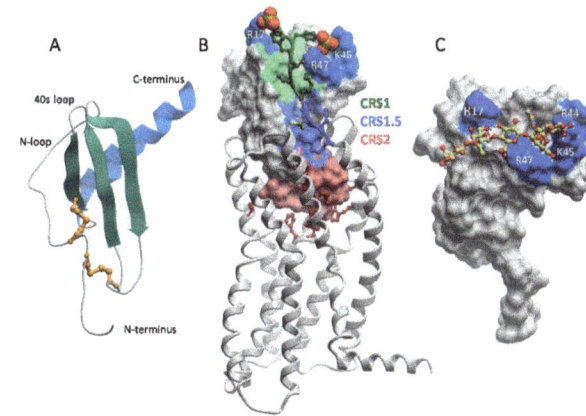

Figure 2. Chemokine tertiary structure, chemokine–receptor interactions, and chemokine–glycosaminoglycan interactions. (**A**) Structure of a typical chemokine, illustrated by a monomeric subunit of CXCL8 (PDB ID 1IL8 [48]). (**B**) Structure of CCR5 bound to a variant of CCL5 with a modified N-terminus (PDB ID 5UIW [52]). Chemokine recognition sites 1, 1.5 and 2 (CRS1, CRS1.5 and CRS2) are highlighted in green, blue and salmon. In CRS1, residues that contribute to GAG binding are highlighted in dark blue (R17 and 40s-loop BBXB motif residues R44 (not visible), K45 and R47). Tyrosine sulfates are highlighted as orange and yellow spheres interacting with the 40s-loop cluster and R17. (**C**) Model of CCL5 in complex with a chondroitin sulfate (CS) hexasaccharide from paramagnetic relaxation enhancement and intra- and intermolecular nuclear Overhauser effect constraints (supplementary data to [56]). GAG binding residues R17, R44, K45 and R47 are highlighted in dark blue. Comparison with (**B**) shows that GAG and receptor utilize similar epitopes on the chemokine core domain (CRS1) and sulfation is involved in both cases. Consequently, binding of GAGs and receptors to chemokines are generally mutually exclusive. Panels (**A–C**) are not to scale.

With the exception of CCL3/MIP-1α and CCL4/MIP-1β, which are acidic, chemokines are highly basic proteins. As a consequence, they tend to have the highest affinity for HS and heparin over GAGs with lower sulfate content (e.g., chondroitin sulfate (CS), dermatan sulfate (DS) [35]). The GAG-binding epitopes for many chemokines have been identified and unsurprisingly are dominated by basic residues [17,49,53,55,57–63]. In several chemokines, GAG binding motifs are defined by characteristic "BBXB" sequence motifs (where B is a basic and X is any amino acid). Taking the example of CCL5, the 40s-loop BBXB cluster, [44]RKNR[47], was originally shown to be the most important GAG binding epitope by in vitro and in vivo experiments [47,58] (Figure 2C). In the case of CCL2, the main contributors are non-BBXB residues R18, K19, R24 and K49, which form a basic patch on the chemokine core domain [55]. In both CCL2 and CCL5, these basic residues are also important for receptor binding, and interestingly, involve interactions with sulfate groups on both the GAG and the receptors (which are modified by tyrosine sulfation [64,65]). In general there is a great deal of overlap between GAG binding residues and receptor binding residues on the chemokine core domain, which suggests that a single chemokine subunit cannot simultaneously interact with receptors and GAGs [54–56,61] (Figure 2B,C).

3.2. Chemokines Bind Receptors as Monomers but Many Chemokines Bind GAGs as Oligomers

Numerous chemokine structures have now been solved and show the tendency of many chemokines to oligomerize [16,49,66]. CXCL8 and other CXC chemokines form a characteristic "CXC dimer" driven by the antiparallel association of β1 strands from two separate subunits of chemokine monomers (Figure 3A) [48]. CC chemokines such as CCL2/MCP-1 adopt the canonical tertiary structure (Figure 2A), but have a different quaternary fold (Figure 3B) [67,68]. They form elongated "CC dimers", stabilized by the formation of an antiparallel β-sheet between residues proximal to the first two Cys residues of the component dimer subunits. At first, chemokine dimers were thought to contribute to the selectivity of CXC chemokines for CXC receptors and CC chemokines for CC receptors [67]. However, it was subsequently shown with oligomerization-impaired mutants that chemokines bind and activate receptors as monomers, which was confirmed by cell based studies [69–71] and by recent X-ray structures of intact chemokine–receptor complexes [50–52] (Figure 2B). Moreover, when the first structure of a chemokine–receptor complex was determined, it was clear that CC dimers cannot bind receptors due to steric incompatibility [50] (Figure 3C), which is consistent with experimental studies [72,73]. Disulfide cross-linked CXC chemokine dimers are compatible with receptor binding (Figure 3D) and have been shown to be functional in vitro and in vivo; however, these engineered dimers typically show lower affinity and partial agonism compared to their WT counterparts in vitro [74–78]. In summary, chemokine monomers function as full agonists of receptors, CC chemokine dimers cannot bind receptors and while CXC dimers are sterically compatible with receptor binding, the role of such complexes in vivo is not known.

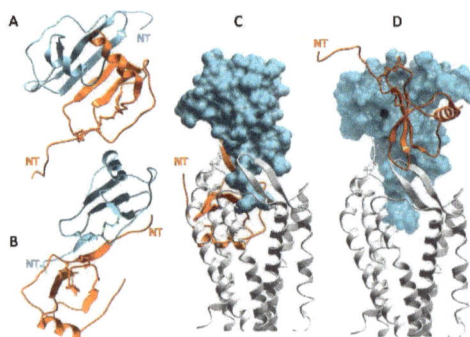

Figure 3. Chemokine oligomers and their ability to bind chemokine receptors, or not. (**A**) Structure of a typical CXC dimer, illustrated by CXCL12 (PDB ID 3GV3) with individual subunits colored in blue and orange. (**B**) Structure of a typical CC dimer, illustrated by vMIP-II (PDB ID 2FHT) with individual subunits colored in blue and orange. (**C**) Docked model of the vMIP-II dimer to CXCR4 shows that CC dimers are sterically incompatible to bind receptor; the orange subunit completely overlaps and clashes with the receptor. (**D**) Docked model of the CXCL12 dimer with CXCR4 shows that CXC dimers are compatible with receptor binding. Models from (**C,D**) are reported in [50].

By contrast, chemokine oligomers are important for the interactions of many (but not all) chemokines with GAGs. In vitro biochemical and biophysical studies showed that chemokines oligomerize on GAGs and that GAGs stabilize dimers and higher order chemokine oligomers [45,55,79,80]. This suggests that binding of chemokines to GAGs and chemokine oligomerization are mutually re-enforcing processes, which would provide a mechanism for concentrating chemokines near inflammatory sites. Importantly, in vivo studies of chemokine-induced cell migration also demonstrated the importance of chemokine oligomerization and GAG binding [81]; in these studies GAG-binding deficient mutants and monomeric mutants of CC chemokines failed to stimulate cell migration into the peritoneal cavity of mice. In similar in vivo peritoneal recruitment assays, obligate CXC chemokine monomers were active; nevertheless, since they were less active than their WT counterparts, the data also support the importance of chemokine oligomerization [74,75]. Taken together, the studies collectively suggest that for many chemokines, both oligomerization and GAG binding are critical for regulating cell migration in vivo [27,74,75,81,82].

3.3. Chemokines Have a Wide Range of Oligomerization Propensities and Affinities for GAGs

Chemokine oligomerization is not restricted to dimers; instead they adopt a spectrum of oligomerization states from monomers (e.g., CCL7/MCP-3) to tetramers and polymers (e.g., CXCL4 and CCL5, respectively) [45,83–85] (Figure 4). For those that do self-assemble, the ability to oligomerize has been show to be important for their GAG-binding affinities. This has been demonstrated with oligomerization-deficient variants, which have markedly reduced affinities for heparin and HS in vitro, and corresponding reduced abilities to accumulate on cell surfaces compared to WT chemokines [31,45,81]. By contrast, although CCL7/MCP-3 does not oligomerize, it still binds GAGs because it has a high density of GAG binding epitopes within its tertiary structure compared to the highly homologous but oligomerizing chemokine, CCL2 [83].

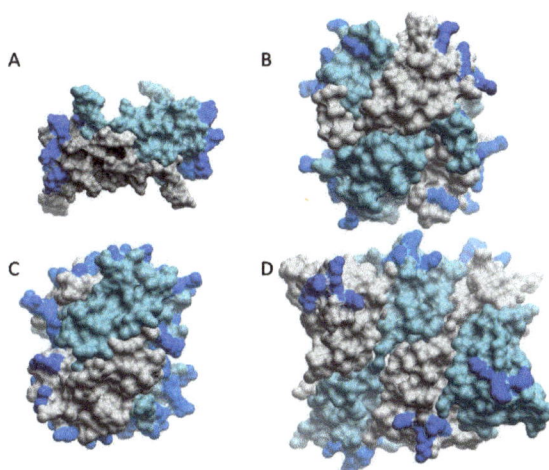

Figure 4. Chemokines adopt a wide range of oligomeric structures, sometimes in response to different GAGs. Structures are shown with the different chemokine subunits color-coded in sky blue and gray, and the main GAG binding residues highlighted in dark blue. (**A**) The CCL2 dimer, which binds to HS (PDB ID 1DOM [68]); residues highlighted include R18, K19, R24, K49. K58, H66 [55]. (**B**) The CCL2 tetramer, which binds to heparin (PDB ID 1DOL [86]); residues highlighted include R18, K19, R24, K49. K58, H66 [55]. (**C**) The CXCL4 tetramer, which binds to heparin (PDB ID 1RHP [85]); residues highlighted include R20, R22, K46, R49, K61, K62, K65, K66 [87]. (**D**) The CCL5 polymer (PDB ID 5DNF [84]); residues highlighted include K55, K56 and R59 [58,88].

Chemokines also have a wide range of affinities for GAGs. CXCL4, CXCL11, CCL5 and CCL21 have very high affinities for GAGs whereas CCL2 and CXCL8 have intermediate affinities, and the affinities of CCL3 and CCL4, the two uniquely acidic chemokines, are weak [45,89]. This is consistent with studies which suggest that only a subset of chemokines bind efficiently to cell surface and ECM GAGs [89]. Together, the GAG-binding affinities of chemokines coupled with their different oligomerization propensities affect the amount of chemokine that accumulates on GAGs, as well as the persistence of the chemokines on GAGs [31,45]. The expectation is that these in vitro results should translate into differences in the nature, shape and duration of chemokine–glycosaminoglycan gradients in vivo [28,29].

3.4. Some Chemokines Bind GAGs through C-Terminal Tail Interactions

Whereas CXCL12α, the most well-characterized of the CXCL12 isoforms, forms dimers and polymers [90,91], the CXCL12 splice variant, CXCL12γ, is not known to oligomerize. Instead, CXCL12γ disordered, approximately 30 amino acid C-terminal extension with a tight array of BBXB motifs that confers even higher affinity for GAGs than CXCL12α [62,92]. Similarly, the CCR7 ligand, CCL21, has an extended, basic C-terminal region of approximately 40 residues, which is required for its immobilization on GAGs and the recruitment of dendritic cells [14]. Along with diverse oligomers formed by chemokines, these alternative GAG-interaction mechanisms imply chemokine-specific and GAG-specific control of cell migration [92].

3.5. Specificity and Structural Plasticity in Chemokine–GAG Interactions

An important but challenging problem is identifying the structure of GAGs that are recognized by specific chemokines. Given the diversity of GAG sequences, it is likely that chemokines recognize numerous GAGs. As reviewed by Monneau and coworkers [19], little is known about this topic, because GAGs are not as easily isolated and analytically characterized, or amenable to structure-function analysis as routinely performed for proteins. However, some generalizations are worth noting. First, longer GAGs (e.g., roughly 18–20 monosaccharides for CCL3 and CXCL12) tend to have higher affinity for chemokines than short GAGs. This is expected since longer GAGs would be able to bridge multiple GAG-binding epitopes including those between different chemokine subunits on oligomers [35,36,93] (Figure 4). As described above, GAG sulfation is also important. For example, 2-O-desulfation of heparin causes a significant loss of affinity for many chemokines. However, the distribution of sulfates appears to be more important than the actual average sulfate content. In a study by Dyer and coworkers [45], a panel of chemokines was shown to have similar affinities for heparin (characterized as having an average of 2.3 sulfate groups per disaccharide, where >90% of the disaccharides have at least one sulfate) and HS (characterized as having an average of 0.8 sulfates per disaccharide, where 55% of the disaccharides were unsulfated). By contrast, chondroitin sulfate-A (CS-A), which has a relatively low content and uniform distribution of sulfates (characterized as having ~0.7 sulfates per disaccharide, similar to HS, where ~84% of the disaccharides are sulfated, similar to heparin), had a significantly reduced affinity for chemokines compared to HS and heparin. In fact, only the subset of chemokines with the highest affinity for HS and heparin were able to bind CS-A [45]. Even the precise position of a single sulfate can be important, as demonstrated in a study where the presence or absence of a 6-O-sulfate interchanged the ability of a dodecasaccharide to inhibit the biological function of CXCL8 vs. CXCL12 [94]. These and other data suggest that there is significant specificity in chemokine–GAG recognition [19,94,95].

Despite evidence for specificity, it is becoming clear from structural data that chemokine–GAG interactions are not defined by single structures; instead, these complexes are characterized by structural plasticity which may enable a single chemokine to recognize multiple GAG sequences. For example, different oligomeric structures of the same chemokine can present different spatial geometries of its GAG binding residues, enabling recognition of different GAGs. Along these lines, HS prefers CCL2 dimers, whereas heparin binds and stabilizes CCL2 tetramers [55,83]. These preferences can be rationalized in terms of the distribution of GAG-binding epitopes on the chemokine oligomers, and the corresponding pattern of sulfation on the GAGs [55,57,93]. In the CCL2 dimer, the basic GAG binding clusters are separated by ~45 Å, while HS typically consists of highly sulfated regions connected by intervening N-acetylated regions (e.g., SAS domains) [19,40]. By associating with the CCL2 dimer, the spacing of the sulfated domains on HS presumably overlap with the basic epitopes of CCL2, thereby stabilizing the complex [55] (Figure 4A), similar to complexes of CCL3 with HS (90). By contrast, in the tetrameric arrangement of CCL2, the GAG-binding residues form an almost continuous basic epitope that wraps around the chemokine surface and would better complement the more uniformly sulfated nature of heparin than the epitope distribution in the chemokine dimer [55] (Figure 4B). A similar continuous distribution of epitopes on the CXCL4 tetramer has also been suggested to facilitate its interaction with heparin [87] (Figure 4C). Other chemokines such as CXCL10 and CXCL12, have been captured in different oligomerization states by crystallography [90,96,97], which may reflect an ability of these chemokines to bind different GAGs by adopting different oligomer forms.

Structural plasticity, whereby different epitopes are involved in GAG binding, depending on the oligomerization state of the chemokine, is also apparent from studies of CCL5 [56,58,98,99]. Three structures of a CCL5 dimer with sulfated disaccharides showed contacts between the disaccharides and the 40s-loop BBXB cluster, as well unexpected interactions with the 30s-loop and N-terminus of the chemokine [58,98]. The 40s-loop and N-terminal interactions of the dimer were also observed in the structure of the CCL5 dimer with a CS hexasaccharide [56] (Figure 3C). However, in the structure of a polymeric CCL5 complex containing a heparin hexasaccharide, the 50s-loop basic motif, ^{55}KKWVR^{59}, was shown to be the main binding site for heparin while the 40s-loop motif was largely buried [84] (Figure 4D). These data suggest oligomerization-dependent specificity in chemokine–GAG interactions, with the 40s-loop and 50s-loop playing roles in different contexts. In fact, one study attributes different functions to the 40s-loop and 50s-loop GAG interactions, and emphasizes the importance of chemokine presentation in mediating these different functional roles [88].

Certain chemokines that utilize unstructured C-terminal tails for GAG binding (e.g., CCL21, CXCL12γ) may be particularly promiscuous in their ability to bind numerous GAGs because of the likelihood that the tails adopt multiple geometries. Chemokines with high-density GAG binding domains (e.g., CCL7) may also have a high degree of structural plasticity even if they do not oligomerize [83]. Structural plasticity has the potential to expand the range of chemokine interactions beyond what might be expected for these small proteins, and enable chemokines to adapt to local GAG environments, potentially with differentiating functional consequences, as suggested by the CCL5 study [88].

3.6. Heterodimerization and Post-Translational Modifications of Chemokines–Mechanisms for Regulating Chemokine–GAG Interactions

In addition to forming homo-oligomers, chemokines have been shown to heterodimerize [100–105]. Since multiple chemokines are frequently expressed at sites of inflammation, heterodimerization would offer a potential mechanism for regulating GAG binding, and indirectly, receptor activation. Using NMR, Nesmelova and coworkers demonstrated that incubating CXCL4 tetramers and CXCL8 dimers together resulted in subunit exchange and the formation of CXCL4:CXCL8 heterodimers [104]. Similarly, incubation of CCL2 with CCL8 resulted in a strong preference for CCL2:CCL8 heterodimers over the corresponding homodimers [100]. CC:CXC heterocomplexes involving CCL5 and CXCL4 have also been observed and are thought to have functional consequences in amplifying leukocyte arrest responses to CCL5 [102]. As shown by Crown and coworkers, GAGs can also stabilize the formation of chemokine heterocomplexes [100], and in principle heterocomplexes can modulate GAG-binding affinity [100,106] and possibly even specificity. For example, the isolation of GAG-bound heterocomplexes containing CCL3, CCL4 and CCL5 with sulfated proteoglycans [106] may represent an example where the high affinity of CCL5 dominates the weak affinities of CCL3 and CCL4 such that CCL3 and CCL4 assemble with CCL5 in a GAG complex that might not otherwise form for CCL3 or CCL4 alone.

Post-translational modifications (PTMs) of chemokines also affect GAG interactions. Citrullination of Arg5 in CXCL8 by peptidylarginine deiminase reduces its affinity for GAGs [107] as does nitration of Tyr13, Tyr28 and Trp59 in CCL2 [108]. Since Tyr13 is important for CCL2 dimerization [70,86] while Tyr28 is involved in the tetramer interface [86], nitration of these residues almost certainly disrupts GAG binding by destabilizing CCL2 oligomers. Thus, modulating the interaction of chemokine–GAG interactions via PTMs adds yet another mechanism for regulating cell migration in a chemokine-dependent manner.

4. Are Chemokine Receptors Activated by GAG-Immobilized Chemokine, Soluble Chemokine, or Both?

Despite the emphasis on haptotactic gradients, a long-standing issue has been the role of immobilized versus soluble gradients of chemokines, as well as if, and how, GAG-bound chemokines activate receptors. Specifically: (i) Are receptors on leukocytes activated by chemokines simultaneously bound to GAGs on endothelial cells or the ECM (i.e., immobilized haptotactic gradients)? (ii) Are chemokines concentrated in immobilized depots by GAGs but released in soluble form to activate receptors and cause cell migration close to the source (a hybrid haptotactic/chemotactic gradient)? (iii) Do some chemokines have little or no interaction with GAGs and simply create a gradient by diffusion from the source (e.g., chemotaxis)? This issue awaits a definitive answer, but current data suggest that all three scenarios may be relevant depending on chemokine, and that different types of gradients may function together to control cell migration in vivo [28,29]. It is clear that cell migration to soluble chemokines is feasible since simple Boyden chambers that rely on soluble gradients are routinely used by most laboratories to monitor cell migration. Migration to essentially immobilized chemokine has also been observed in some [28] but not other [109] experiments where differences may reflect the completely different experimental setups and/or chemokine systems under study. The development of sophisticated microfluidic devices and biomimetic surfaces that enable precise control over the composition, shape and stability of chemokine gradients [28,109,110], will undoubtedly lead to a deeper understanding of this complex issue and complement in vivo studies where achieving such precise control would be much more challenging.

In the meantime, one can hypothesize based on structural and affinity information, what types of gradients might be feasible for different chemokines. Simultaneous binding of chemokine to receptor and GAG should be possible for CCL21 and CXCL12γ since the extended C-terminal tails of these chemokines is expected to orient away from the receptor in the receptor–chemokine complex, making it accessible to GAG. This hypothesis is supported by the fact that a CCL21 variant, immobilized through a PEG-biotin tag to a streptavidin-biotin surface and patterned in a gradient, promotes dendritic cell (DC) adhesion and migration [28]. Whether this happens in vivo, or the chemokine is released from GAGs prior to receptor engagement, remains to be seen. However, in vitro results clearly support the idea that soluble and haptotactic gradients of CCL19 and CCL21, respectively, work together to recruit CCR7 expressing DCs [14,25,28,111].

For other chemokines lacking a tail, simultaneous interactions of chemokine with receptor and GAG seems less likely. As described above, the extensive overlap between GAG binding sites and receptor binding sites on the surface of chemokine monomers, suggests that the interactions are mutually exclusive (Figure 2B,C). Arguments could be made that the N-terminus of the chemokine can bind in the receptor binding pocket (CRS2) while the chemokine core domain (CRS1) binds to glycosaminoglycans prior to engaging the receptor N-terminus. However, given the low affinity of monomeric forms of oligomerizing chemokines for GAGs [45], this scenario seems highly unlikely. It has also been suggested that oligomerized chemokines might be able to simultaneously interact with receptors and GAGs using different subunits of the oligomers [55]; however, this is not possible for CC chemokines because CC dimers cannot physically bind receptors [50,72,73] (Figure 3C). While CXC chemokine dimers are compatible with receptor binding (Figure 3D) [50,74–77,80], again, the affinity of a single subunit of a chemokine dimer for GAG is low [45]; thus simultaneous interaction seems unlikely. We are also unaware of higher order CXC chemokine oligomers that would be physically compatible with receptor binding. Majumdar and colleagues suggested that while chemokines may remain bound to GAGs while being sensed by receptor, that it is also possible that GAGs attract dense "clouds" of chemokines, which are then sensed in their soluble state [29]. Structural data are most consistent with this explanation for the majority of chemokines; in other words, GAG interactions provide a mechanism for concentrating and localizing chemokines, but chemokines most likely dissociate before interacting with receptor. This contradicts a previous hypothesis proposed by the authors suggesting that the bound form might be the active form [55,81]. However, it is consistent with studies of a neutralizing anti-CXCL10 antibody (described below) that supports the concept of a cloud of chemokine released from a GAG-bound cluster [37].

As suggested in early studies [89], some chemokines may only form soluble gradients which is consistent with their low affinities measured in vitro [45]. Recent studies also suggest that endothelial presentation is not necessary for some chemokines and cells. As demonstrated by Stoler-Barak and colleagues, activated T cells can obtain transmigration cues directly from intra-endothelial chemokine stores [112].

5. Beyond Chemokine Gradients: Functional Effects of Chemokine–GAG Interactions

Most literature reports discuss the role of chemokine–GAG interactions in the context of gradient formation. However, GAG interactions are involved in many other aspects of chemokine biology, as reviewed in this section.

5.1. Positive and Negative Regulation of Receptor-Mediated Functional Responses

Several reports have documented the ability of soluble, exogenously added GAGs, to inhibit the function of many chemokines in assays of receptor binding and activation [35,94]. Now that structures are available, the reason is clear—the GAG binding epitopes and receptor binding epitopes of chemokines overlap heavily [54–56,61], as illustrated in Figure 2B,C. This means that while GAGs and receptors work together to promote cell migration, they can also have opposing functions. Cells shed GAGs during many pathological situations [40], which, in principle, could inhibit chemokine–receptor interactions and consequently inflammatory responses. On the other hand, soluble HS has been reported to act as a coreceptor for CCL21 [113] and to enhance neutrophil responses to CXCL8 [11]. Inhibition of chemokine function is the more commonly documented result, however, and this has inspired efforts to develop small GAG mimetics as receptor antagonists [114,115], which is discussed in Section 6.

Several studies have reported that combinations of chemokines, including chemokines from different subfamilies, and those that activate different receptors, can potentiate the functional responses of individual chemokines. For example, chemokines CCL2, CCL3 and CCL8 (all monocyte chemoattractant proteins) were shown to function cooperatively with CXCL8 in an assay of neutrophil chemotaxis, when none of the CC chemokines showed any function on their own. CXCL8 also showed synergy with CXCL4 and CXCL12, in neutrophil migration [116]. Similarly, CCL19 and CCL21, which do not have receptors on monocytes, caused migration and cellular responses of CCR2 agonists at much lower concentrations than the CCR2 agonists alone [117]. These and many additional examples of synergistic chemokine activities [102,118–121] led to the hypothesis that in inflammatory situations, an abundance of different chemokines could produce a reduction in the threshold for cell migration and activation [122], thereby invoking more robust cell responses at lower chemokine concentrations than would be anticipated from single chemokine–receptor pairs.

In some reports, this functional synergy has been attributed to positive crosstalk between intracellular signaling pathways downstream of receptors [116,119] or by formation of hetero-complexes between a receptor, its cognate chemokine, and a non-cognate chemokine [102,122].

However, other reports suggest that interactions with GAGs can produce synergistic effects of chemokines on receptor activation [32]. In the latter scenario, chemokines that do not activate a given receptor, potentiate the activity of a bona fide receptor agonist by displacing the agonist from GAGs, and increasing its effective concentration for binding receptor. In support of this competitive binding mechanism, functional cooperativity was demonstrated for many chemokine combinations, whereas GAG-binding deficient chemokines (still able to activate receptor) were incapable of reproducing the same synergy.

Although not a subject of the above study, CXCL4 might be expected to show synergy with other chemokines due to its exceptionally high affinity for GAGs, and corresponding ability to competitively displace many chemokines. Since it is a weak chemoattractant [123] but a strong GAG-binder [45], having a significant role in regulating chemokine function by modulating chemokine–GAG interactions is intuitively appealing. On the other hand, competitive displacement of certain chemokines from GAGs could also lead to functional inhibition by disrupting chemokine gradients, and CXCL4 could certainly also negatively regulate more weakly binding chemokines in this manner. In this regard, a negative regulatory role was postulated for CCL18, another chemokine with weak chemoattractant properties [124]. CCL18 is found at high levels in the circulation, and is further upregulated in many diseases [125,126]. Along with its ability to inhibit the function of several chemokine/receptor pairs through competitive receptor interactions, it was found to displace chemokines from heparin in vitro, which could also translate into gradient disruption in vivo [124]. Finally, since many cytokines and growth factors also rely on GAG binding, it is possible that chemokines could regulate other cytokines as well, and visa versa, through competitive displacement from GAGs.

5.2. GAGs Protect Chemokines from Proteolysis

Proteolysis of chemokines is a well documented mechanism for regulating the inflammatory response [127], which can be rich in proteases in addition to inflammatory stimuli. The role of chemokine N-termini as the crucial mediators of signaling makes them natural targets for proteolytic processing, where even single amino acid changes can alter the pharmacological activity of chemokines [127]. For example, limited proteolytic processing of the N-termini of CXCL8 and CCL3L1 results in enhanced chemokine activity, while it results in reduced activity of CCL7 and CCL11 [128–131] and inactivation of CXCL12 [132]. Chemokines are also proteolytically cleaved internally and at their C-termini, which regulates their activity. For example, the extended GAG-binding domain of CCL21 is cleaved by a dendritic cell-associated protease, and this modification produces a soluble version of CCL21 that can no longer induce leukocyte arrest [14,25]. GAGs can modulate these regulatory processes by protecting chemokines from proteolytic degradation [33,36,133]. The protection may be due to steric blockade of the chemokine from the protease active site in some cases. However, stabilization of chemokine oligomers may also play a role [36,84]. In the context of the CCL5 polymer, for example, the chemokine N-terminus is buried and unavailable for modification. Thus, in principle, chemokine protection from proteolysis through interactions with GAGs could regulate the intensity and duration of an inflammatory response.

5.3. Chemokines Modulate the Mechanical Properties of Heparan Sulfate and May Contribute to Glycocalyx Remodeling

In addition to providing a substrate for the localized accumulation and slow release of chemokines to guide leukocytes to inflammatory sites, the GAG chains of endothelial cell surface proteoglycans contribute to the physical adhesion-resistant barrier function of the glycocalyx [134–136]. By virtue of its physicochemical properties and thickness, the glycocalyx inhibits contact between key molecules (e.g., selectins, integrins and their ligands) that mediate cell–cell interactions required for leukocyte adhesion and transmigration [137] (Figure 5A). The molecular mechanisms that control this barrier are poorly understood but the glycocalyx is known to undergo remodeling in the context of disease and inflammation to permit close approach of endothelial cells and leukocytes [136,138,139]. Inflammatory mediators like TNF play a role in reducing the barrier thickness to promote cell adhesion and subsequent transmigration [140]. This suggests that chemokines may also play a role [31], although, at a nascent stage of understanding, novel biophysical techniques that report on the fluidity and diffusion of HS chains have shown that chemokines differentially crosslink and rigidify HS in biomimetic surrogates of cell surface proteoglycan layers [30,31]. Notably, high affinity chemokines showed the greatest propensity to crosslink and remain associated with HS chains, which was also significantly enhanced by their ability to oligomerize. Although the implications of these findings are speculative at this point, it has been suggested that HS clustering may be involved in receptor-independent signaling of chemokine through proteoglycans (Figure 5B), as has been observed for CXCL12 and CCL5 [31,34,141]. HS remodeling may also prepare the endothelial surface for localized leukocyte-endothelial adhesion events prior to leukocyte transmigration (Figure 5C) [31]. Consistent with this concept, CXCL12 and CCL5 have been shown to stimulate proteoglycan (syndecan) clustering and shedding, an important mechanism for reducing the glycocalyx barrier thickness and density to permit cell–cell contact [142,143]. This clustering may be a consequence of the ability of these chemokines to crosslink proteoglycan HS chains as demonstrated by the above in vitro experiments [30,31]. If relevant, HS/glycocalyx remodeling would likely occur concomitantly with chemokine gradient formation, and represent yet another critical role for chemokine–GAG interactions in cell migration.

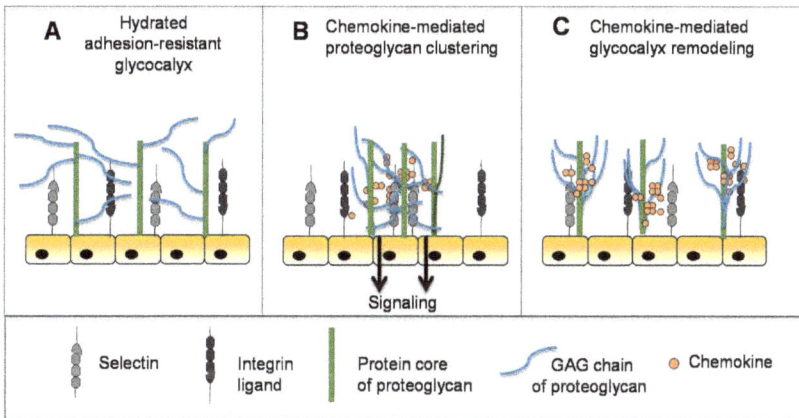

Figure 5. Functional effects of chemokine–GAG interactions. (**A**) The GAG chains of proteoglycans form a hydrated adhesion-resistant surface on endothelial cells that inhibits leukocyte transmigration. (**B,C**) Binding of chemokines to the HS chains of proteoglycans may promote: clustering of the syndecans and chemokine–receptor independent signaling (**B**); or remodeling of the endothelial glycocalyx to enable leukocyte transmigration (**C**). Figure adapted from [31].

6. Exploiting Chemokine–GAG Interactions for Therapeutic Applications

Targeting the chemokine system for therapeutic applications has almost exclusively focused on inhibiting chemokine–receptor interactions, either with small molecules interacting with receptors, or with antibodies neutralizing the receptors or the chemokines themselves. However, in view of the essential nature of chemokine–GAG interactions for cell migration and activation, alternative strategies targeting these interactions can be envisioned to disrupt the function of the chemokine system, as described below.

6.1. Protein-Based Strategies

In one approach, non-signaling chemokine variants were created by mutating residues that activate receptor, concomitant with mutations that increase the strength of the GAG interaction [144,145]. Such non-signaling super-GAG-binding variants have been tested in several disease models and found to reduce inflammation in preclinical models (for example a CXCL8 variant reduced inflammation in an antigen-induced arthritis model [146]). This approach, trademarked as the CellJammer® technology, is in clinical development [147].

An alternative approach was discovered by serendipity in the process of defining the GAG-binding pharmacophores of CCL5 and several other chemokines. Mutation of the BBXB motif ([44]RKNR[47] to[44]AANA[47]) produced a CCL5 mutant incapable of recruiting cells in vivo, thereby highlighting the essential role that this interaction plays in directing cell migration [58,81]. Other chemokines with abrogated GAG binding such as CCL2, CCL7 and CXCL11 were also unable to recruit cells in vivo [55,148,149]. While these observations were important for elucidating the biological relevance of chemokine–GAG interactions, the most surprising result was that these variants had anti-inflammatory properties. Essentially, pre-treatment with these mutated proteins blocked the ability of the wild type chemokines to induce cell recruitment in vivo, which translated into reduced inflammatory symptoms in several pre-clinical disease models. For example, the [44]AANA[47]-CCL5 variant reduced inflammatory and clinical symptoms in experimental autoimmune encephalitis (EAE), as well as in models of liver injury and fibrosis, myocardial reperfusion and atherosclerosis [47,150–152], and a CCL7 GAG binding mutant prolonged skin allografts [149]. However, these variants were partial or full agonists that retained some ability to activate their receptors, which in the case of CCL5, ultimately halted a discovery program prior to Phase I clinical studies.

Subsequent studies of the mechanistic basis for the inhibitory properties of [44]AANA[47]-CCL5 re-enforced the interrelationship between GAG binding and oligomerization of chemokines, suggesting that oligomerization-deficient mutants might also be functional antagonists. Specifically, the BBXB mutation not only disrupted the ability of CCL5 to bind GAGs, but limited it to the formation of dimers rather than the polymers. Furthermore, [44]AANA[47]-CCL5 was shown to act as a "dominant-negative" inhibitor of WT CCL5 by forming non-functional (i.e., GAG-binding deficient) heterodimers [47]. Following this observation, oligomerization-impaired mutants of CCL2, CCL4 and CCL5 were then tested and shown to be inactive in vivo [81]. As was the case for the GAG mutants, inhibition of WT proteins by the oligomerization-deficient mutant of CCL2, P8A-CCL2, was also observed. The P8A-CCL2 variant demonstrated anti-inflammatory properties in a murine model of EAE [153] as well as in a rat model of arthritis [154].

The inability of GAG-binding deficient and oligomerization deficient chemokines to recruit cells in vivo, does not hold for all chemokines. When administered into the lungs of mice, CXCL8 GAG mutants recruited more neutrophils than WT CXCL8 [82]. The result was attributed to the appearance of the mutants in plasma at significantly higher concentrations than WT CXCL8, due to more rapid diffusion across the extracellular matrix. Disulfide-crosslinked obligate monomers of CXCL1 and CXCL8 were also shown to be active in vivo, although less so than their WT counterparts [74,75]. Furthermore, different results have been observed when the same chemokine variant was administered in different tissue compartments (i.e., recruitment in the lung versus the peritoneal cavity [74]. Thus, a major take home message is that the GAG interactions and oligomeric properties of chemokines are finely tuned to regulate cell migration in a chemokine-specific and tissue-specific manner [27,74,75,82].

In addition to the potential of chemokines with modified GAG-binding properties as therapeutics, chemokine–GAG interactions can be exploited for stabilization and delivery purposes. An N-terminally modified variant of CCL5 was developed as a potent CCR5 antagonist and inhibitor of HIV infection [155,156]. Encapsulation of the chemokine in GAG-containing hydrogels was shown to significantly preserve its activity and facilitate its controlled released over the course of a month [157]. Other therapeutic applications of GAG-based hydrogels have been reported such as their use in sequestering chemokines to promote wound healing [158].

6.2. Small Molecule-Based Strategies

In view of the facts that chemokine–GAG interactions often involve binding epitopes defined by small clusters of basic residues on the chemokine, and that soluble GAGs inhibit receptors, it was hypothesized that small molecule inhibitors targeting these clusters, could be identified. Earlier proof of concept studies showed that small heparin derived saccharides could indeed block CCL5-mediated cell migration in vivo [114]. However, a tetrasaccharide was the minimum-sized fragment to show an effect, and a 15-fold excess of GAG over chemokine was needed to observe statistically significant inhibition; in other words it was not very effective. Subsequent studies explored the use of small persulfated oligosacharrides, which also showed anti-inflammatory results in some disease models [114]. However, for reasons that are unclear, these molecules induced pro-inflammatory responses in a CCL5-mediated peritoneal recruitment model.

In contrast to small molecules directed against CCL5, promising results were obtained from a study targeting CCL20. A GAG microarray, designed to explore the specificity of various chemokines for different GAGs revealed that a synthetic monosaccharide, 2,4-O-di-sulfated iduronic acid (Di-S-IdoA), had high affinity for CCL20 but not for seven other chemokines [115]. When tested in a mouse model of allergic asthma, the monosaccharide caused attenuated leukocyte recruitment into the lungs and bronchoalveolar lavage fluid. Moreover, the reduced leukocyte accumulation was associated with a lack of CCL20 on the vascular endothelial cells in the treated mice, whereas robust CCL20 expression was observed in the untreated mice. What is most striking about the results is that Di-S-IdoA is only a monosaccharide, which bodes well for the potential of blocking chemokine-mediated disease with small molecule carbohydrate mimics. It may be that some chemokines and some disease contexts are easier to block than others. For example, CCL20 interactions with GAGs may be more amenable to inhibition than CCL5 interactions due to the fact that CCL20 is a weakly oligomerizing chemokine [159] whereas CCL5 interacts with GAGs as a high affinity polymer with multiple redundant epitopes. In any case, success will be dependent on synthetic feasibility, and, fortunately, there has been enormous progress in carbohydrate chemistry in recent years [43,160–162], which may help position GAG mimetics as viable therapeutic entities.

6.3. Antibody-Based Strategies

Although the majority of approaches for therapeutics targeting the chemokine system have been small molecules, several programs have aimed to develop antibodies against chemokines or their receptors. However, the only successful anti-chemokine antibody developed thus far is a topical anti-CXCL8 monoclonal antibody for psoriasis (Abcream, a product of Anogen), which was approved in China. Examples of failures include an anti-CXCL8 antibody produced by Abgenix [163], which did not meet its endpoints in phase II trials for chronic obstructive pulmonary disease and psoriasis, and anti-CCL2 antibodies for rheumatoid arthritis [164] and metastatic prostate cancer [165] which also failed due to lack of efficacy [37]. Many possible reasons for efficacy failures have been proposed. For example, the anti-CXCL8 antibody did not recognize GAG bound CXCL8, which could be hypothesized to be the cause of its failure [163], and the anti-CCL2 caused dose dependent increases of systemic CCL2 [164]. Additionally, the CCL2/CCR2 axis is now considered an inappropriate target for rheumatoid arthritis, which would account for clinical trial failures [166,167].

Other potential reasons may relate to whether the form of a chemokine recognized by an antibody is the appropriate target. As described above, chemokines may be soluble or bound to GAG, and in response to prior anti-chemokine antibody failures, it had been suggested that antibodies targeting both the GAG-bound form and the soluble form of a given chemokine might be most effective [37] (Figure 6A). A comparison of two anti-murine CXCL10 antibodies that recognize soluble CXCL10 (antibody 1B11) versus GAG-bound CXCL10 (antibody 1B6) illustrated how this is indeed an important parameter that needs to be considered, and which form might be most efficacious for blocking the chemokine–receptor interaction [37,168]. In vitro chemotaxis studies showed that 1B6 (recognizing GAG-bound CXCL10) was considerably more potent than 1B11 (recognizing soluble

CXCL10). Surprisingly, however, in several in vivo disease models, the less potent 1B11 showed efficacy, whereas 1B6 showed little effect [37]. After ruling out other reasons for the failure of 1B6, it was concluded that complexation of the antibody with GAG-bound chemokine causes target-mediated drug disposition (TMDD) and rapid clearance from the circulation. Furthermore since the amount of the GAG-bound form significantly exceeds that of the soluble form, most of the antibody would be depleted leaving little to neutralize soluble CXCL10. By contrast, binding of 1B11 to soluble CXCL10 inhibits chemokine interactions with both GAGs, required for forming a gradient, and with receptor CXCR3 (Figure 6B) [37]. These data illustrate how the complexities introduced by chemokine–GAG interactions need to be carefully considered when developing antibodies, with special attention to those chemokines that are particularly abundant and avid GAG binders. The data are also most consistent with the "cloud" concept—that CXCL10 must be released from GAGs to bind its receptor on leukocytes in soluble—and they provide further evidence that GAG-bound CXCL10 is not "the active form".

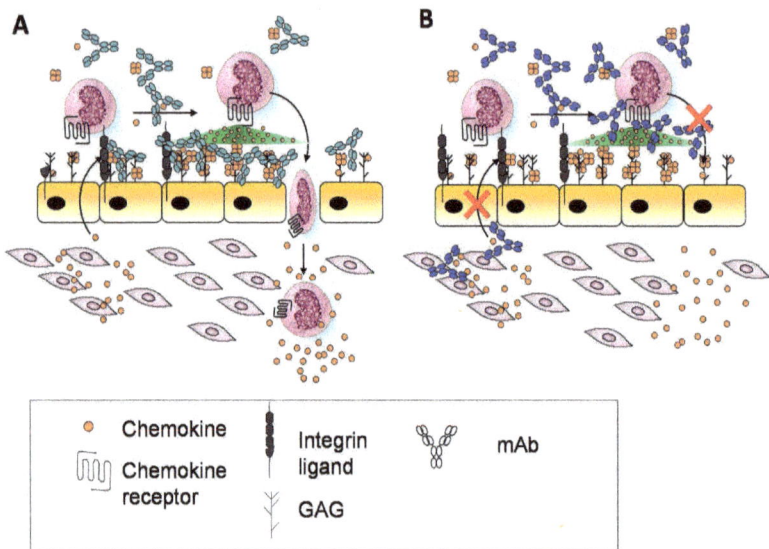

Figure 6. Proposed modes of action of antibodies 1B6 and 1F11. In the updated model of chemokine activity the directional signal is produced by a localized cloud of soluble chemokine. (**A**) The majority of 1B6 molecules are bound to GAG-displayed CXCL10 and free chemokines in the soluble gradient are not inhibited. (**B**) The binding of the antibody to soluble chemokines inhibits cell migration induced by the soluble chemokine cloud and may interfere with the formation of the chemokine gradient.

7. Conclusions

Chemokine–receptor interactions are often described as "redundant", because many chemokines interact with the same receptor and many receptors interact with multiple chemokine [169]. While this may be true to some extent, there are now many examples where GAGs break this otherwise functional redundancy. Although precise in vivo GAG partners for chemokines are not known, it is clear that chemokines have a wide range of affinities for GAGs, ranging from extremely weak binders (e.g., CCL3 and CCL4) to extremely strong nanomolar and subnanomolar binders (CCL5, CCL21, CXCL4, CXCL11). Chemokines also have a wide range of propensities to oligomerize in solution or on GAGs, while others have unstructured C-terminal tails as GAG-binding domains. Similarly, they also have a wide range of propensities to heterodimerize. Without even considering impacts on other functions described in this review, all of these parameters will effect the size, shape and duration of chemokine gradients and whether they are haptotactic or soluble. CCL19 and CCL21 are the most well studied examples of non-redundant ligands of the same receptor, CCR7. Whereas CCL21 has a C-terminal tail that enables it to bind GAGs with high affinity and to form haptotactic gradients, CCL19 lacks the tail and is considered a soluble chemokine. Of the CCR5 ligands, all of which form stable polymers, CCL5 is basic and has high affinity for GAGs whereas CCL3 and CCL4 are acidic and have low affinity for GAGs. CXCL4L1, like CXCL4 is a ligand of CXCR3; however it differs by three amino acids, which is sufficient to make it essentially a soluble chemokine in contrast to the exceptional high affinity of CXCL4 for GAGs [170].

From these and other examples, it has become clear that there is a great deal of diversity in chemokine–GAG interactions. However, most of the observations have been made from in vitro studies. Going forward, it will be critical to understand their functional significance in vivo. If this can be done, it may be possible to exploit this information to make better therapeutics, as illustrated by the anti-CXCL10 antibody story where understanding whether one should target soluble versus GAG-bound chemokine was the difference between success and failure in an animal model.

Acknowledgments: AEIP received funding from the European Union FP6 (INNOCHEM, grant number LSHB-CT-2005-518167) and the European Union FP7 (TIMER, grant agreement No. HEALTH-F4-2011-281608). TMH acknowledges funding from the National Institutes of Health (grants R01 AI118985 and R01 GM117424).

Conflicts of Interest: The authors declare no conflicts of interest.

References

1. Rosenberg, R.D.; Damus, P.S. The purification and mechanism of action of human antithrombin-heparin cofactor. *J. Biol. Chem.* **1973**, *248*, 6490–6505. [PubMed]
2. Handin, R.I.; Cohen, H.J. Purification and binding properties of human platelet factor four. *J. Biol. Chem.* **1976**, *251*, 4273–4282. [PubMed]
3. Luster, A.D.; Unkeless, J.C.; Ravetch, J.V. Gamma-interferon transcriptionally regulates an early-response gene containing homology to platelet proteins. *Nature* **1985**, *315*, 672–676. [CrossRef]
4. Begg, G.S.; Pepper, D.S.; Chesterman, C.N.; Morgan, F.J. Complete covalent structure of human beta-thromboglobulin. *Biochemistry* **1978**, *17*, 1739–1744. [CrossRef] [PubMed]
5. Baggiolini, M. CXCL8—The First Chemokine. *Front. Immunol.* **2015**, *6*, 285. [CrossRef] [PubMed]
6. Yoshimura, T. Discovery of IL-8/CXCL8 (The Story from Frederick). *Front. Immunol.* **2015**, *6*, 278. [CrossRef] [PubMed]
7. Scholten, D.J.; Canals, M.; Maussang, D.; Roumen, L.; Smit, M.J.; Wijtmans, M.; de Graaf, C.; Vischer, H.F.; Leurs, R. Pharmacological modulation of chemokine receptor function. *Br. J. Pharmacol.* **2012**, *165*, 1617–1643. [CrossRef] [PubMed]
8. Stone, M.J.; Hayward, J.A.; Huang, C.; E. Huma, Z.; Sanchez, J. Mechanisms of Regulation of the Chemokine-Receptor Network. *Int. J. Mol. Sci.* **2017**, *18*, 342. [CrossRef] [PubMed]
9. Rot, A. Binding of neutrophil attractant/activation protein-1 (interleukin 8) to resident dermal cells. *Cytokine* **1992**, *4*, 347–352. [CrossRef]
10. Rot, A. Endothelial cell binding of NAP-1/IL-8: Role in neutrophil emigration. *Immunol. Today* **1992**, *13*, 291–294. [CrossRef]
11. Webb, L.M.; Ehrengruber, M.U.; Clark-Lewis, I.; Baggiolini, M.; Rot, A. Binding to heparan sulfate or heparin enhances neutrophil responses to interleukin 8. *Proc. Natl. Acad. Sci. USA* **1993**, *90*, 7158–7162. [CrossRef] [PubMed]
12. Middleton, J.; Neil, S.; Wintle, J.; Clark-Lewis, I.; Moore, H.; Lam, C.; Auer, M.; Hub, E.; Rot, A. Transcytosis and surface presentation of IL-8 by venular endothelial cells. *Cell* **1997**, *91*, 385–395. [CrossRef]
13. Sarris, M.; Masson, J.B.; Maurin, D.; van der Aa, L.M.; Boudinot, P.; Lortat-Jacob, H.; Herbomel, P. Inflammatory chemokines direct and restrict leukocyte migration within live tissues as glycan-bound gradients. *Curr. Biol.* **2012**, *22*, 2375–2382. [CrossRef] [PubMed]

14. Weber, M.; Hauschild, R.; Schwarz, J.; Moussion, C.; de Vries, I.; Legler, D.F.; Luther, S.A.; Bollenbach, T.; Sixt, M. Interstitial dendritic cell guidance by haptotactic chemokine gradients. *Science* **2013**, *339*, 328–332. [CrossRef] [PubMed]

15. Proudfoot, A.E. The biological relevance of chemokine-proteoglycan interactions. *Biochem. Soc. Trans.* **2006**, *34 Pt 3*, 422–426. [CrossRef] [PubMed]

16. Salanga, C.L.; Handel, T.M. Chemokine oligomerization and interactions with receptors and glycosaminoglycans: The role of structural dynamics in function. *Exp. Cell. Res.* **2011**, *317*, 590–601. [CrossRef] [PubMed]

17. Handel, T.M.; Johnson, Z.; Crown, S.E.; Lau, E.K.; Proudfoot, A.E. Regulation of protein function by glycosaminoglycans—As exemplified by chemokines. *Annu. Rev. Biochem.* **2005**, *74*, 385–410. [CrossRef] [PubMed]

18. Johnson, Z.; Proudfoot, A.E.; Handel, T.M. Interaction of chemokines and glycosaminoglycans: A new twist in the regulation of chemokine function with opportunities for therapeutic intervention. *Cytokine Growth Factor Rev.* **2005**, *16*, 625–636. [CrossRef] [PubMed]

19. Monneau, Y.; Arenzana-Seisdedos, F.; Lortat-Jacob, H. The sweet spot: How GAGs help chemokines guide migrating cells. *J. Leukoc. Biol.* **2016**, *99*, 935–953. [CrossRef] [PubMed]

20. Springer, T.A. Traffic signals for lymphocyte recirculation and leukocyte emigration: The multistep paradigm. *Cell* **1994**, *76*, 301–314. [CrossRef]

21. Springer, T.A. Traffic signals on endothelium for lymphocyte recirculation and leukocyte emigration. *Annu. Rev. Physiol.* **1995**, *57*, 827–872. [CrossRef] [PubMed]

22. Laudanna, C.; Kim, J.Y.; Constantin, G.; Butcher, E. Rapid leukocyte integrin activation by chemokines. *Immunol. Rev.* **2002**, *186*, 37–46. [CrossRef] [PubMed]

23. Volpe, S.; Cameroni, E.; Moepps, B.; Thelen, S.; Apuzzo, T.; Thelen, M. CCR2 acts as scavenger for CCL2 during monocyte chemotaxis. *PLoS ONE* **2012**, *7*, e37208. [CrossRef] [PubMed]

24. Baggiolini, M. Chemokines in pathology and medicine. *J. Intern. Med.* **2001**, *250*, 91–104. [CrossRef] [PubMed]

25. Schumann, K.; Lammermann, T.; Bruckner, M.; Legler, D.F.; Polleux, J.; Spatz, J.P.; Schuler, G.; Forster, R.; Lutz, M.B.; Sorokin, L.; et al. Immobilized chemokine fields and soluble chemokine gradients cooperatively shape migration patterns of dendritic cells. *Immunity* **2010**, *32*, 703–713. [CrossRef] [PubMed]

26. Schwarz, J.; Bierbaum, V.; Vaahtomeri, K.; Hauschild, R.; Brown, M.; de Vries, I.; Leithner, A.; Reversat, A.; Merrin, J.; Tarrant, T.; et al. Dendritic Cells Interpret Haptotactic Chemokine Gradients in a Manner Governed by Signal-to-Noise Ratio and Dependent on GRK6. *Curr. Biol.* **2017**, *27*, 1314–1325. [CrossRef] [PubMed]

27. Das, S.T.; Rajagopalan, L.; Guerrero-Plata, A.; Sai, J.; Richmond, A.; Garofalo, R.P.; Rajarathnam, K. Monomeric and dimeric CXCL8 are both essential for in vivo neutrophil recruitment. *PLoS ONE* **2010**, *5*, e11754. [CrossRef] [PubMed]

28. Schwarz, J.; Bierbaum, V.; Merrin, J.; Frank, T.; Hauschild, R.; Bollenbach, T.; Tay, S.; Sixt, M.; Mehling, M. A microfluidic device for measuring cell migration towards substrate-bound and soluble chemokine gradients. *Sci. Rep.* **2016**, *6*, 36440. [CrossRef] [PubMed]

29. Majumdar, R.; Sixt, M.; Parent, C.A. New paradigms in the establishment and maintenance of gradients during directed cell migration. *Curr. Opin. Cell. Biol.* **2014**, *30*, 33–40. [CrossRef] [PubMed]

30. Migliorini, E.; Thakar, D.; Kuhnle, J.; Sadir, R.; Dyer, D.P.; Li, Y.; Sun, C.; Volkman, B.F.; Handel, T.M.; Coche-Guerente, L.; et al. Cytokines and growth factors cross-link heparan sulfate. *Open Biol.* **2015**, *5*, 150046. [CrossRef] [PubMed]

31. Dyer, D.P.; Migliorini, E.; Salanga, C.L.; Thakar, D.; Handel, T.M.; Richter, R.P. Differential structural remodelling of heparan sulfate by chemokines: The role of chemokine oligomerization. *Open Biol.* **2017**, *7*, 160286. [CrossRef] [PubMed]

32. Verkaar, F.; van Offenbeek, J.; van der Lee, M.M.; van Lith, L.H.; Watts, A.O.; Rops, A.L.; Aguilar, D.C.; Ziarek, J.J.; van der Vlag, J.; Handel, T.M.; et al. Chemokine cooperativity is caused by competitive glycosaminoglycan binding. *J. Immunol.* **2014**, *192*, 3908–3914. [CrossRef] [PubMed]

33. Sadir, R.; Imberty, A.; Baleux, F.; Lortat-Jacob, H. Heparan sulfate/heparin oligosaccharides protect stromal cell-derived factor-1 (SDF-1)/CXCL12 against proteolysis induced by CD26/dipeptidyl peptidase IV. *J. Biol. Chem.* **2004**, *279*, 43854–43860. [CrossRef] [PubMed]

34. Roscic-Mrkic, B.; Fischer, M.; Leemann, C.; Manrique, A.; Gordon, C.J.; Moore, J.P.; Proudfoot, A.E.; Trkola, A. RANTES (CCL5) uses the proteoglycan CD44 as an auxiliary receptor to mediate cellular activation signals and HIV-1 enhancement. *Blood* **2003**, *102*, 1169–1177. [CrossRef] [PubMed]

35. Kuschert, G.S.; Coulin, F.; Power, C.A.; Proudfoot, A.E.; Hubbard, R.E.; Hoogewerf, A.J.; Wells, T.N. Glycosaminoglycans interact selectively with chemokines and modulate receptor binding and cellular responses. *Biochemistry* **1999**, *38*, 12959–12968. [CrossRef] [PubMed]

36. Ziarek, J.J.; Veldkamp, C.T.; Zhang, F.; Murray, N.J.; Kartz, G.A.; Liang, X.; Su, J.; Baker, J.E.; Linhardt, R.J.; Volkman, B.F. Heparin oligosaccharides inhibit chemokine (CXC motif) ligand 12 (CXCL12) cardioprotection by binding orthogonal to the dimerization interface, promoting oligomerization, and competing with the chemokine (CXC motif) receptor 4 (CXCR4) N terminus. *J. Biol. Chem.* **2013**, *288*, 737–746. [CrossRef] [PubMed]

37. Bonvin, P.; Gueneau, F.; Buatois, V.; Charreton-Galby, M.; Lasch, S.; Messmer, M.; Christen, U.; Luster, A.D.; Johnson, Z.; Ferlin, W.; et al. Antibody Neutralization of CXCL10 in Vivo Is Dependent on Binding to Free and Not Endothelial-bound Chemokine: Implications for the design of a new generation of anti-chemokine therapeutic antibodies. *J. Biol. Chem.* **2017**, *292*, 4185–4197. [CrossRef] [PubMed]

38. Bonecchi, R.; Graham, G.J. Atypical Chemokine Receptors and Their Roles in the Resolution of the Inflammatory Response. *Front. Immunol.* **2016**, *7*, 224. [CrossRef] [PubMed]

39. Graham, G.J.; Locati, M.; Mantovani, A.; Rot, A.; Thelen, M. The biochemistry and biology of the atypical chemokine receptors. *Immunol. Lett.* **2012**, *145*, 30–38. [CrossRef] [PubMed]

40. Sarrazin, S.; Lamanna, W.C.; Esko, J.D. Heparan sulfate proteoglycans. *Cold Spring Harb. Perspect. Biol.* **2011**, *3*, a004952. [CrossRef] [PubMed]

41. Shriver, Z.; Liu, D.; Sasisekharan, R. Emerging views of heparan sulfate glycosaminoglycan structure/activity relationships modulating dynamic biological functions. *Trends Cardiovasc. Med.* **2002**, *12*, 71–77. [CrossRef]

42. Guerrini, M.; Raman, R.; Venkataraman, G.; Torri, G.; Sasisekharan, R.; Casu, B. A novel computational approach to integrate NMR spectroscopy and capillary electrophoresis for structure assignment of heparin and heparan sulfate oligosaccharides. *Glycobiology* **2002**, *12*, 713–719. [CrossRef] [PubMed]

43. DeAngelis, P.L.; Liu, J.; Linhardt, R.J. Chemoenzymatic synthesis of glycosaminoglycans: Re-creating, re-modeling and re-designing nature's longest or most complex carbohydrate chains. *Glycobiology* **2013**, *23*, 764–777. [CrossRef] [PubMed]

44. Liu, J.; Linhardt, R.J. Chemoenzymatic synthesis of heparan sulfate and heparin. *Nat. Prod. Rep.* **2014**, *31*, 1676–1685. [CrossRef] [PubMed]

45. Dyer, D.P.; Salanga, C.L.; Volkman, B.F.; Kawamura, T.; Handel, T.M. The dependence of chemokine-glycosaminoglycan interactions on chemokine oligomerization. *Glycobiology* **2016**, *26*, 312–326. [CrossRef] [PubMed]

46. Hamel, D.J.; Sielaff, I.; Proudfoot, A.E.; Handel, T.M. Chapter 4. Interactions of chemokines with glycosaminoglycans. *Methods Enzymol.* **2009**, *461*, 71–102. [PubMed]

47. Johnson, Z.; Kosco-Vilbois, M.H.; Herren, S.; Cirillo, R.; Muzio, V.; Zaratin, P.; Carbonatto, M.; Mack, M.; Smailbegovic, A.; Rose, M.; et al. Interference with heparin binding and oligomerization creates a novel anti-inflammatory strategy targeting the chemokine system. *J. Immunol.* **2004**, *173*, 5776–5785. [CrossRef] [PubMed]

48. Clore, G.M.; Appella, E.; Yamada, M.; Matsushima, K.; Gronenborn, A.M. Three-dimensional structure of interleukin 8 in solution. *Biochemistry* **1990**, *29*, 1689–1696. [CrossRef] [PubMed]

49. Kufareva, I.; Salanga, C.L.; Handel, T.M. Chemokine and chemokine receptor structure and interactions: Implications for therapeutic strategies. *Immunol. Cell. Biol.* **2015**, *93*, 372–383. [CrossRef] [PubMed]

50. Qin, L.; Kufareva, I.; Holden, L.G.; Wang, C.; Zheng, Y.; Zhao, C.; Fenalti, G.; Wu, H.; Han, G.W.; Cherezov, V.; et al. Structural biology. Crystal structure of the chemokine receptor CXCR4 in complex with a viral chemokine. *Science* **2015**, *347*, 1117–1122. [CrossRef] [PubMed]

51. Burg, J.S.; Ingram, J.R.; Venkatakrishnan, A.J.; Jude, K.M.; Dukkipati, A.; Feinberg, E.N.; Angelini, A.; Waghray, D.; Dror, R.O.; Ploegh, H.L.; et al. Structural biology. Structural basis for chemokine recognition and activation of a viral G protein-coupled receptor. *Science* **2015**, *347*, 1113–1117. [CrossRef] [PubMed]

52. Zheng, Y.; Han, G.W.; Abagyan, R.; Wu, B.; Stevens, R.C.; Cherezov, V.; Kufareva, I.; Handel, T.M. Structure of CC Chemokine Receptor 5 with a Potent Chemokine Antagonist Reveals Mechanisms of Chemokine Recognition and Molecular Mimicry by HIV. *Immunity* **2017**, *46*, 1005–1017. [CrossRef] [PubMed]

53. Sepuru, K.M.; Rajarathnam, K. CXCL1/MGSA Is a Novel Glycosaminoglycan (GAG)-binding Chemokine: Structural evidence for two distinct non-overlapping binding domains. *J. Biol. Chem.* **2016**, *291*, 4247–4255. [CrossRef] [PubMed]

54. Kufareva, I.; Gustavsson, M.; Zheng, Y.; Stephens, B.S.; Handel, T.M. What Do Structures Tell Us About Chemokine Receptor Function and Antagonism? *Annu. Rev. Biophys.* **2017**, *46*, 175–198. [CrossRef] [PubMed]

55. Lau, E.K.; Paavola, C.D.; Johnson, Z.; Gaudry, J.P.; Geretti, E.; Borlat, F.; Kungl, A.J.; Proudfoot, A.E.; Handel, T.M. Identification of the glycosaminoglycan binding site of the CC chemokine, MCP-1: Implications for structure and function in vivo. *J. Biol. Chem.* **2004**, *279*, 22294–22305. [CrossRef] [PubMed]

56. Deshauer, C.; Morgan, A.M.; Ryan, E.O.; Handel, T.M.; Prestegard, J.H.; Wang, X. Interactions of the Chemokine CCL5/RANTES with Medium-Sized Chondroitin Sulfate Ligands. *Structure* **2015**, *23*, 1066–1077. [CrossRef] [PubMed]

57. Kuschert, G.S.; Hoogewerf, A.J.; Proudfoot, A.E.; Chung, C.W.; Cooke, R.M.; Hubbard, R.E.; Wells, T.N.; Sanderson, P.N. Identification of a glycosaminoglycan binding surface on human interleukin-8. *Biochemistry* **1998**, *37*, 11193–11201. [CrossRef] [PubMed]

58. Proudfoot, A.E.; Fritchley, S.; Borlat, F.; Shaw, J.P.; Vilbois, F.; Zwahlen, C.; Trkola, A.; Marchant, D.; Clapham, P.R.; Wells, T.N. The BBXB motif of RANTES is the principal site for heparin binding and controls receptor selectivity. *J. Biol. Chem.* **2001**, *276*, 10620–10626. [CrossRef] [PubMed]

59. Fox, J.C.; Tyler, R.C.; Peterson, F.C.; Dyer, D.P.; Zhang, F.; Linhardt, R.J.; Handel, T.M.; Volkman, B.F. Examination of Glycosaminoglycan Binding Sites on the XCL1 Dimer. *Biochemistry* **2016**, *55*, 1214–1225. [CrossRef] [PubMed]

60. Laurence, J.S.; Blanpain, C.; de Leener, A.; Parmentier, M.; LiWang, P.J. Importance of basic residues and quaternary structure in the function of MIP-1 beta: CCR5 binding and cell surface sugar interactions. *Biochemistry* **2001**, *40*, 4990–4999. [CrossRef] [PubMed]

61. Sepuru, K.M.; Nagarajan, B.; Desai, U.R.; Rajarathnam, K. Molecular Basis of Chemokine CXCL5-Glycosaminoglycan Interactions. *J. Biol. Chem.* **2016**, *291*, 20539–20550. [CrossRef] [PubMed]

62. Rueda, P.; Balabanian, K.; Lagane, B.; Staropoli, I.; Chow, K.; Levoye, A.; Laguri, C.; Sadir, R.; Delaunay, T.; Izquierdo, E.; et al. The CXCL12gamma chemokine displays unprecedented structural and functional properties that make it a paradigm of chemoattractant proteins. *PLoS ONE* **2008**, *3*, e2543. [CrossRef] [PubMed]

63. Koopmann, W.; Krangel, M.S. Identification of a glycosaminoglycan-binding site in chemokine macrophage inflammatory protein-1alpha. *J. Biol. Chem.* **1997**, *272*, 10103–10109. [CrossRef] [PubMed]

64. Farzan, M.; Mirzabekov, T.; Kolchinsky, P.; Wyatt, R.; Cayabyab, M.; Gerard, N.P.; Gerard, C.; Sodroski, J.; Choe, H. Tyrosine sulfation of the amino terminus of CCR5 facilitates HIV-1 entry. *Cell* **1999**, *96*, 667–676. [CrossRef]

65. Preobrazhensky, A.A.; Dragan, S.; Kawano, T.; Gavrilin, M.A.; Gulina, I.V.; Chakravarty, L.; Kolattukudy, P.E. Monocyte chemotactic protein-1 receptor CCR2B is a glycoprotein that has tyrosine sulfation in a conserved extracellular N-terminal region. *J. Immunol.* **2000**, *165*, 5295–5303. [CrossRef] [PubMed]

66. Fernandez, E.J.; Lolis, E. Structure, function, and inhibition of chemokines. *Annu. Rev. Pharmacol. Toxicol.* **2002**, *42*, 469–499. [CrossRef] [PubMed]

67. Lodi, P.J.; Garrett, D.S.; Kuszewski, J.; Tsang, M.L.; Weatherbee, J.A.; Leonard, W.J.; Gronenborn, A.M.; Clore, G.M. High-resolution solution structure of the beta chemokine hMIP-1 beta by multidimensional NMR. *Science* **1994**, *263*, 1762–1767. [CrossRef] [PubMed]

68. Handel, T.M.; Domaille, P.J. Heteronuclear (^{1}H, ^{13}C, ^{15}N) NMR assignments and solution structure of the monocyte chemoattractant protein-1 (MCP-1) dimer. *Biochemistry* **1996**, *35*, 6569–6584. [CrossRef] [PubMed]

69. Rajarathnam, K.; Sykes, B.D.; Kay, C.M.; Dewald, B.; Geiser, T.; Baggiolini, M.; Clark-Lewis, I. Neutrophil activation by monomeric interleukin-8. *Science* **1994**, *264*, 90–92. [CrossRef] [PubMed]

70. Paavola, C.D.; Hemmerich, S.; Grunberger, D.; Polsky, I.; Bloom, A.; Freedman, R.; Mulkins, M.; Bhakta, S.; McCarley, D.; Wiesent, L.; et al. Monomeric monocyte chemoattractant protein-1 (MCP-1) binds and activates the MCP-1 receptor CCR2B. *J. Biol. Chem.* **1998**, *273*, 33157–33165. [CrossRef] [PubMed]

71. Laurence, J.S.; Blanpain, C.; Burgner, J.W.; Parmentier, M.; LiWang, P.J. CC chemokine MIP-1 beta can function as a monomer and depends on Phe13 for receptor binding. *Biochemistry* **2000**, *39*, 3401–3409. [CrossRef] [PubMed]

72. Jin, H.; Shen, X.; Baggett, B.R.; Kong, X.; LiWang, P.J. The human CC chemokine MIP-1beta dimer is not competent to bind to the CCR5 receptor. *J. Biol. Chem.* **2007**, *282*, 27976–27983. [CrossRef] [PubMed]
73. Hemmerich, S.; Paavola, C.; Bloom, A.; Bhakta, S.; Freedman, R.; Grunberger, D.; Krstenansky, J.; Lee, S.; McCarley, D.; Mulkins, M.; et al. Identification of residues in the monocyte chemotactic protein-1 that contact the MCP-1 receptor, CCR2. *Biochemistry* **1999**, *38*, 13013–13025. [CrossRef] [PubMed]
74. Gangavarapu, P.; Rajagopalan, L.; Kolli, D.; Guerrero-Plata, A.; Garofalo, R.P.; Rajarathnam, K. The monomer-dimer equilibrium and glycosaminoglycan interactions of chemokine CXCL8 regulate tissue-specific neutrophil recruitment. *J. Leukoc. Biol.* **2012**, *91*, 259–265. [CrossRef] [PubMed]
75. Sawant, K.V.; Poluri, K.M.; Dutta, A.K.; Sepuru, K.M.; Troshkina, A.; Garofalo, R.P.; Rajarathnam, K. Chemokine CXCL1 mediated neutrophil recruitment: Role of glycosaminoglycan interactions. *Sci. Rep.* **2016**, *6*, 33123. [CrossRef] [PubMed]
76. Nasser, M.W.; Raghuwanshi, S.K.; Grant, D.J.; Jala, V.R.; Rajarathnam, K.; Richardson, R.M. Differential activation and regulation of CXCR1 and CXCR2 by CXCL8 monomer and dimer. *J. Immunol.* **2009**, *183*, 3425–3432. [CrossRef] [PubMed]
77. Veldkamp, C.T.; Seibert, C.; Peterson, F.C.; de la Cruz, N.B.; Haugner, J.C., 3rd; Basnet, H.; Sakmar, T.P.; Volkman, B.F. Structural basis of CXCR4 sulfotyrosine recognition by the chemokine SDF-1/CXCL12. *Sci. Signal.* **2008**, *1*, ra4. [CrossRef] [PubMed]
78. Leong, S.R.; Lowman, H.B.; Liu, J.; Shire, S.; Deforge, L.E.; Gillece-Castro, B.L.; McDowell, R.; Hebert, C.A. IL-8 single-chain homodimers and heterodimers: Interactions with chemokine receptors CXCR1, CXCR2, and DARC. *Protein Sci.* **1997**, *6*, 609–617. [CrossRef] [PubMed]
79. Hoogewerf, A.J.; Kuschert, G.S.; Proudfoot, A.E.; Borlat, F.; Clark-Lewis, I.; Power, C.A.; Wells, T.N. Glycosaminoglycans mediate cell surface oligomerization of chemokines. *Biochemistry* **1997**, *36*, 13570–13578. [CrossRef] [PubMed]
80. Veldkamp, C.T.; Peterson, F.C.; Pelzek, A.J.; Volkman, B.F. The monomer-dimer equilibrium of stromal cell-derived factor-1 (CXCL 12) is altered by pH, phosphate, sulfate, and heparin. *Protein Sci.* **2005**, *14*, 1071–1081. [CrossRef] [PubMed]
81. Proudfoot, A.E.; Handel, T.M.; Johnson, Z.; Lau, E.K.; LiWang, P.; Clark-Lewis, I.; Borlat, F.; Wells, T.N.; Kosco-Vilbois, M.H. Glycosaminoglycan binding and oligomerization are essential for the in vivo activity of certain chemokines. *Proc. Natl. Acad. Sci. USA* **2003**, *100*, 1885–1890. [CrossRef] [PubMed]
82. Tanino, Y.; Coombe, D.R.; Gill, S.E.; Kett, W.C.; Kajikawa, O.; Proudfoot, A.E.; Wells, T.N.; Parks, W.C.; Wight, T.N.; Martin, T.R.; et al. Kinetics of chemokine-glycosaminoglycan interactions control neutrophil migration into the airspaces of the lungs. *J. Immunol.* **2010**, *184*, 2677–2685. [CrossRef] [PubMed]
83. Salanga, C.L.; Dyer, D.P.; Kiselar, J.G.; Gupta, S.; Chance, M.R.; Handel, T.M. Multiple glycosaminoglycan-binding epitopes of monocyte chemoattractant protein-3/CCL7 enable it to function as a non-oligomerizing chemokine. *J. Biol. Chem.* **2014**, *289*, 14896–14912. [CrossRef] [PubMed]
84. Liang, W.G.; Triandafillou, C.G.; Huang, T.Y.; Zulueta, M.M.; Banerjee, S.; Dinner, A.R.; Hung, S.C.; Tang, W.J. Structural basis for oligomerization and glycosaminoglycan binding of CCL5 and CCL3. *Proc. Natl. Acad. Sci. USA* **2016**, *113*, 5000–5005. [CrossRef] [PubMed]
85. Zhang, X.; Chen, L.; Bancroft, D.P.; Lai, C.K.; Maione, T.E. Crystal structure of recombinant human platelet factor 4. *Biochemistry* **1994**, *33*, 8361–8366. [CrossRef] [PubMed]
86. Lubkowski, J.; Bujacz, G.; Boque, L.; Domaille, P.J.; Handel, T.M.; Wlodawer, A. The structure of MCP-1 in two crystal forms provides a rare example of variable quaternary interactions. *Nat. Struct. Biol.* **1997**, *4*, 64–69. [CrossRef] [PubMed]
87. Mayo, K.H.; Ilyina, E.; Roongta, V.; Dundas, M.; Joseph, J.; Lai, C.K.; Maione, T.; Daly, T.J. Heparin binding to platelet factor-4. An NMR and site-directed mutagenesis study: Arginine residues are crucial for binding. *Biochem. J.* **1995**, *312 Pt 2*, 357–365. [CrossRef] [PubMed]
88. Segerer, S.; Johnson, Z.; Rek, A.; Baltus, T.; von Hundelshausen, P.; Kungl, A.J.; Proudfoot, A.E.; Weber, C.; Nelson, P.J. The basic residue cluster (55)KKWVR(59) in CCL5 is required for in vivo biologic function. *Mol. Immunol.* **2009**, *46*, 2533–2538. [CrossRef] [PubMed]
89. Patel, D.D.; Koopmann, W.; Imai, T.; Whichard, L.P.; Yoshie, O.; Krangel, M.S. Chemokines have diverse abilities to form solid phase gradients. *Clin. Immunol.* **2001**, *99*, 43–52. [CrossRef] [PubMed]
90. Murphy, J.W.; Yuan, H.; Kong, Y.; Xiong, Y.; Lolis, E.J. Heterologous quaternary structure of CXCL12 and its relationship to the CC chemokine family. *Proteins* **2010**, *78*, 1331–1337. [CrossRef] [PubMed]

91. Murphy, J.W.; Cho, Y.; Sachpatzidis, A.; Fan, C.; Hodsdon, M.E.; Lolis, E. Structural and functional basis of CXCL12 (stromal cell-derived factor-1 alpha) binding to heparin. *J. Biol. Chem.* **2007**, *282*, 10018–10027. [CrossRef] [PubMed]

92. Chang, S.L.; Cavnar, S.P.; Takayama, S.; Luker, G.D.; Linderman, J.J. Cell, isoform, and environment factors shape gradients and modulate chemotaxis. *PLoS ONE* **2015**, *10*, e0123450. [CrossRef] [PubMed]

93. Stringer, S.E.; Forster, M.J.; Mulloy, B.; Bishop, C.R.; Graham, G.J.; Gallagher, J.T. Characterization of the binding site on heparan sulfate for macrophage inflammatory protein 1alpha. *Blood* **2002**, *100*, 1543–1550. [PubMed]

94. Jayson, G.C.; Hansen, S.U.; Miller, G.J.; Cole, C.L.; Rushton, G.; Avizienyte, E.; Gardiner, J.M. Synthetic heparan sulfate dodecasaccharides reveal single sulfation site interconverts CXCL8 and CXCL12 chemokine biology. *Chem. Commun. Camb.* **2015**, *51*, 13846–13849. [CrossRef] [PubMed]

95. De Paz, J.L.; Moseman, E.A.; Noti, C.; Polito, L.; von Andrian, U.H.; Seeberger, P.H. Profiling heparin-chemokine interactions using synthetic tools. *ACS Chem. Biol.* **2007**, *2*, 735–744. [CrossRef] [PubMed]

96. Jabeen, T.; Leonard, P.; Jamaluddin, H.; Acharya, K.R. Structure of mouse IP-10, a chemokine. *Acta Crystallogr. D Biol. Crystallogr.* **2008**, *64*, 6611–6619. [CrossRef] [PubMed]

97. Swaminathan, G.J.; Holloway, D.E.; Colvin, R.A.; Campanella, G.K.; Papageorgiou, A.C.; Luster, A.D.; Acharya, K.R. Crystal structures of oligomeric forms of the IP-10/CXCL10 chemokine. *Structure* **2003**, *11*, 521–532. [CrossRef]

98. Shaw, J.P.; Johnson, Z.; Borlat, F.; Zwahlen, C.; Kungl, A.; Roulin, K.; Harrenga, A.; Wells, T.N.; Proudfoot, A.E. The X-ray structure of RANTES: Heparin-derived disaccharides allows the rational design of chemokine inhibitors. *Structure* **2004**, *12*, 2081–2093. [CrossRef] [PubMed]

99. Joseph, P.R.; Mosier, P.D.; Desai, U.R.; Rajarathnam, K. Solution NMR characterization of chemokine CXCL8/IL-8 monomer and dimer binding to glycosaminoglycans: Structural plasticity mediates differential binding interactions. *Biochem. J.* **2015**, *472*, 121–133. [CrossRef] [PubMed]

100. Crown, S.E.; Yu, Y.; Sweeney, M.D.; Leary, J.A.; Handel, T.M. Heterodimerization of CCR2 chemokines and regulation by glycosaminoglycan binding. *J. Biol. Chem.* **2006**, *281*, 25438–25446. [CrossRef] [PubMed]

101. Kramp, B.K.; Sarabi, A.; Koenen, R.R.; Weber, C. Heterophilic chemokine receptor interactions in chemokine signaling and biology. *Exp. Cell. Res.* **2011**, *317*, 655–663. [CrossRef] [PubMed]

102. Von Hundelshausen, P.; Koenen, R.R.; Sack, M.; Mause, S.F.; Adriaens, W.; Proudfoot, A.E.; Hackeng, T.M.; Weber, C. Heterophilic interactions of platelet factor 4 and RANTES promote monocyte arrest on endothelium. *Blood* **2005**, *105*, 924–930. [CrossRef] [PubMed]

103. Carlson, J.; Baxter, S.A.; Dreau, D.; Nesmelova, I.V. The heterodimerization of platelet-derived chemokines. *Biochim. Biophys. Acta* **2013**, *1834*, 158–168. [CrossRef] [PubMed]

104. Nesmelova, I.V.; Sham, Y.; Dudek, A.Z.; van Eijk, L.I.; Wu, G.; Slungaard, A.; Mortari, F.; Griffioen, A.W.; Mayo, K.H. Platelet factor 4 and interleukin-8 CXC chemokine heterodimer formation modulates function at the quaternary structural level. *J. Biol. Chem.* **2005**, *280*, 4948–4958. [CrossRef] [PubMed]

105. Nesmelova, I.V.; Sham, Y.; Gao, J.; Mayo, K.H. CXC and CC chemokines form mixed heterodimers: Association free energies from molecular dynamics simulations and experimental correlations. *J. Biol. Chem.* **2008**, *283*, 24155–24166. [CrossRef] [PubMed]

106. Wagner, L.; Yang, O.O.; Garcia-Zepeda, E.A.; Ge, Y.; Kalams, S.A.; Walker, B.D.; Pasternack, M.S.; Luster, A.D. Beta-chemokines are released from HIV-1-specific cytolytic T-cell granules complexed to proteoglycans. *Nature* **1998**, *391*, 908–911. [CrossRef] [PubMed]

107. Proost, P.; Loos, T.; Mortier, A.; Schutyser, E.; Gouwy, M.; Noppen, S.; Dillen, C.; Ronsse, I.; Conings, R.; Struyf, S.; et al. Citrullination of CXCL8 by peptidylarginine deiminase alters receptor usage, prevents proteolysis, and dampens tissue inflammation. *J. Exp. Med.* **2008**, *205*, 2085–2097. [CrossRef] [PubMed]

108. Barker, C.E.; Thompson, S.; O'Boyle, G.; Lortat-Jacob, H.; Sheerin, N.S.; Ali, S.; Kirby, J.A. CCL2 nitration is a negative regulator of chemokine-mediated inflammation. *Sci. Rep.* **2017**, *7*, 44384. [CrossRef] [PubMed]

109. Thakar, D.; Dalonneau, F.; Migliorini, E.; Lortat-Jacob, H.; Boturyn, D.; Albiges-Rizo, C.; Coche-Guerente, L.; Picart, C.; Richter, R.P. Binding of the chemokine CXCL12alpha to its natural extracellular matrix ligand heparan sulfate enables myoblast adhesion and facilitates cell motility. *Biomaterials* **2017**, *123*, 24–38. [CrossRef] [PubMed]

110. Haessler, U.; Pisano, M.; Wu, M.; Swartz, M.A. Dendritic cell chemotaxis in 3D under defined chemokine gradients reveals differential response to ligands CCL21 and CCL19. *Proc. Natl. Acad. Sci. USA* **2011**, *108*, 5614–5619. [CrossRef] [PubMed]

111. Vaahtomeri, K.; Brown, M.; Hauschild, R.; de Vries, I.; Leithner, A.F.; Mehling, M.; Kaufmann, W.A.; Sixt, M. Locally Triggered Release of the Chemokine CCL21 Promotes Dendritic Cell Transmigration across Lymphatic Endothelia. *Cell Rep.* **2017**, *19*, 902–909. [CrossRef] [PubMed]

112. Stoler-Barak, L.; Barzilai, S.; Zauberman, A.; Alon, R. Transendothelial migration of effector T cells across inflamed endothelial barriers does not require heparan sulfate proteoglycans. *Int. Immunol.* **2014**, *26*, 315–324. [CrossRef] [PubMed]

113. Yin, X.; Truty, J.; Lawrence, R.; Johns, S.C.; Srinivasan, R.S.; Handel, T.M.; Fuster, M.M. A critical role for lymphatic endothelial heparan sulfate in lymph node metastasis. *Mol. Cancer* **2010**, *9*, 316. [CrossRef] [PubMed]

114. Severin, I.C.; Soares, A.; Hantson, J.; Teixeira, M.; Sachs, D.; Valognes, D.; Scheer, A.; Schwarz, M.K.; Wells, T.N.; Proudfoot, A.E.; et al. Glycosaminoglycan analogs as a novel anti-inflammatory strategy. *Front. Immunol.* **2012**, *3*, 293. [CrossRef] [PubMed]

115. Nonaka, M.; Bao, X.; Matsumura, F.; Gotze, S.; Kandasamy, J.; Kononov, A.; Broide, D.H.; Nakayama, J.; Seeberger, P.H.; Fukuda, M. Synthetic di-sulfated iduronic acid attenuates asthmatic response by blocking T-cell recruitment to inflammatory sites. *Proc. Natl. Acad. Sci. USA* **2014**, *111*, 8173–8178. [CrossRef] [PubMed]

116. Gouwy, M.; Struyf, S.; Catusse, J.; Proost, P.; van Damme, J. Synergy between proinflammatory ligands of G protein-coupled receptors in neutrophil activation and migration. *J. Leukoc. Biol.* **2004**, *76*, 185–194. [CrossRef] [PubMed]

117. Kuscher, K.; Danelon, G.; Paoletti, S.; Stefano, L.; Schiraldi, M.; Petkovic, V.; Locati, M.; Gerber, B.O.; Uguccioni, M. Synergy-inducing chemokines enhance CCR2 ligand activities on monocytes. *Eur. J. Immunol.* **2009**, *39*, 1118–1128. [CrossRef] [PubMed]

118. Sebastiani, S.; Danelon, G.; Gerber, B.; Uguccioni, M. CCL22-induced responses are powerfully enhanced by synergy inducing chemokines via CCR4: Evidence for the involvement of first beta-strand of chemokine. *Eur. J. Immunol.* **2005**, *35*, 746–756. [CrossRef] [PubMed]

119. Vanbervliet, B.; Bendriss-Vermare, N.; Massacrier, C.; Homey, B.; de Bouteiller, O.; Briere, F.; Trinchieri, G.; Caux, C. The inducible CXCR3 ligands control plasmacytoid dendritic cell responsiveness to the constitutive chemokine stromal cell-derived factor 1 (SDF-1)/CXCL12. *J. Exp. Med.* **2003**, *198*, 823–830. [CrossRef] [PubMed]

120. Bai, Z.; Hayasaka, H.; Kobayashi, M.; Li, W.; Guo, Z.; Jang, M.H.; Kondo, A.; Choi, B.I.; Iwakura, Y.; Miyasaka, M. CXC chemokine ligand 12 promotes CCR7-dependent naive T cell trafficking to lymph nodes and Peyer's patches. *J. Immunol.* **2009**, *182*, 1287–1295. [CrossRef] [PubMed]

121. Proudfoot, A.E.; Uguccioni, M. Modulation of Chemokine Responses: Synergy and Cooperativity. *Front. Immunol.* **2016**, *7*, 183. [CrossRef] [PubMed]

122. Paoletti, S.; Petkovic, V.; Sebastiani, S.; Danelon, M.G.; Uguccioni, M.; Gerber, B.O. A rich chemokine environment strongly enhances leukocyte migration and activities. *Blood* **2005**, *105*, 3405–3412. [CrossRef] [PubMed]

123. Mueller, A.; Meiser, A.; McDonagh, E.M.; Fox, J.M.; Petit, S.J.; Xanthou, G.; Williams, T.J.; Pease, J.E. CXCL4-induced migration of activated T lymphocytes is mediated by the chemokine receptor CXCR3. *J. Leukoc. Biol.* **2008**, *83*, 875–882. [CrossRef] [PubMed]

124. Krohn, S.C.; Bonvin, P.; Proudfoot, A.E. CCL18 exhibits a regulatory role through inhibition of receptor and glycosaminoglycan binding. *PLoS ONE* **2013**, *8*, e72321. [CrossRef] [PubMed]

125. Schutyser, E.; Richmond, A.; van Damme, J. Involvement of CC chemokine ligand 18 (CCL18) in normal and pathological processes. *J. Leukoc. Biol.* **2005**, *78*, 14–26. [CrossRef] [PubMed]

126. Struyf, S.; Schutyser, E.; Gouwy, M.; Gijsbers, K.; Proost, P.; Benoit, Y.; Opdenakker, G.; van Damme, J.; Laureys, G. PARC/CCL18 is a plasma CC chemokine with increased levels in childhood acute lymphoblastic leukemia. *Am. J. Pathol.* **2003**, *163*, 2065–2075. [CrossRef]

127. Moelants, E.A.; Mortier, A.; van Damme, J.; Proost, P. In vivo regulation of chemokine activity by post-translational modification. *Immunol. Cell Biol.* **2013**, *91*, 402–427. [CrossRef] [PubMed]

128. Van den Steen, P.E.; Proost, P.; Wuyts, A.; van Damme, J.; Opdenakker, G. Neutrophil gelatinase B potentiates interleukin-8 tenfold by aminoterminal processing, whereas it degrades CTAP-III, PF-4, and GRO-alpha and leaves RANTES and MCP-2 intact. *Blood* **2000**, *96*, 2673–2681. [PubMed]
129. McQuibban, G.A.; Gong, J.H.; Tam, E.M.; McCulloch, C.A.; Clark-Lewis, I.; Overall, C.M. Inflammation dampened by gelatinase A cleavage of monocyte chemoattractant protein-3. *Science* **2000**, *289*, 1202–1206. [CrossRef] [PubMed]
130. Proost, P.; Menten, P.; Struyf, S.; Schutyser, E.; de Meester, I.; van Damme, J. Cleavage by CD26/dipeptidyl peptidase IV converts the chemokine LD78beta into a most efficient monocyte attractant and CCR1 agonist. *Blood* **2000**, *96*, 1674–1680. [PubMed]
131. Struyf, S.; Proost, P.; Schols, D.; de Clercq, E.; Opdenakker, G.; Lenaerts, J.P.; Detheux, M.; Parmentier, M.; de Meester, I.; Scharpe, S.; et al. CD26/dipeptidyl-peptidase IV down-regulates the eosinophil chemotactic potency, but not the anti-HIV activity of human eotaxin by affecting its interaction with CC chemokine receptor 3. *J. Immunol.* **1999**, *162*, 4903–4909. [PubMed]
132. Valenzuela-Fernandez, A.; Planchenault, T.; Baleux, F.; Staropoli, I.; Le-Barillec, K.; Leduc, D.; Delaunay, T.; Lazarini, F.; Virelizier, J.L.; Chignard, M.; et al. Leukocyte elastase negatively regulates Stromal cell-derived factor-1 (SDF-1)/CXCR4 binding and functions by amino-terminal processing of SDF-1 and CXCR4. *J. Biol. Chem.* **2002**, *277*, 15677–15689. [CrossRef] [PubMed]
133. Ellyard, J.I.; Simson, L.; Bezos, A.; Johnston, K.; Freeman, C.; Parish, C.R. Eotaxin selectively binds heparin. An interaction that protects eotaxin from proteolysis and potentiates chemotactic activity in vivo. *J. Biol. Chem.* **2007**, *282*, 15238–15247. [CrossRef] [PubMed]
134. Van den Berg, B.M.; Vink, H.; Spaan, J.A. The endothelial glycocalyx protects against myocardial edema. *Circ. Res.* **2003**, *92*, 592–594. [CrossRef] [PubMed]
135. Van den Berg, B.M.; Spaan, J.A.; Vink, H. Impaired glycocalyx barrier properties contribute to enhanced intimal low-density lipoprotein accumulation at the carotid artery bifurcation in mice. *Pflugers Arch.* **2009**, *457*, 1199–1206. [CrossRef] [PubMed]
136. Marki, A.; Esko, J.D.; Pries, A.R.; Ley, K. Role of the endothelial surface layer in neutrophil recruitment. *J. Leukoc. Biol.* **2015**, *98*, 503–515. [CrossRef] [PubMed]
137. Constantinescu, A.A.; Vink, H.; Spaan, J.A. Endothelial cell glycocalyx modulates immobilization of leukocytes at the endothelial surface. *Arterioscler. Thromb. Vasc. Biol.* **2003**, *23*, 1541–1547. [CrossRef] [PubMed]
138. Schmidt, E.P.; Yang, Y.; Janssen, W.J.; Gandjeva, A.; Perez, M.J.; Barthel, L.; Zemans, R.L.; Bowman, J.C.; Koyanagi, D.E.; Yunt, Z.X.; et al. The pulmonary endothelial glycocalyx regulates neutrophil adhesion and lung injury during experimental sepsis. *Nat. Med.* **2012**, *18*, 1217–1223. [CrossRef] [PubMed]
139. Wiesinger, A.; Peters, W.; Chappell, D.; Kentrup, D.; Reuter, S.; Pavenstadt, H.; Oberleithner, H.; Kumpers, P. Nanomechanics of the endothelial glycocalyx in experimental sepsis. *PLoS ONE* **2013**, *8*, e80905. [CrossRef] [PubMed]
140. Henry, C.B.; Duling, B.R. TNF-alpha increases entry of macromolecules into luminal endothelial cell glycocalyx. *Am. J. Physiol. Heart Circ. Physiol.* **2000**, *279*, H2815–H2823. [PubMed]
141. Charnaux, N.; Brule, S.; Hamon, M.; Chaigneau, T.; Saffar, L.; Prost, C.; Lievre, N.; Gattegno, L. Syndecan-4 is a signaling molecule for stromal cell-derived factor-1 (SDF-1)/CXCL12. *FEBS J.* **2005**, *272*, 1937–1951. [CrossRef] [PubMed]
142. Brule, S.; Charnaux, N.; Sutton, A.; Ledoux, D.; Chaigneau, T.; Saffar, L.; Gattegno, L. The shedding of syndecan-4 and syndecan-1 from HeLa cells and human primary macrophages is accelerated by SDF-1/CXCL12 and mediated by the matrix metalloproteinase-9. *Glycobiology* **2006**, *16*, 488–501. [CrossRef] [PubMed]
143. Charnaux, N.; Brule, S.; Chaigneau, T.; Saffar, L.; Sutton, A.; Hamon, M.; Prost, C.; Lievre, N.; Vita, C.; Gattegno, L. RANTES (CCL5) induces a CCR5-dependent accelerated shedding of syndecan-1 (CD138) and syndecan-4 from HeLa cells and forms complexes with the shed ectodomains of these proteoglycans as well as with those of CD44. *Glycobiology* **2005**, *15*, 119–130. [CrossRef] [PubMed]
144. Piccinini, A.M.; Knebl, K.; Rek, A.; Wildner, G.; Diedrichs-Mohring, M.; Kungl, A.J. Rationally evolving MCP-1/CCL2 into a decoy protein with potent anti-inflammatory activity in vivo. *J. Biol. Chem.* **2010**, *285*, 8782–8792. [CrossRef] [PubMed]

145. Brandner, B.; Rek, A.; Diedrichs-Mohring, M.; Wildner, G.; Kungl, A.J. Engineering the glycosaminoglycan-binding affinity, kinetics and oligomerization behavior of RANTES: A tool for generating chemokine-based glycosaminoglycan antagonists. *Protein Eng. Des. Sel.* **2009**, *22*, 367–373. [CrossRef] [PubMed]

146. Falsone, A.; Wabitsch, V.; Geretti, E.; Potzinger, H.; Gerlza, T.; Robinson, J.; Adage, T.; Teixeira, M.M.; Kungl, A.J. Designing CXCL8-based decoy proteins with strong anti-inflammatory activity in vivo. *Biosci. Rep.* **2013**, *33*, e00068. [CrossRef] [PubMed]

147. Adage, T.; Piccinini, A.M.; Falsone, A.; Trinker, M.; Robinson, J.; Gesslbauer, B.; Kungl, A.J. Structure-based design of decoy chemokines as a way to explore the pharmacological potential of glycosaminoglycans. *Br. J. Pharmacol.* **2012**, *167*, 1195–1205. [CrossRef] [PubMed]

148. Severin, I.C.; Gaudry, J.P.; Johnson, Z.; Kungl, A.; Jansma, A.; Gesslbauer, B.; Mulloy, B.; Power, C.; Proudfoot, A.E.; Handel, T. Characterization of the chemokine CXCL11-heparin interaction suggests two different affinities for glycosaminoglycans. *J. Biol. Chem.* **2010**, *285*, 17713–17724. [CrossRef] [PubMed]

149. Ali, S.; O'Boyle, G.; Hepplewhite, P.; Tyler, J.R.; Robertson, H.; Kirby, J.A. Therapy with nonglycosaminoglycan-binding mutant CCL7: A novel strategy to limit allograft inflammation. *Am. J. Transplant.* **2010**, *10*, 47–58. [CrossRef] [PubMed]

150. Braunersreuther, V.; Pellieux, C.; Pelli, G.; Burger, F.; Steffens, S.; Montessuit, C.; Weber, C.; Proudfoot, A.; Mach, F.; Arnaud, C. Chemokine CCL5/RANTES inhibition reduces myocardial reperfusion injury in atherosclerotic mice. *J. Mol. Cell. Cardiol.* **2010**, *48*, 789–798. [CrossRef] [PubMed]

151. Braunersreuther, V.; Steffens, S.; Arnaud, C.; Pelli, G.; Burger, F.; Proudfoot, A.; Mach, F. A novel RANTES antagonist prevents progression of established atherosclerotic lesions in mice. *Arterioscler. Thromb. Vasc. Biol.* **2008**, *28*, 1090–1096. [CrossRef] [PubMed]

152. Nellen, A.; Heinrichs, D.; Berres, M.L.; Sahin, H.; Schmitz, P.; Proudfoot, A.E.; Trautwein, C.; Wasmuth, H.E. Interference with oligomerization and glycosaminoglycan binding of the chemokine CCL5 improves experimental liver injury. *PLoS ONE* **2012**, *7*, e36614. [CrossRef] [PubMed]

153. Handel, T.M.; Johnson, Z.; Rodrigues, D.H.; Santos, A.C.D.; Cirillo, R.; Muzio, V.; Riva, S.; Mack, M.; Deruaz, M.; Borlat, F.; et al. An engineered monomer of CCL2 has anti-inflammatory properties emphasizing the importance of oligomerization for chemokine activity in vivo. *J. Leukoc. Biol.* **2008**, *84*, 1101–1108. [CrossRef] [PubMed]

154. Shahrara, S.; Proudfoot, A.E.; Park, C.C.; Volin, M.V.; Haines, G.K.; Woods, J.M.; Aikens, C.H.; Handel, T.M.; Pope, R.M. Inhibition of monocyte chemoattractant protein-1 ameliorates rat adjuvant-induced arthritis. *J. Immunol.* **2008**, *180*, 3447–3456. [CrossRef] [PubMed]

155. Gaertner, H.; Cerini, F.; Escola, J.M.; Kuenzi, G.; Melotti, A.; Offord, R.; Rossitto-Borlat, I.; Nedellec, R.; Salkowitz, J.; Gorochov, G.; et al. Highly potent, fully recombinant anti-HIV chemokines: Reengineering a low-cost microbicide. *Proc. Natl. Acad. Sci. USA* **2008**, *105*, 17706–17711. [CrossRef] [PubMed]

156. Cerini, F.; Gaertner, H.; Madden, K.; Tolstorukov, I.; Brown, S.; Laukens, B.; Callewaert, N.; Harner, J.C.; Oommen, A.M.; Harms, J.T.; et al. A scalable low-cost cGMP process for clinical grade production of the HIV inhibitor 5P12-RANTES in Pichia pastoris. *Protein Expr. Purif.* **2016**, *119*, 1–10. [CrossRef] [PubMed]

157. Wang, N.X.; Sieg, S.F.; Lederman, M.M.; Offord, R.E.; Hartley, O.; von Recum, H.A. Using glycosaminoglycan/chemokine interactions for the long-term delivery of 5P12-RANTES in HIV prevention. *Mol. Pharm.* **2013**, *10*, 3564–3573. [CrossRef] [PubMed]

158. Lohmann, N.; Schirmer, L.; Atallah, P.; Wandel, E.; Ferrer, R.A.; Werner, C.; Simon, J.C.; Franz, S.; Freudenberg, U. Glycosaminoglycan-based hydrogels capture inflammatory chemokines and rescue defective wound healing in mice. *Sci. Transl. Med.* **2017**, *9*, eaai9044. [CrossRef] [PubMed]

159. Hoover, D.M.; Boulegue, C.; Yang, D.; Oppenheim, J.J.; Tucker, K.; Lu, W.; Lubkowski, J. The structure of human macrophage inflammatory protein-3alpha /CCL20. Linking antimicrobial and CC chemokine receptor-6-binding activities with human beta-defensins. *J. Biol. Chem.* **2002**, *277*, 37647–37654. [CrossRef] [PubMed]

160. Fu, L.; Suflita, M.; Linhardt, R.J. Bioengineered heparins and heparan sulfates. *Adv. Drug Deliv. Rev.* **2016**, *97*, 237–249. [CrossRef] [PubMed]

161. Ricard-Blum, S.; Lisacek, F. Glycosaminoglycanomics: Where we are. *Glycoconj. J.* **2017**, *34*, 339–349. [CrossRef] [PubMed]

162. Hahm, H.S.; Schlegel, M.K.; Hurevich, M.; Eller, S.; Schuhmacher, F.; Hofmann, J.; Pagel, K.; Seeberger, P.H. Automated glycan assembly using the Glyconeer 2.1 synthesizer. *Proc. Natl. Acad. Sci. USA* **2017**, *114*, E3385–E3389. [CrossRef] [PubMed]

163. Yang, X.D.; Corvalan, J.R.; Wang, P.; Roy, C.M.; Davis, C.G. Fully human anti-interleukin-8 monoclonal antibodies: Potential therapeutics for the treatment of inflammatory disease states. *J. Leukoc. Biol.* **1999**, *66*, 401–410. [PubMed]

164. Haringman, J.J.; Gerlag, D.M.; Smeets, T.J.; Baeten, D.; van den Bosch, F.; Bresnihan, B.; Breedveld, F.C.; Dinant, H.J.; Legay, F.; Gram, H.; et al. A randomized controlled trial with an anti-CCL2 (anti-monocyte chemotactic protein 1) monoclonal antibody in patients with rheumatoid arthritis. *Arthritis Rheumatol.* **2006**, *54*, 2387–2392. [CrossRef] [PubMed]

165. Pienta, K.J.; Machiels, J.P.; Schrijvers, D.; Alekseev, B.; Shkolnik, M.; Crabb, S.J.; Li, S.; Seetharam, S.; Puchalski, T.A.; Takimoto, C.; et al. Phase 2 study of carlumab (CNTO 888), a human monoclonal antibody against CC-chemokine ligand 2 (CCL2), in metastatic castration-resistant prostate cancer. *Investig. New Drugs* **2013**, *31*, 760–768. [CrossRef] [PubMed]

166. Schall, T.J.; Proudfoot, A.E. Overcoming hurdles in developing successful drugs targeting chemokine receptors. *Nat. Rev. Immunol.* **2011**, *11*, 355–363. [CrossRef] [PubMed]

167. Struthers, M.; Pasternak, A. CCR2 antagonists. *Curr. Top. Med. Chem.* **2010**, *10*, 1278–1298. [CrossRef] [PubMed]

168. De Graaf, K.L.; Kosco-Vilbois, M.H.; Fischer, N. Therapeutic targeting of chemokines with monoclonal antibodies. *Curr. Immunol. Rev.* **2012**, *8*, 141–148. [CrossRef]

169. Baggiolini, M. Chemokines and leukocyte traffic. *Nature* **1998**, *392*, 565–568. [CrossRef] [PubMed]

170. Dubrac, A.; Quemener, C.; Lacazette, E.; Lopez, F.; Zanibellato, C.; Wu, W.G.; Bikfalvi, A.; Prats, H. Functional divergence between 2 chemokines is conferred by single amino acid change. *Blood* **2010**, *116*, 4703–4711. [CrossRef] [PubMed]

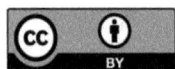

pharmaceuticals

MDPI

Article

Development of a Glycosaminoglycan Derived, Selectin Targeting Anti-Adhesive Coating to Treat Endothelial Cell Dysfunction

James R. Wodicka [1,2], Andrea M. Chambers [1], Gurneet S. Sangha [1], Craig J. Goergen [1] and Alyssa Panitch [1,3,*]

[1] Weldon School of Biomedical Engineering, Purdue University, West Lafayette, IN 47907, USA; jwodicka@purdue.edu (J.R.W.); chambe48@purdue.edu (A.M.C.); gsangha@purdue.edu (G.S.S.); cgoergen@purdue.edu (C.J.G.)
[2] Indiana University School of Medicine, Indianapolis, IN 46202, USA
[3] Department of Biomedical Engineering, University of California—Davis, Davis, CA 95616, USA
* Correspondence: apanitch@ucdavis.edu

Academic Editor: Barbara Mulloy
Received: 24 January 2017; Accepted: 24 March 2017; Published: 29 March 2017

Abstract: Endothelial cell (EC) dysfunction is associated with many disease states including deep vein thrombosis (DVT), chronic kidney disease, sepsis and diabetes. Loss of the glycocalyx, a thin glycosaminoglycan (GAG)-rich layer on the EC surface, is a key feature of endothelial dysfunction and increases exposure of EC adhesion molecules such as selectins, which are involved in platelet binding to ECs. Once bound, platelets cause thrombus formation and an increased inflammatory response. We have developed a GAG derived, selectin targeting anti-adhesive coating (termed EC-SEAL) consisting of a dermatan sulfate backbone and multiple selectin-binding peptides designed to bind to inflamed endothelium and prevent platelet binding to create a more quiescent endothelial state. Multiple EC-SEAL variants were evaluated and the lead variant was found to preferentially bind to selectin-expressing ECs and smooth muscle cells (SMCs) and inhibit platelet binding and activation in a dose-dependent manner. In an in vivo model of DVT, treatment with the lead variant resulted in reduced thrombus formation. These results indicate that EC-SEAL has promise as a potential therapeutic in the treatment of endothelial dysfunction.

Keywords: glycocalyx; endothelial cell; dysfunction; selectin; dermatan sulfate; deep vein thrombosis

1. Introduction

Deep vein thrombosis (DVT) affects approximately 900,000 individuals annually in the United States, and pulmonary emboli, a severe complication of DVT, are often observed in these patients [1]. Unlike in arterial thrombus, which is observed to initiate upon exposed extracellular matrix (ECM), venous thrombus initiates from dysfunctional endothelium, in part due to platelet binding to and activation on endothelium [1]. The binding and activation of platelets not only supports thrombus formation, but also further contributes to the inflammatory state of the venous endothelium, thus exacerbating the diseased vessel state [2].

Vascular endothelial cells (ECs) line the entire cardiovascular system in the human body. As the innermost layer of the blood vessel lumen, ECs are in constant contact with the blood and perform many critical functions. These include involvement in metabolism, regulating blood vessel tone, permeability and growth, vascular smooth muscle cell (SMC) proliferation, inflammation, platelet and leukocyte interactions, thrombosis and fibrinolysis [3–5]. Given these overlapping and wide-ranging activities, it is not surprising that disruption of normal EC function is associated with many different disease states. Indeed, EC dysfunction has been shown to play a role in DVT, atherosclerosis, myocardial infarction, peripheral vascular disease, stroke, hypertension, diabetes, chronic kidney disease, infections including sepsis, and even cancer [3,4,6–11].

In general, characteristics of endothelial dysfunction include a reduction in ability of vessels to vasodilate, along with increases in inflammation and prothrombotic properties [3,12]. Additionally, loss of the glycocalyx, an anionic layer comprised primarily of glycosaminoglycans (GAGs) that lines the endothelium, is a key feature of EC dysfunction [13,14]. The loss of this delicate layer causes a significant increase in vascular wall permeability and subsequent migration of fluid, protein and other cell types into the vessel [15]. Lack of a glycocalyx layer also results in exposure of EC adhesion molecules such as E-selectin, P-selectin, intracellular adhesion molecule 1 (ICAM-1), vascular cell adhesion molecule 1 (VCAM-1) and platelet-endothelial cell adhesion molecule 1 (PECAM-1) [13,16], some of which are known to play a role in platelet binding to the endothelial cell surface. Once bound, platelets release cytokines, chemokines and platelet activation factors, such as platelet activating factor (PAF), neutrophil-activating peptide-2 (NAP-2) and platelet factor-4 (PF-4), which leads to thrombus formation and a further increase in inflammatory cell recruitment to the site [17–20].

Endothelial dysfunction is likely a reversible disorder as eliminating cardiovascular risk factors through such means as smoking cessation, hypertension control, cholesterol lowering and physical activity have been shown to improve endothelial health [10]. Angiotensin converting enzyme (ACE) inhibitors, N-acetylcysteine (NAC), ascorbic acid (Vitamin C), vitamin E, and erythropoietin (EPO) have all been studied as potential therapeutics for EC dysfunction [21–24]. While some positive outcomes have been observed, they have often displayed a minimal effect on overall endothelial health or resulted in unintended cardiovascular events [4,23]. Therefore, additional means of targeting and effectively treating EC dysfunction and reducing associated cardiovascular events are needed.

Targeting EC adhesion molecules, such as selectins, for therapeutic or diagnostic purposes has been relatively well studied. Examples include microparticle drug delivery [25], therapeutic gene delivery [26,27], inflammation reduction [28–30], cancer metastasis prevention [31] and in vivo diagnostic imaging [32,33]. Specifically, antibodies and peptides have been utilized to target selectin receptors on EC surfaces to prevent platelet and leukocyte binding and the subsequent inflammatory response that occurs [28–30,34]. Therefore, our laboratory has recently developed several variants of a GAG derived, selectin targeting anti-adhesive coating (termed EC-SEAL) designed to utilize overexpressed selectins in EC dysfunction to prevent platelet binding and subsequent thrombus formation and restore a more quiescent endothelial state. Each variant consists of a dermatan sulfate (GAG component of the glycocalyx) [13] backbone with multiple selectin-binding peptides attached. EC-SEAL variants differing in type and number of peptides attached were investigated to determine highest binding affinities to inflamed ECs and assess ability to prevent platelet binding along the EC surface. Results indicated effective molecule binding to inflamed ECs and subsequent prevention of platelet binding and activation, as well as suppression of thrombus formation in a murine model of DVT, highlighting the possibility of EC-SEAL as a therapeutic to treat EC dysfunction.

2. Results

2.1. Selectin Expression

To measure levels of selectin expression on SMCs and ECs under various conditions, antibodies designed to target E-selectin were utilized. ECs were stimulated with 5 or 25 ng/mL tumor necrosis factor (TNF)-α or control (unstimulated) media, and SMCs were stimulated with only control (unstimulated) media. While all cultures showed selectin expression compared to the background (No Cells), there was no difference in expression between cultures that contained TNF-α stimulated and control media (Figure 1). Since antibodies are likely cross-reactive with P-selectin, these data suggest SMCs, which have been shown to express P-selectin [35,36] but not E-selectin [37], also exhibited selectin expression. Both lower and higher concentrations of TNF-α (Supplementary Figure S1) and other proinflammatory cytokines (interleukin (IL)-1β, IL-6, lipopolysaccharide (LPS)) at varying concentrations (10–100 ng/mL) (Supplementary Figure S2) were tested in an attempt to upregulate selectin expression compared to unstimulated ECs. All proinflammatory stimuli failed to show any upregulation in selectin expression, indicating that EC cultures likely exhibited a basal upregulation of selectin receptors. Additionally, ECs were unable to form fully intact monolayers despite a lack of proinflammatory stimuli present, as indicated by their permeability to fluorescently-labeled dextran (Supplementary Figure S3). This lack of cell–cell junctions under normal conditions is another indication that the cultured ECs were likely in a constitutively activated state.

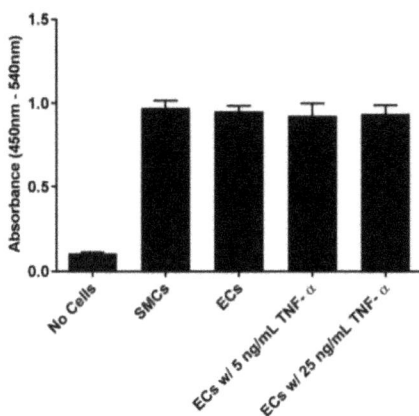

Figure 1. Selectin expression on SMCs and ECs under various conditions. Expression was quantified using primary anti-E-selectin and secondary horseradish peroxidase (HRP)-conjugated antibodies. All cultures exhibited significant selectin expression; however, selectin levels did not change when stimulated with TNF-α. $n = 3$; $p < 0.05$.

2.2. EC-SEAL Binding (Cells)

Each selectin-binding peptide being examined (IDLMQARGC (IDL), IELLQARGC (IEL) and QITWAQLWNMMKGC (QIT)) was used to synthesize EC-SEAL variants containing 10, 15, 20 and 30 peptides per dermatan sulfate (DS) backbone (with, on average, one biotinylated peptide per DS molecule). To test the binding ability of these EC-SEAL molecules varying in both type and number of peptides, binding to SMCs and ECs (with and without 5 ng/mL TNF-α) was examined. Results of our first analysis are shown in Figure 2. Overall, both the peptide itself and the number of peptides attached to each molecule affected binding affinity. We observed that none of the variants tested displayed a difference in binding when added to ECs in control (unstimulated) media versus ECs stimulated with 5 ng/mL TNF-α (Figure 2C). This was consistent with data presented in Figure 1 in which ECs exhibited the same level of selectin expression with or without TNF-α stimulation. In addition, all variants (except DS-IDL$_{10}$) exhibited a higher affinity for ECs than SMCs (Figure 2B,C). EC-SEAL variants containing the IDL peptide appeared to have increased nonspecific binding, particularly in molecules with a low number of peptides, as indicated by the relatively high binding in the absence of cells (Figure 2A). Additionally, variants containing the peptide IEL displayed the highest level of binding to ECs with and without TNF-α stimulation (Figure 2C). It should be noted that QIT variants with 15, 20 and 30 peptides per DS were also tested in other studies and showed similar binding as DS-QIT$_{10}$, but due to solubility issues leading to difficulty in molecule synthesis, use of these variants was discontinued.

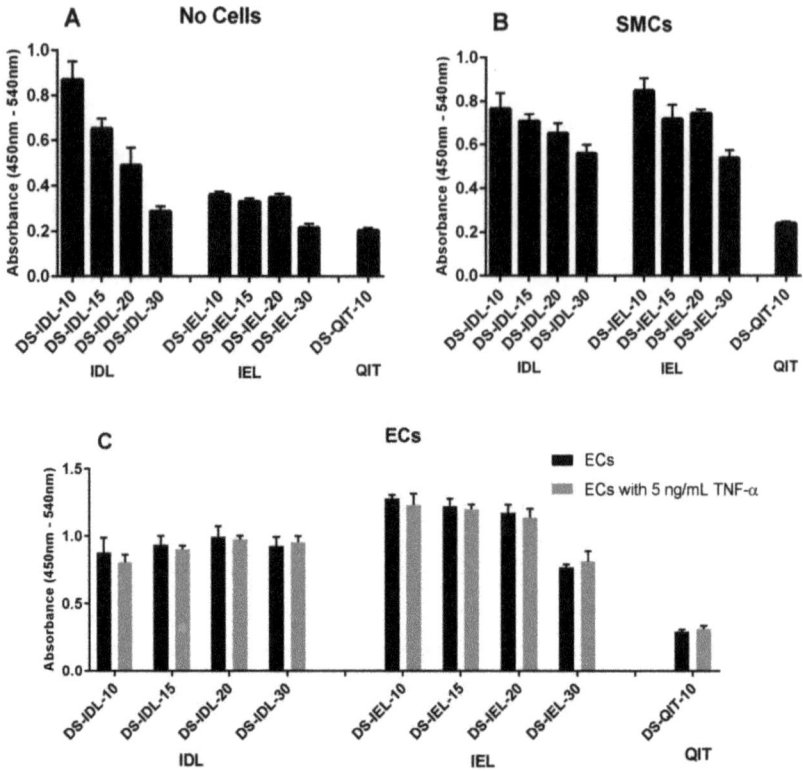

Figure 2. EC-SEAL variant binding to No Cells, SMCs and ECs (with and without 5 ng/mL TNF-α). (**A**) No Cells; (**B**) SMCs; and (**C**) ECs with and without 5 ng/mL TNF-α were treated with 3 μM of each EC-SEAL variant. Absorbance was measured using a streptavidin-HRP assay to quantify biotinylated peptides on each molecule bound to the surface. None of the EC-SEAL variants displayed a significant difference in binding to unstimulated ECs and ECs stimulated with TNF-α. Variants containing the peptide IEL showed the highest binding affinity to ECs. $n = 3$; $p < 0.05$.

Given its superior ability to bind to ECs, further investigations focused on EC-SEAL variants containing the peptide IEL. Since DS-IEL$_{10}$ displayed some of the highest levels of binding during initial testing, variants with even fewer peptides were synthesized and evaluated. Figure 3 depicts a comparison of two controls (No Treatment and DS-Biotin Tag Only) and all synthesized IEL variants ranging from 2 to 30 peptides per DS backbone. There was again no difference between binding to unstimulated ECs versus ECs stimulated with 5 ng/mL TNF-α, regardless of treatment applied. All variants demonstrated an increased binding affinity to ECs over SMCs (with the exception of DS-IEL$_{30}$) and all IEL variants showed increased binding compared to the DS-Biotin Tag Only control. As indicated in Figure 3, DS-IEL$_4$, DS-IEL$_7$ and DS-IEL$_{10}$ had the highest number of molecules bound to ECs and were statistically equivalent to each other. Therefore, DS-IEL$_{10}$ was chosen as the molecule for further testing given that it contained the most selectin-binding peptides among the highest binding group.

2.3. Platelet Activation and Binding

After confirming EC-SEAL variants not only bound to cell surfaces, but also their binding was dependent on type and number of peptides attached, their ability to prevent platelet binding and subsequent activation was quantified. We first investigated DS-IEL$_{10}$ because, based on its increased level of binding to endothelial cells (Figure 3), we expected that it would best inhibit platelet binding as compared to the other variants we examined. DS-IEL$_{30}$ was included to verify that the IEL peptide would not enhance platelet binding to the activated endothelium due to its interaction with the P-selectin receptor that is present on platelets. Levels of NAP-2 and PF-4, released from platelets during activation [18,20,38], were used as platelet activation markers to compare various treatment conditions. Surprisingly, treating ECs with DS-IEL$_{10}$ prior to platelet rich plasma (PRP) incubation had no effect on NAP-2 and PF-4 release as compared to the control (No Treatment), regardless of concentration of DS-IEL$_{10}$ applied (Figure 4). However, treating with 30 μM DS-IEL$_{30}$ showed a significant decrease in NAP-2 and PF-4 levels when compared to the control and all other treatment groups.

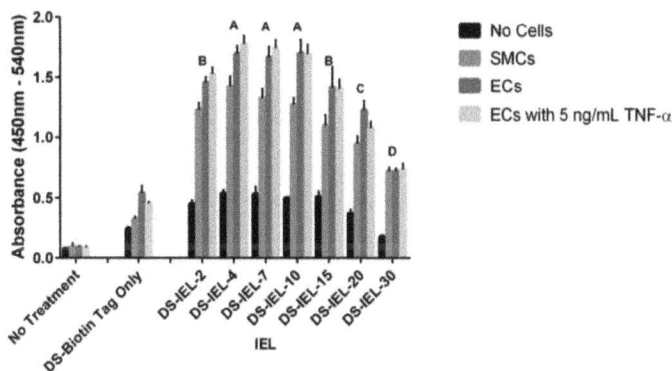

Figure 3. IEL variant binding to No Cells, SMCs and ECs (with and without 5 ng/mL TNF-α). Concentration of IEL variants = 3 μM. Absorbance was measured using a streptavidin-HRP assay to quantify biotinylated peptides on each molecule remaining bound to the surface. Each letter represents groups that exhibited statistically equivalent binding to ECs. Number of molecules bound to EC surface: A > B > C > D. $n = 2$; $p < 0.05$.

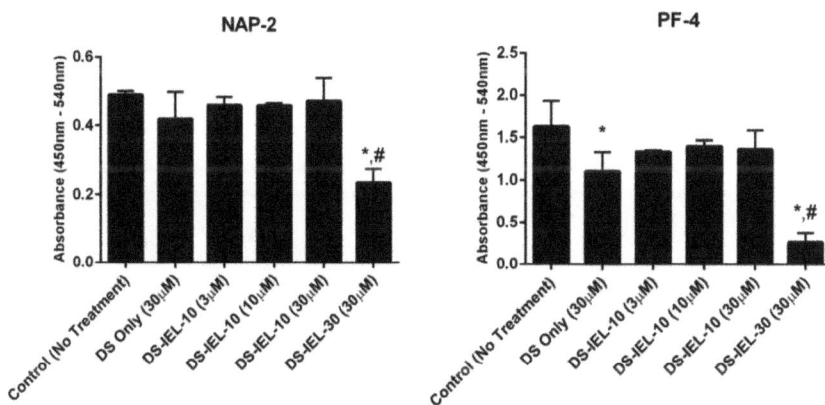

Figure 4. Impact of DS-IEL$_{10}$ and DS-IEL$_{30}$ on platelet activation markers NAP-2 and PF-4. ECs were stimulated with 5 ng/mL TNF-α and treated with 3–30 μM EC-SEAL variants or control (No Treatment). PRP was added and NAP-2 and PF-4 levels in the collected PRP were recorded using sandwich ELISAs. DS-IEL$_{30}$ showed the greatest reduction in platelet activation. * represents a significant difference from the control (No Treatment); # represents a significant difference when compared to all other treatment groups. $n = 3$; $p < 0.05$.

Next, various concentrations of DS-IEL$_{30}$ were tested to determine an effective dose. As shown in Figure 5, DS-IEL$_{30}$ decreases platelet activation markers at 10 μM compared to the control (No Treatment), however, treating with 30 μM DS-IEL$_{30}$ results in a greater decrease in both NAP-2 and PF-4 compared to the control and all other treatment groups. The individual components of DS-IEL$_{30}$, DS only (30 μM) and free IEL peptide (0.9 mM), were also tested at concentrations equivalent to 30 μM DS-IEL$_{30}$. While both components decreased platelet activation markers compared to the control, neither did so as effectively as 30 μM DS-IEL$_{30}$.

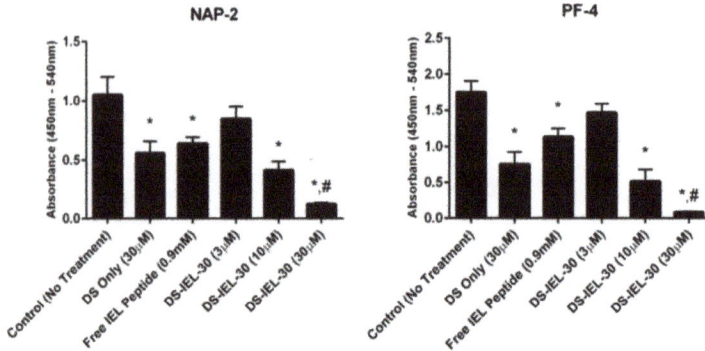

Figure 5. Dose-dependent response of DS-IEL$_{30}$ on platelet activation. ECs were stimulated with 5 ng/mL TNF-α and treated with 3–30 μM DS-IEL$_{30}$ or control (No Treatment). PRP was added and NAP-2 and PF-4 levels in the collected PRP were recorded using sandwich ELISAs. DS-IEL$_{30}$ at 30 μM proved to be the most effective dose to reduce platelet activation. * represents a significant difference from the control (No Treatment); # represents a significant difference when compared to all other treatment groups. $n = 2$; $p < 0.05$.

In addition to reducing platelet activation, DS-IEL$_{30}$ was also shown to prevent platelet binding to ECs (Figure 6). Labeled with membrane bound CellTrackers, platelets (red) were added to ECs (green) with and without prior 30 μM DS-IEL$_{30}$ treatment. Treated EC cultures (Figure 6B) displayed a decrease in overall platelet binding, particularly directly on ECs, compared to untreated cultures (Figure 6A). In addition, the limited number of platelets that did bind to cultures treated with DS-IEL$_{30}$ appeared to bind in areas not covered by ECs, indicating that DS-IEL$_{30}$ was preferentially targeting ECs (and not the underlying tissue culture plastic) and subsequently preventing platelet binding and activation.

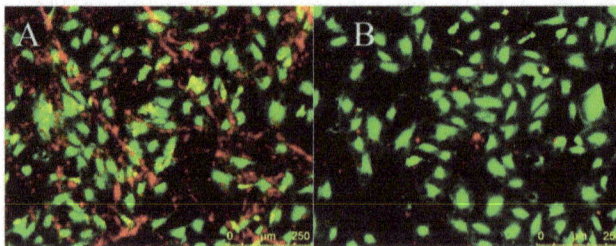

Figure 6. Platelets binding to ECs in the presence of EC-SEAL. ECs (green) were stimulated with 5 ng/mL TNF-α and treated with: control media (A); or 30 μM DS-IEL$_{30}$ (B). Platelets (red) were isolated from human whole blood and incubated on ECs. Cultures treated with DS-IEL$_{30}$ showed less platelet binding, particularly on EC surfaces. The 10× images were acquired using a fluorescent microscope. Scale bar = 250 μm. $n = 3$.

2.4. EC-SEAL Binding (Selectin Protein)

To confirm that the observed interactions between EC-SEAL variants and cells were through a selectin binding process, the ability of DS-IEL$_{30}$ to preferentially bind to selectin protein was studied. Increasing concentrations of human recombinant E-selectin were coated on a high bind plate and 1% bovine serum albumin (BSA) was added to eliminate nonspecific binding. A single concentration of DS-IEL$_{30}$ (3 μM) was incubated and the amount bound to the surface was quantified (Figure 7). Initially, DS-IEL$_{30}$ binding increases with increased concentrations of E-selectin. Then, at 50 μg/mL E-selectin, DS-IEL$_{30}$ binding falls off slightly, but is overcome with further increases in E-selectin concentration (100 μg/mL).

A similar trend is observed when the binding of antibodies (primary mouse monoclonal anti-E-selectin IgG$_{2a}$ with secondary goat anti-mouse IgG HRP-conjugated) are quantified under the same conditions (Figure 8). There is also an initial increase in antibody binding with increased concentrations of E-selectin. Then, at 10 μg/mL E-selectin, antibody binding falls off significantly, but is also overcome with increasing concentrations of E-selectin (25–100 μg/mL).

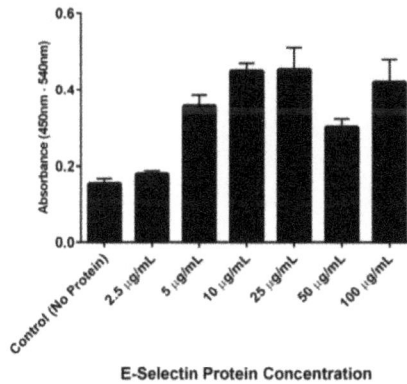

Figure 7. EC-SEAL binding to recombinant human E-selectin. Absorbance was measured using a streptavidin-HRP assay to quantify biotinylated peptides on DS-IEL$_{30}$ bound to the surface. DS-IEL$_{30}$ exhibits preferential binding to selectin over BSA and is dependent upon the concentration of selectin protein present. $n = 3$; $p < 0.05$.

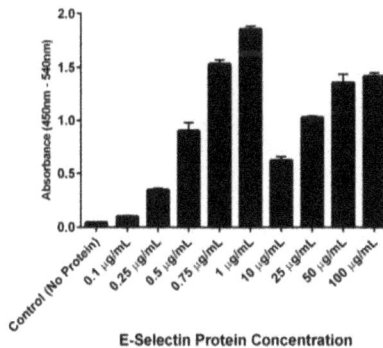

Figure 8. Antibody binding to recombinant human E-selectin. Expression was quantified using primary anti-E-selectin and secondary HRP-conjugated antibodies. Antibodies display preferential binding to selectin over BSA and binding is dependent upon the concentration of selectin protein present. $n = 2$; $p < 0.05$.

2.5. DVT Mouse Model

To assess the effects of DS-IEL$_{30}$ in vivo, a study utilizing a mouse model of DVT was conducted. Partial ligation of the inferior vena cava (IVC) was performed and tail vein injections of saline ($n = 6$), 200 IU/kg heparin ($n = 6$), or 30 μM DS-IEL$_{30}$ ($n = 4$) were administered. Ultrasound images were obtained at 6 h post-ligation for each mouse (Figure 9). The thrombus volume (expressed as mean ± standard error of the mean) was 12.3 ± 1.6 mm^3 for saline, 5.0 ± 2.2 mm^3 for heparin, and 4.3 ± 2.2 mm^3 for DS-IEL$_{30}$. The mean thrombus percentage (defined as thrombus volume/total IVC volume between the ligation suture and iliac bifurcation) was 63% ± 5% for saline, 26% ± 11% for heparin, and 26% ± 11% for DS-IEL$_{30}$ (Figure 10). Both heparin and DS-IEL$_{30}$ significantly decreased thrombus percentage compared to the saline controls ($p < 0.05$).

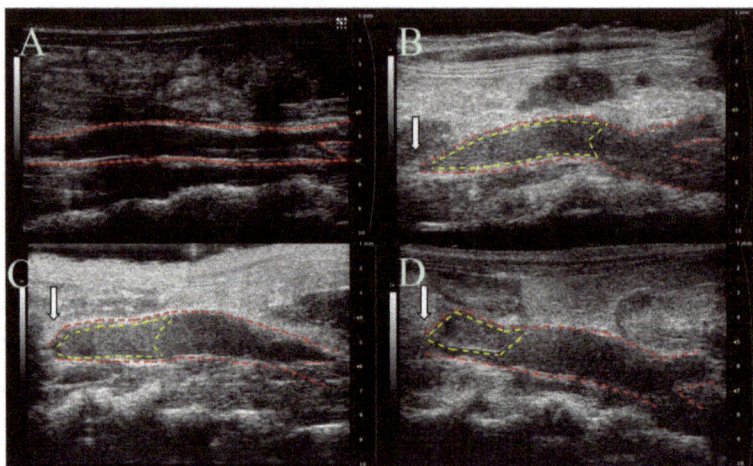

Figure 9. B-Mode ultrasound images of the IVC before and after partial ligation surgery. Representative images from: (**A**) Baseline (pre-surgery); (**B**) Saline; (**C**) Heparin; and (**D**) EC-SEAL (DS-IEL$_{30}$) at 6 h after partial ligation are shown. IVC is outlined in red and thrombus is outlined in yellow. White arrows represent the location of the 6-0 silk suture creating the partial ligation.

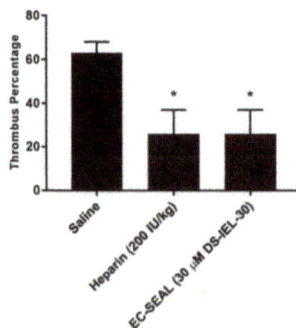

Figure 10. Thrombus percentage in DVT mouse model. Ultrasound images were utilized to calculate thrombus percentage by dividing thrombus volume by total IVC volume between the partial ligation suture and iliac bifurcation. Both heparin ($n = 6$) and EC-SEAL ($n = 4$) decreased thrombus percentage compared to saline controls ($n = 6$). * represents a significant difference from the control group (Saline). $p < 0.05$.

2.6. Clotting Time (aPTT)

Although heparin and EC-SEAL (DS-IEL$_{30}$) showed statistically equivalent outcomes with respect to thrombus percentage in the DVT mouse model, it is believed these effects are achieved through different mechanisms. Therefore, clotting times (activated partial thromboplastin time (aPTT)) were obtained for various concentrations of heparin and EC-SEAL (Figure 11). It should be noted that the highest concentration of both heparin and EC-SEAL depicted in Figure 11 were equivalent to the doses administered to mice in vivo. Heparin displayed a substantial effect, causing a nearly four-fold increase in aPTT at the highest dose compared to saline controls. Comparatively, EC-SEAL exhibited a relatively small effect on aPTT (e.g., 23% increase at the highest concentration compared to saline controls).

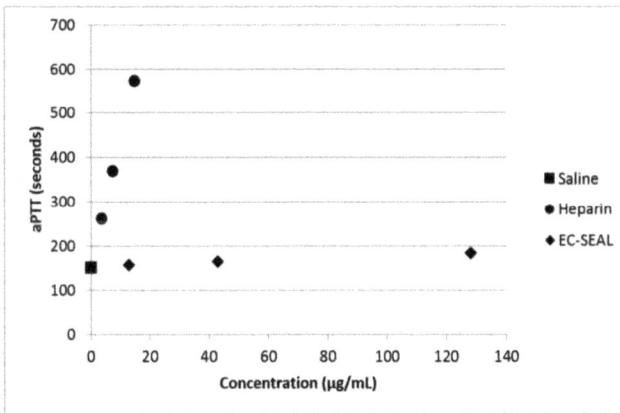

Figure 11. Whole blood clotting time (aPTT) in the presence of heparin and EC-SEAL. aPTT measurements were recorded with varying concentrations of heparin and EC-SEAL. Heparin exhibited a much greater effect on aPTT than EC-SEAL, likely indicating different mechanisms of reducing thrombus formation in vivo. $n = 2$; $p < 0.05$.

3. Discussion

Loss of the glycocalyx is a key characteristic of EC dysfunction [13,14]. Removal of this glycosaminoglycan (GAG)-rich layer results in the exposure and upregulation of EC adhesion molecules, including selectins [13,16]. Selectins and their ligands, located on both ECs and platelets, play a key role in the binding of platelets to inflamed endothelium. In the context of endothelial dysfunction, this process can lead to complications in a myriad of disease states including DVT, atherosclerosis, diabetes, chronic kidney disease and sepsis [3,4,6,8,39]. Masking these selectins with antibodies or peptides to prevent platelet binding presents a possible avenue of treatment [28–30]. We sought to develop and test multiple variants of a GAG derived, selectin-binding anti-adhesive coating (termed EC-SEAL) utilizing selectin-binding peptides to bind to an inflamed endothelial surface. We demonstrate the ability to successfully synthesize variants ranging from 2 to 30 peptides per dermatan sulfate molecule that bind to E-selectin and cells expressing selectins, and prevent platelet binding and activation in a dose-dependent manner. Additionally, we present evidence that the lead variant reduces thrombus size in vivo while exhibiting minimal effects on clotting time.

In order to examine the binding of EC-SEAL variants to vascular cells, we first established that selectin was present on the cell surfaces. As shown in Figure 1 and Supplementary Figures S1 and S2, ECs (which express both E and P-selectin) did not increase selectin levels following TNF-α stimulation or any other proinflammatory stimulants used. Although not anticipated because it has been shown previously that adding TNF-α to human aortic ECs leads to an increase in E-selectin expression 3–6 h after stimulation [40–42], there is also evidence that many different factors including number of cell passages, seeding density, certain growth factors present in media, and even the culture substrate can lead to increased basal levels of adhesion molecules on cultured ECs [43–46]. It is also possible that the rinsing and manipulation of the live ECs throughout the experiments contributed to the observed basal selectin expression. The presence of selectins on the EC surface in the unstimulated cultures, the lack of response to multiple proinflammatory cytokines (TNF-α, LPS, IL-1β and IL-6), and the inability to form intact monolayers (Supplementary Figure S3), all suggest that the EC cultures were in a constitutively activated state. SMCs, known to express P-selectin [35,36], but not E-selectin [37], demonstrated P-selectin cross-reactivity with the anti-E-selectin antibody.

The selectin-expressing cells were then used to test and compare EC-SEAL variant binding. Both the type and number of peptides attached to the DS backbone had a significant impact on binding affinity (Figures 2 and 3). There was no difference in binding to unstimulated ECs or ECs stimulated with TNF-α for any EC-SEAL variant, which is consistent with the selectin expression data discussed previously. Although nearly all variants had a higher binding affinity to ECs, they also adhered to SMCs, presumably through P-selectin. Prior studies on IDL and IEL peptides indeed indicated binding to both E and P-selectin [31]. QIT was previously shown to have a significantly higher preference for E-selectin over P-selectin [47], but in our hands the binding observed in the DS-QIT$_x$ variants was primarily due to nonspecific interactions as indicated by the (relatively) high level of binding with no cells present compared to both SMCs and ECs (Figure 2). IEL was selected as the peptide to examine further due to its increased binding to ECs and reduced nonspecific interactions when no cells were present. This is consistent with a previous study that showed IEL had a higher binding affinity to E-selectin expressing bacteria than IDL [31]. Importantly, all DS-IEL$_x$ variants showed increased levels of binding compared to only DS, which as a native glycocalyx component will interact with the EC surface, indicating the benefit of the selectin-binding peptides. The apparent ability to bind to both E and P-selectin is also viewed as advantageous as it may allow for more complete coverage of: (1) ECs expressing both E and P-selectin; and (2) SMCs expressing P-selectin should they become exposed following EC injury or denudation.

DS-IEL$_{10}$ was originally chosen for platelet binding and activation testing given that it possessed the greatest number of selectin-binding peptides among the highest binding group of DS-IEL$_x$ variants (Figure 3.) However, using NAP-2 and PF-4 as platelet activation markers, DS-IEL$_{10}$ did not reduce platelet activation at any treatment concentration compared to untreated controls (Figure 4). DS-IEL$_{30}$ was also studied because the high density of selectin-binding peptide per backbone presented the possibility that some peptide would not be bound to the endothelial cell surface and might in fact bind to P-selectin on platelets and increase platelet binding. Importantly, there was no evidence for platelet-peptide interactions in these studies; in fact, DS-IEL$_{30}$ showed a dose-dependent response in reducing platelet activation compared to untreated controls (Figure 5). Additionally, 30 μM DS-IEL$_{30}$ proved to be an extremely effective dose even when compared to equivalent amounts of its individual components (30 μM DS Only and 0.9 mM Free IEL Peptide). We believe that the apparent discrepancy between the binding studies (where DS-IEL$_{10}$ was believed to be best) and platelet activation results (where DS-IEL$_{30}$ was most effective) lies in how the binding was quantified. Since each DS backbone has one biotinylated peptide, the streptavidin-HRP assay will quantify each DS molecule attached regardless of the number of selectin-binding peptides bound to the surface. Therefore, despite DS-IEL$_{10}$ showing a slightly more than two-fold increase in number of molecules bound compared to DS-IEL$_{30}$, there are three times the number of selectin-binding peptides on each molecule of DS-IEL$_{30}$, resulting in a higher number of peptides available to bind to the cell surface and block interaction with platelets. Furthermore, increasing the number of peptides per molecule appeared to decrease nonspecific interactions (Figures 2 and 3) and therefore, more of the molecules likely reached and bound to their targeted site. This suggests that despite fewer molecules present, the higher local peptide density of DS-IEL$_{30}$ supports more efficient binding to the EC surface to prevent platelet binding and activation.

The ability of DS-IEL$_{30}$ to preferentially bind to recombinant human E-selectin over BSA was observed by incubating a single concentration of DS-IEL$_{30}$ on plates coated with increasing concentrations of E-selectin. DS-IEL$_{30}$ binding increased with initial increases in E-selectin concentration, but dropped off at a certain point, only to increase again upon a further increase in E-selectin concentration (Figure 7). Interestingly, anti-E-selectin antibodies exhibited a similar binding trend, although at different concentrations of E-selectin (Figure 8). We hypothesize that these binding characteristics are due to a potential selectin conformational change that is dependent upon concentration of both receptor (E-selectin) and ligand (DS-IEL$_{30}$ or antibody) and their respective binding affinities. Ligand binding itself is known to cause conformational changes at the binding site [48,49], including that of E-selectin [50,51]. It is also possible that the concentration of E-selectin protein coated on the plate's surface influences the orientation in which the protein adsorbs and therefore, the exposure (or lack thereof) of ligand binding sites. Given that DS-IEL$_{30}$ and anti-E-selectin antibody may have different binding sites and affinities to E-selectin, it is not surprising that the drop off and subsequent rise in binding occur at different concentrations of plated E-selectin protein.

Given the vast number of vascular disease states associated with endothelial dysfunction, animal models in this area are wide-ranging. The utilization of mouse models has proven to be an extremely useful tool allowing for the study of underlying mechanisms and initial screenings of therapeutics [52]. Thus, we employed a mouse model of deep vein thrombosis mediated endothelial dysfunction to observe the anti-thrombotic effects of EC-SEAL in vivo. This inferior vena cava (IVC) partial ligation model provides valuable information regarding vessel wall-blood interactions during thrombus formation and has been used previously to evaluate therapeutic agents [52,53]. Study results, obtained via ultrasound imaging, indicate that DS-IEL$_{30}$ significantly decreases thrombus formation at six hours following IVC partial ligation (Figure 10) and highlight the potential for DS-IEL$_{30}$ to act locally following systemic administration. It is believed that these therapeutic effects are due to DS-IEL$_{30}$ binding to the vessel wall and subsequently preventing platelet binding and not through direct anticoagulant properties. Dermatan sulfate from porcine origin (which is the type used for EC-SEAL synthesis) has been shown to have very minimal anticoagulant properties depending on the concentration [54]. By measuring aPTT of whole blood that had been incubated with varying concentrations of both heparin and DS-IEL$_{30}$, we have confirmed the minimal effect of DS-IEL$_{30}$ on clotting time (Figure 11). Therefore, EC-SEAL has the potential to be utilized as a treatment for DVT without the negative side effects of current standard of care anticoagulant therapies such as heparin.

Since DS-IEL$_{30}$ proved to be the most effective EC-SEAL variant and no variants were synthesized with greater than 30 peptides per DS molecule, it is possible that further increases to the number of peptides per molecule may be beneficial. Previous work has shown, however, that excessive oxidation of GAGs can lead to chain scission [55,56], so a balance between number of selectin-binding peptides and DS backbone integrity will need to be considered. It is also possible that targeting additional EC adhesion molecules, such as ICAM-1 or VCAM-1, may further increase binding and therapeutic effect. Future studies on DS-IEL$_{30}$ and any additional EC-SEAL variants can focus on prevention of leukocyte binding and subsequent diapedesis. Additional experiments further assessing the specificity of EC-SEAL binding as well as observing the binding characteristics of EC-SEAL over time and under flow conditions to account for shear forces would be valuable.

4. Materials and Methods

4.1. GAG Dervied, Selectin Targeting Anti-Adhesive Coating (EC-SEAL) Synthesis

The synthesis of the GAG derived, selectin targeting anti-adhesive coating variants (Scheme 1) was performed at room temperature as follows: vicinal diol groups on dermatan sulfate (DS, MW$_{avg}$ 46,275 Da, Celsus Laboratories, Cincinnati, OH, USA) were oxidized to aldehydes using sodium meta-periodate (Thermo Fisher Scientific, Waltham, MA, USA) in 0.1 M acetate buffer. The ratio of DS to sodium meta-periodate varied depending on the desired degree of oxidation. Following oxidation, the modified DS was isolated via size exclusion chromatography (SEC) (AKTA Purifier FPLC, GE Healthcare). An excess of N-[β-maleimidopropionic acid] hydrazide, trifluoroacetic acid salt (BMPH, Thermo Fisher Scientific), was then conjugated via the hydrazide to the DS aldehyde groups in 1× phosphate buffered saline (PBS, 1.05 mM KH_2PO_4, 155.17 mM NaCl, 2.97 Na_2HPO_4-$7H_2O$; pH 7.4, Thermo Fisher Scientific) to form DS-BMPH$_x$. Unbound BMPH was removed via SEC and quantified by calculating the area under the peak to determine the average number (x) of BMPH molecules bound to each DS backbone. Next, biotinylated peptide was added at a 1:1 molar ratio of DS:biotinylated peptide in 1× PBS to conjugate an average of one biotinylated peptide per molecule of DS, and then an excess of one of three selectin-binding peptides (Genscript, Piscataway, NJ, USA) was conjugated via the cysteine thiol to the maleimide groups on DS-BMPH$_x$ in 1× PBS. The three peptide sequences used were as follows: IDLMQARGC (IDL) [31], IELLQARGC (IEL) [31,32,34,57], and QITWAQLWNMMKGC (QIT) [47]. After the peptide reaction was complete, semicarbazide hydrochloride (Sigma-Aldrich, St. Louis, MO, USA) was added directly to the solution to reduce any unreacted aldehyde groups. Subsequent SEC isolation and lyophilization resulted in the purified sixteen variants containing from one to thirty peptides per DS backbone of DS-BMPH$_x$-Peptide$_{x, biotin}$ (hereby simply referred to in the form of DS-Peptide$_x$, ex: DS-IEL$_{20}$).

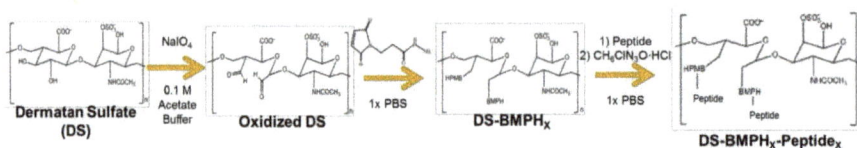

Scheme 1. GAG-derived, selectin targeting anti-adhesive coating (EC-SEAL) synthesis.

4.2. Cell Cultures

Human aortic endothelial cells (ECs, Thermo Fisher Scientific) were cultured in Medium 200 (M 200, Thermo Fisher Scientific) with low serum growth supplement (LSGS, Thermo Fisher Scientific). Human coronary artery smooth muscle cells (SMCs, Thermo Fisher Scientific) were cultured in Medium 231 (M 231, Thermo Fisher Scientific) with smooth muscle growth supplement (SMGS, Thermo Fisher Scientific). Cells were maintained at 37 °C and 5% CO_2. Unless otherwise noted, passage 3–7 cells were seeded at a density of 1×10^5 cells/cm^2 on tissue culture polystyrene and allowed to adhere for 24 h prior to any stimulation or treatment.

4.3. Selectin Expression

Monolayers of SMCs and ECs were seeded separately on Biocoat Collagen I Cellware 96-well plates (Corning, Corning, NY, USA). ECs were stimulated for four hours with 0.05–50 ng/mL tumor necrosis factor-α (TNF-α, Thermo Fisher Scientific), 10–100 ng/mL interleukin-1β (IL-1β, PeproTech, Rocky Hill, NJ, USA), 10–100 ng/mL interleukin-6 (IL-6, PeproTech), 10–100 ng/mL lipopolysaccharide (LPS, Sigma-Aldrich) or control (unstimulated) media. SMCs were cultured with only control (unstimulated) media. To block nonspecific binding, cells were treated with 1% bovine serum albumin (BSA, Sigma-Aldrich) in 0.05 M tris-buffered saline (TBS, 0.138 M NaCl, 0.0027 M KCl; pH 8.0, Sigma-Aldrich) for 30 min at room temperature with shaking. Primary rabbit polyclonal anti-E-selectin IgG (Santa Cruz Biotechnology, Dallas, TX, USA) or mouse monoclonal anti-E-selectin IgG$_{2a}$ (Santa Cruz Biotechnology) antibody was added (1:50 dilution of initial 200 μg/mL in 1% BSA in TBS) for one hour at 4 °C with shaking. Cells were rinsed three times with 1% BSA in TBS and secondary donkey anti-rabbit IgG HRP-conjugated (Thermo Fisher Scientific) or goat anti-mouse IgG HRP-conjugated (Thermo Fisher Scientific) antibody was added (1:1000 dilution of initial 0.5 mg/mL in 1% BSA in TBS) for 30 min at room temperature with shaking. Cells were rinsed three times with 1% BSA in TBS and colorimetric change was induced with 1:1 hydrogen peroxide: tetramethylbenzidine

(R&D Systems, Minneapolis, MN, USA). Following 20 min of incubation with shaking, 2N sulfuric acid was added to cease the reaction and absorbance was measured at 450 nm and 540 nm using a SpectraMax M5 plate reader (Molecular Devices, Sunnyvale, CA, USA). For each individual well, 540 nm was subtracted from 450 nm to obtain final absorbance reading.

4.4. EC Monolayer Permeability

ECs were seeded in control (unstimulated) media on tissue culture treated Transwell polyester membrane inserts with 3.0 μm pores on a 24-well plate (Corning) and cultured for 48 h to form monolayers. Cell culture media in both the upper and lower chambers was then changed with fresh, unstimulated media, and Rhodamine B isothiocyanate (RITC)-dextran (Sigma-Aldrich) was added to obtain a final concentration of 3 mg/mL in the upper chamber. The monolayers were incubated at 37 °C and 5% CO_2 for four hours, then the media in the lower chamber was removed and fluorescence was read using an M5 plate reader (Ex: 520 nm; Em: 590 nm).

4.5. EC-SEAL Binding to Cells

Monolayers of SMCs and ECs were seeded separately on Biocoat Collagen I Cellware 96-well plates or CellBIND surface 96-well plates (Corning). ECs were stimulated for four hours with 5 ng/mL TNF-α or control (unstimulated) media, and SMCs were treated with only control (unstimulated) media. Nonspecific binding was blocked using 1% BSA in TBS with 150 mM $CaCl_2$ for 20 min at room temperature with shaking. Cells were then treated with EC-SEAL variants (3 μM in 1% BSA in TBS with 150 mM $CaCl_2$) for one hour at 37 °C and 5% CO_2. After rinsing three times with 1% BSA in TBS with 150 mM $CaCl_2$, streptavidin-HRP (R&D Systems) was diluted 1:200 in 1% BSA in TBS with 150 mM $CaCl_2$ and added for 20 min at room temperature with shaking. After three more rinses in TBS with 150 mM $CaCl_2$, a 1:1 hydrogen peroxide: tetramethylbenzidine solution was added to induce colorimetric change. After 20 min of incubation with shaking, 2N sulfuric acid was used to stop the reaction and an M5 plate reader was utilized to measure absorbance at 450 nm and 540 nm as described above.

4.6. Platelet Activation

EC monolayers were seeded on Biocoat Collagen I Cellware 96-well plates and stimulated with 5 ng/mL TNF-α for four hours. One-percent BSA in TBS with 150 mM $CaCl_2$ was added for 15 min at room temperature to decrease nonspecific binding. ECs were then treated with 3–30 μM EC-SEAL variants for 1 h at 37 °C and 5% CO_2. Whole blood was obtained from healthy volunteers in collection vials containing sodium citrate and centrifuged for 20 min at $200 \times g$ and 25 °C. Platelet rich plasma (PRP) was isolated and after EC-SEAL treatments, ECs were rinsed three times with TBS with 150 mM $CaCl_2$ and 100 μL of PRP was added to each well. After 1 h of incubation at room temperature, 45 μL of PRP was then removed and added to tubes containing 5 μL of ETP (107 mM Ethylenediaminetetraacetic acid, disodium salt (EDTA, Promega, Madison, WI, USA), 12 mM Theophylline (Sigma-Aldrich) and 2.8 mM Prostaglandin E1 (Enzo Life Sciences, Farmingdale, NY, USA) in water). Samples were then centrifuged for 30 min at $2000 \times g$ and 4 °C and supernatant was collected and stored at −80 °C for use in subsequent assays.

4.7. NAP-2 and PF-4 ELISA

To quantify platelet activation, neutrophil activating peptide-2 (NAP-2) and platelet factor-4 (PF-4) levels in PRP collected from platelet activation experiments were measured utilizing sandwich ELISAs. Mouse monoclonal anti-hNAP-2 IgG and anti-hPF-4 IgG_{2B} capture antibodies (R&D Systems) were coated on 96-well EIA/RIA high binding plates (Corning) at 2 μg/mL in $1\times$ phosphate buffered saline (PBS) and incubated at 4 °C overnight. After rinsing three times with $1\times$ PBS + 0.05% Tween and blocking with 1% BSA in $1\times$ PBS for 1 h at room temperature with shaking, previously collected PRP samples were thawed, diluted 1:10,000 in 1% BSA in $1\times$ PBS and added for 2 h at room temperature with shaking. Samples were removed, wells were triple rinsed with $1 \times$ PBS + 0.05% Tween and biotinylated polyclonal goat anti-hNAP-2 IgG and anti-hPF-4 IgG detection antibodies (R&D Systems) were added at 0.2 $\mu g/mL$ in $1 \times$ PBS for 2 h at room temperature with shaking. After three rinses in $1 \times$ PBS + 0.05% Tween, streptavidin-HRP (diluted 1:200 in 1% BSA in $1 \times$ PBS) was added and detected as described above.

4.8. Platelet Binding

EC monolayers were seeded on CellBIND surface 96-well plates and stimulated with 5 ng/mL TNF-α for four hours to create a proinflammatory environment. CellTracker Green CMFDA (5-chloromethylfluorescein diacetate) (Thermo Fisher Scientific) was dissolved in dimethyl sulfoxide (DMSO), diluted in EC media and added to ECs for 20 min at 37 °C and 5% CO_2. Cells were then rinsed three times in TBS with 150 mM $CaCl_2$ and 1% BSA in TBS with 150 mM $CaCl_2$ was added to ECs for 10 min at room temperature to decrease nonspecific binding. ECs were then treated with 30 μM EC-SEAL variants for 1 h at 37 °C and 5% CO_2. PRP was isolated from human whole blood as described above and labeled with CellTracker Orange CMRA (Thermo Fisher Scientific) (which was previously dissolved in DMSO) for 25 min at 37 °C and 5% CO_2. Platelets were then pelleted via centrifugation for 10 min at $900 \times g$ and 25 °C, supernatant was removed and remaining platelets were suspended in EC media. Following EC-SEAL treatments and rinsing three times in TBS with 150 mM $CaCl_2$, labeled platelets in EC media were added to ECs for 1 h at 37 °C and 5% CO_2. After incubation, media was removed and the cells were rinsed in TBS with 150 mM $CaCl_2$ and then fixed with 3% paraformaldehyde for 20 min at room temperature. Three final rinses with TBS with 150 mM $CaCl_2$ were performed and cells were imaged using a Leica DMI6000 B microscope with EL6000 external light source (Leica Microsystems, Wetzler, Germany) and CoolSNAP HQ^2 camera (Photometrics, Tucson, AZ, USA). Leica application suite (LAS) AF6000 software (Leica Microsystems) was utilized for image acquisition. Excitation/emission spectra used were 460–500 nm/512–542 nm for ECs (green) and 540–552 nm/580–620 nm for platelets (orange). Contrast and brightness editing of acquired images was accomplished using the program ImageJ (National Institutes of Health, Bethesda, MD, USA) and identical settings were applied to all images.

4.9. EC-SEAL Binding (Selectin Protein)

Recombinant human E-selectin (PeproTech) was dissolved in water and added to a 96-well EIA/RIA high binding plate at 0.1–100 $\mu g/mL$. Following overnight incubation at 4 °C, the plate was rinsed three times with TBS with 150 mM $CaCl_2$ and blocked with 1% BSA in TBS with 150 mM $CaCl_2$ for 1 h at room temperature with shaking. The plate was then rinsed three more times with TBS with 150 mM $CaCl_2$. In experiments observing EC-SEAL binding, 3 μM EC-SEAL (in 1%BSA in TBS with 150 mM $CaCl_2$) was added for 1 h at room temperature with shaking. Following three rinses with TBS with 150 mM $CaCl_2$, streptavidin-HRP (1:200 in 1% BSA in TBS with 150 mM $CaCl_2$) was added for 20 min at room temperature with shaking. For experiments observing antibody binding, primary mouse monoclonal anti-E-selectin IgG$_{2a}$ antibody was added (1:50 dilution of initial 200 $\mu g/mL$ in 1% BSA in TBS) for two hours at room temperature with shaking. Following three rinses with TBS with 150 mM $CaCl_2$, secondary goat anti-mouse IgG HRP-conjugated antibody was added (1:1000 dilution of initial 0.5 mg/mL in 1% BSA in TBS) for 1 h at room temperature with shaking. HRP activity was detected as described above.

4.10. DVT Mouse Model

Ten-week-old C57BL/6 male mice (average weight: 26.4 g) were utilized in a model of surgically-induced deep vein thrombosis (DVT). All animals used in this study were obtained from Jackson Laboratory (Bar Harbor, ME) and fed standard chow diet. A well-established model of DVT caused by a significant inferior vena cava (IVC) flow restriction was utilized following a protocol (1505001247) approved by the institutional animal care and use committee at Purdue University. Mice were anesthetized using 1%–3% isoflurane and oxygen at a flow rate of 225 mL/min [58]; toe pinch was be used to determine sufficient anesthetic induction. Buprenorphine (0.03 mg/mL) was subcutaneously injected near the incision site at 0.05 mg/kg for pain management. Using aseptic technique, a small incision was made in the abdomen and the entrails were carefully exteriorized onto a sterile saline soaked gauze pad to prevent desiccation. The skin and organs were further retracted to fully expose the IVC, its branching vessels, and the infrarenal aorta. The aorta was then carefully separated from the IVC directly below the left renal vein. In an attempt to ligate all side and back branching vessels of the IVC, 6-0 black silk-braided sutures and a low power cautery pen (Bovie Medical, Purchase, NY, USA) were used, respectively. To achieve flow restriction, the proximal region of the IVC below the left renal vein was partially ligated by placing a 30-guage needle adjacent to the IVC and then tying a 6-0 black silk-braided suture around both the IVC and needle. The needle was then removed, resulting in an approximate 90% reduction in flow through the vessel. The muscle and skin layer were closed using 5-0 polypropylene sutures. A syringe with a 30-gauge needle was utilized to inject 100 µL of 30 µM EC-SEAL ($n = 4$), 200 IU/kg heparin ($n = 6$), or saline ($n = 6$) via tail vein. Tail vein injections were made approximately 10 min post-partial ligation of the IVC.

4.11. Ultrasound Imaging

Mice were anesthetized using 2%–3% isoflurane in 1.5 L/min oxygen. Cardiac and respiration rates were noninvasively monitored using gold-plated stage electrodes as part of the Vevo imaging station (FUJIFILM VisualSonics Inc., Toronto, ON, Canada). The mice were placed in a supine position on heated animal stage and the temperature was monitored using a rectal probe such that animals remained near 37°C. Depilatory cream was applied to remove hair on the abdomen prior to imaging, and warm ultrasound gel was applied on the skin to the entire abdomen just below the xiphoid process. IVC images were obtained using a Vevo2100 ultrasound imaging system with MS550D (40 MHz center frequency) and MS700 (50 MHz center frequency) transducers (FUJIFILM VisualSonics). The transducers were locked in the adjustable arm of the Vevo integrated rail system (FUJIFILM VisualSonics) for consistent image collection. In order to prevent distortion of the IVC, minimal pressure was applied to the abdomen to maintain original diameter of the vessel. The walls of the IVC were visualized with both long and short axes views. The angle of the stage was adjusted to optimize the view of the IVC and to minimize artifacts due to air and gas. Long and short axis B-mode images of the IVC were acquired at baseline (pre-operation) and at 6 h post-ligation of the IVC. Color Doppler images were used to assess blood flow through the IVC and branching vessels, and 3D scans of sequential slices were used to obtain vessel volumes as described previously [59,60]. Suture placement and the bifurcation of the IVC were used as landmarks to ensure consistent measurements between mice.

4.12. Ultrasound Image Analysis

All vessel measurements were made by the same ultrasonographer using Vevo LAB software (FUJIFILM VisualSonics). Thrombus length and volume and vessel volume were calculated using both the long axis and short axis ultrasound images. To determine the location of the thrombus, Color Doppler flow and B-mode images were utilized to visualize blood flow. The thrombus was also visualized as a hyperechoic region within the vessel lumen. Thrombus length was determined from the suture (point of IVC partial ligation) to the farthest point of thrombus and was calculated using an average of five measurements per image. The length of the thrombus in the 3D scans was compared to the length of thrombus in the long axis B-mode to ensure agreement. Thrombus volume was calculated by lofting together individual 2D segmentations from the first hyperechoic region in the lumen to the suture (where the lumen signal changed from hyperechoic to hypoechoic). Total IVC vessel volume was obtained using these same volumetric images and was measured from the suture to the IVC bifurcation. Percentage of IVC occlusion was obtained by determining the amount of thrombus volume within the total volume of the vessel.

4.13. Clotting Time (aPTT)

Activated partial thromboplastin time (aPTT) was measured using a Hemochron® Response (Accriva Diagnostics, San Diego, CA, USA) with associated reagents. The protocol was run according to manufacturer's instructions. Briefly, whole blood was obtained from healthy volunteers in sodium citrate collection vials and 2 mL was added to the Hemochron® aPTT (citrated blood) test tube. One hundred microliters of saline, heparin or EC-SEAL was then added (final concentrations: 3.75–15 µg/mL heparin; 13–128 µg/mL EC-SEAL), and the test tube was shaken vigorously ten times from end-to-end. The test tube was then placed into the Hemochron® Response device and clotting time was recorded at completion.

4.14. Statistics

Unless otherwise noted, all experiments were performed in triplicate or quadruplicate ($n \geq 2$) and results are presented as mean ± standard deviation. Statistical analysis was performed using GraphPad Prism software (GraphPad Software, Inc., La Jolla, CA, USA). All results were analyzed using ANOVA with post-hoc Tukey test. Statistical significance threshold was set at $p < 0.05$.

5. Conclusions

Here, we present the development of a novel GAG derived, selectin targeting anti-adhesive coating (termed EC-SEAL) consisting of a dermatan sulfate backbone with multiple selectin-binding peptides designed to treat EC dysfunction. We demonstrated the ability of different EC-SEAL variants to successfully bind to selectin-expressing vascular ECs and SMCs. The most effective variants were examined further and DS-IEL$_{30}$ was shown to preferentially bind to selectin protein and inhibit platelet binding and activation on inflamed EC surfaces. Additionally, DS-IEL$_{30}$ reduced thrombus size in vivo in a DVT mouse model while exhibiting a minimal effect on clotting time. Thus, by binding to and pacifying the surface of inflamed endothelium, EC-SEAL has the potential to be utilized as a therapeutic in multiple diseases associated with endothelial dysfunction.

Supplementary Materials: The following are available online at http://www.mdpi.com/1424-8247/10/2/36/s1, Figure S1: Selectin expression on ECs when stimulated with varying concentrations of TNF-α, Figure S2: Selectin expression on ECs when stimulated with varying concentrations of IL-1β, IL-6 and LPS, Figure S3: EC monolayer permeability in unstimulated conditions.

Acknowledgments: This work was funded through NIH R01HL106792 and the Purdue University Executive Vice President for Research and Partnerships (EVPRP) New R01 Program. James R. Wodicka, Andrea M. Chambers and Gurneet S. Sangha were supported by NIH T32DK101001.

Author Contributions: James R. Wodicka contributed to experimental design, synthesized EC-SEAL variants, conducted in vitro experiments, performed data analysis and wrote the majority of the manuscript. Andrea M. Chambers collected and analyzed animal study data and wrote a portion of the manuscript. Gurneet S. Sangha performed animal surgeries and wrote a portion of the manuscript. Craig J. Goergen and Alyssa Panitch coordinated the research project, contributed to experimental design and provided edits of the manuscript.

Conflicts of Interest: EC-SEAL is licensed to Symic Biomedical; Alyssa Panitch is a founder and scientific advisory board member of Symic Biomedical. The authors J.R.W., A.M.C., G.S.S. and C.J.G. declare no conflict of interest.

References

1. Brill, A.; Fuchs, T.A.; Chauhan, A.K.; Yang, J.J.; De Meyer, S.F.; Kollnberger, M.; Wakefield, T.W.; Lammle, B.; Massberg, S.; Wagner, D.D. Von Willebrand factor-mediated platelet adhesion is critical for deep vein thrombosis in mouse models. *Blood* **2011**, *117*, 1400–1407. [PubMed]

2. Gawaz, M.; Langer, H.; May, A.E. Platelets in inflammation and atherogenesis. *J. Clin. Investig.* **2005**, *115*, 3378–3384. [CrossRef] [PubMed]

3. Rajendran, P.; Rengarajan, T.; Thangavel, J.; Nishigaki, Y.; Sakthisekaran, D.; Sethi, G.; Nishigaki, I. The vascular endothelium and human diseases. *In. J. Biol. Sci.* **2013**, *9*, 1057–1069. [CrossRef] [PubMed]

4.   Sena, C.M.; Pereira, A.M.; Seica, R. Endothelial dysfunction—A major mediator of diabetic vascular disease. *Biochim. Biophys. Acta* **2013**, *1832*, 2216–2231. [PubMed]
5.   O'Riordan, E.; Chen, J.; Brodsky, S.V.; Smirnova, I.; Li, H.; Goligorsky, M.S. Endothelial cell dysfunction—The syndrome in making. *Kidney Int.* **2005**, *67*, 1654–1658. [CrossRef] [PubMed]
6.   Davignon, J.; Ganz, P. Role of endothelial dysfunction in atherosclerosis. *Circulation* **2004**, *109*, III27–III32. [CrossRef] [PubMed]
7.   Dharmashankar, K.; Widlansky, M.E. Vascular endothelial function and hypertension: Insights and directions. *Curr. Hypertens. Rep.* **2010**, *12*, 448–455. [CrossRef] [PubMed]
8.   Briet, M.; Burns, K.D. Chronic kidney disease and vascular remodelling: Molecular mechanisms and clinical implications. *Clin. Sci.* **2012**, *123*, 399–416. [CrossRef] [PubMed]
9.   Franses, J.W.; Drosu, N.C.; Gibson, W.J.; Chitalia, V.C.; Edelman, E.R. Dysfunctional endothelial cells directly stimulate cancer inflammation and metastasis. *Int. J. Cancer. J. Int. Cancer* **2013**, *133*, 1334–1344. [CrossRef] [PubMed]
10.   Hadi, H.A.R.; Carr, C.S.; Suwaidi, J.A.I. Endothelial dysfunction—Cardiovascular risk factors, therapy, and outcome. *Vasc. Health Risk Manag.* **2005**, *1*, 183–198. [PubMed]
11.   Wu, K.K.; Thiagarajan, P. Role of Endothelium in Thrombosis and Hemostasis. *Annu. Rev. Med.* **1996**, *47*, 315–331. [PubMed]
12.   Deanfield, J.E.; Halcox, J.P.; Rabelink, T.J. Endothelial function and dysfunction: Testing and clinical relevance. *Circulation* **2007**, *115*, 1285–1295. [PubMed]
13.   Reitsma, S.; Slaaf, D.W.; Vink, H.; van Zandvoort, M.A.; oude Egbrink, M.G. The endothelial glycocalyx: Composition, functions, and visualization. *Pflug. Archiv. Eur. J. Physiol.* **2007**, *454*, 345–359. [CrossRef] [PubMed]
14.   van den Berg, B.M.; Nieuwdorp, M.; Stroes, E.S.G.; Vink, H. Glycocalyx and endothelial (dys) function—From mice to men. *Pharmacol. Rep.* **2006**, *58*, 75–80. [PubMed]
15.   Salmon, A.H.; Satchell, S.C. Endothelial glycocalyx dysfunction in disease: Albuminuria and increased microvascular permeability. *J. Pathol.* **2012**, *226*, 562–574. [CrossRef] [PubMed]
16.   Ait-Oufella, H.; Maury, E.; Lehoux, S.; Guidet, B.; Offenstadt, G. The endothelium: Physiological functions and role in microcirculatory failure during severe sepsis. *Intensive Care Med.* **2010**, *36*, 1286–1298. [CrossRef] [PubMed]
17.   Rumbaut, R.E.; Thiagarajan, P. Chapter 2: General Characteristics of Platelets. In *Platelet-Vessel Wall Interactions in Hemostasis and Thrombosis*; Morgan & Claypool Life Sciences: San Rafael, CA, USA, 2010.
18.   Gurney, D.; Lip, G.Y.H.; Blann, A.D. A Reliable Plasma Marker of Platelet Activation—Does It Exist? *Am. J. Hematol.* **2002**, *70*, 139–144. [CrossRef] [PubMed]
19.   Massberg, S.; Enders, G.; Leiderer, R.; Eisenmenger, S.; Vestweber, D.; Krombach, F.; Messmer, K. Platelet-Endothelial Cell Interactions During Ischemia-Reperfusion—The Role of P-Selectin. *Blood* **1998**, *92*, 507–515. [PubMed]
20.   Smith, C.; Damas, J.K.; Otterdal, K.; Oie, E.; Sandberg, W.J.; Yndestad, A.; Waehre, T.; Scholz, H.; Endresen, K.; Olofsson, P.S.; et al. Increased levels of neutrophil-activating peptide-2 in acute coronary syndromes: Possible role of platelet-mediated vascular inflammation. *J. Am. Coll. Cardiol.* **2006**, *48*, 1591–1599. [PubMed]
21.   Balakumar, P.; Koladiya, R.U.; Ramasamy, S.; Rathinavel, A.; Singh, M. Pharmacological Interventions to Prevent Vascular Endothelial Dysfunction: Future Directions. *J. Health Sci.* **2008**, *54*, 1–16. [CrossRef]
22.   Yu, W.; Akishita, M.; Xi, H.; Nagai, K.; Sudoh, N.; Hasegawa, H.; Kozaki, K.; Toba, K. Angiotensin converting enzyme inhibitor attenuates oxidative stress-induced endothelial cell apoptosis via p38 MAP kinase inhibition. *Clin. Chim. Acta Int. J. Clin. Chem.* **2006**, *364*, 328–334. [CrossRef] [PubMed]
23.   Jourde-Chiche, N.; Dou, L.; Cerini, C.; Dignat-George, F.; Brunet, P. Vascular incompetence in dialysis patients–protein-bound uremic toxins and endothelial dysfunction. *Semin. Dial.* **2011**, *24*, 327–337. [PubMed]
24.   Fliser, D. Perspectives in renal disease progression: The endothelium as a treatment target in chronic kidney disease. *J. Nephrol.* **2010**, *23*, 369–376. [PubMed]
25.   Ma, S.; Tian, X.Y.; Zhang, Y.; Mu, C.; Shen, H.; Bismuth, J.; Pownall, H.J.; Huang, Y.; Wong, W.T. E-selectin-targeting delivery of microRNAs by microparticles ameliorates endothelial inflammation and atherosclerosis. *Sci. Rep.* **2016**, *6*, 22910. [CrossRef] [PubMed]

26. Theoharis, S.; Krueger, U.; Tan, P.H.; Haskard, D.O.; Weber, M.; George, A.J. Targeting gene delivery to activated vascular endothelium using anti E/P-Selectin antibody linked to PAMAM dendrimers. *J. Immunol. Methods* **2009**, *343*, 79–90. [CrossRef] [PubMed]
27. Bachtarzi, H.; Stevenson, M.; Subr, V.; Ulbrich, K.; Seymour, L.W.; Fisher, K.D. Targeting adenovirus gene delivery to activated tumour-associated vasculature via endothelial selectins. *J. Control Release* **2011**, *150*, 196–203. [CrossRef] [PubMed]
28. Barthel, S.R.; Gavino, J.D.; Descheny, L.; Dimitroff, C.J. Targeting selectins and selectin ligands in inflammation and cancer. *Expert Opin. Ther. Targets* **2007**, *11*, 1473–1491. [CrossRef] [PubMed]
29. Haverslag, R.; Pasterkamp, G.; Hoefer, I.E. Targeting Adhesion Molecules in Cardiovascular Disorders. *Cardiovasc. Hematol. Disord. Drug Targets* **2008**, *8*, 252–260. [CrossRef] [PubMed]
30. Muzykantov, V.R. Targeted Drug Delivery to Endothelial Adhesion Molecules. *ISRN Vasc. Med.* **2013**, *2013*, 1–27. [CrossRef]
31. Fukuda, M.N.; Ohyama, C.; Lowitz, K.; Matsuo, O.; Pasqualini, R.; Ruoslahti, E.; Fukuda, M. A Peptide Mimic of E-Selectin Ligand Inhibits Sialyl Lewis X-dependent Lung Colonization of Tumor Cells. *Cancer Res.* **2000**, *60*, 450–456. [PubMed]
32. Fokong, S.; Fragoso, A.; Rix, A.; Curaj, A.; Wu, Z.; Lederle, W.; Iranzo, O.; Gatjens, J.; Kiessling, F.; Palmowski, M. Ultrasound Molecular Imaging of E-Selectin in Tumor Vessels Using Poly *n*-Butyl Cyanoacrylate Microbubbles Covalently Coupled to a Short Targeting Peptide. *Investig. Radiol.* **2013**, *48*, 843–850.
33. Leng, X.; Wang, J.; Carson, A.; Chen, X.; Fu, H.; Ottoboni, S.; Wagner, W.R.; Villanueva, F.S. Ultrasound Detection of Myocardial Ischemic Memory Using an E-Selectin Targeting Peptide Amenable to Human Application. *Mol. Imaging* **2014**, *13*, 1–9. [PubMed]
34. Renkonen, R.; Fukuda, M.N.; Petrov, L.; Paavonen, T.; Renkonen, J.; Hayry, P.; Fukuda, M. A Peptide Mimic of Selectin Ligands Abolishes In Vivo Inflammation But Has No Effect on the Rat Heart Allograft Survival. *Transplantation* **2002**, *74*, 2–6. [CrossRef] [PubMed]
35. Raines, E.W.; Ferri, N. Thematic review series: The immune system and atherogenesis. Cytokines affecting endothelial and smooth muscle cells in vascular disease. *J. Lipid Res.* **2005**, *46*, 1081–1092. [CrossRef] [PubMed]
36. Zeiffer, U.; Schober, A.; Lietz, M.; Liehn, E.A.; Erl, W.; Emans, N.; Yan, Z.Q.; Weber, C. Neointimal smooth muscle cells display a proinflammatory phenotype resulting in increased leukocyte recruitment mediated by P-selectin and chemokines. *Circ. Res.* **2004**, *94*, 776–784. [CrossRef] [PubMed]
37. Yu, G.; Rux, A.H.; Ma, P.; Bdeir, K.; Sachais, B.S. Endothelial expression of E-selectin is induced by the platelet-specific chemokine platelet factor 4 through LRP in an NF-kB-dependent manner. *Blood* **2005**, *105*, 3545–3551. [CrossRef] [PubMed]
38. Cohen, A.B.; Stevens, M.D.; Miller, E.J.; Atkinson, M.A.L.; Mullenbach, G. Generation of the neutrophil-activating peptide-2 by cathepsin G and Cathepsin G-treated human platelets. *Am. J. Physiol. Lung Cell. Mol. Physiol.* **1992**, *263*, L249–L256.
39. Schouten, M.; Wiersinga, W.J.; Levi, M.; van der Poll, T. Inflammation, endothelium, and coagulation in sepsis. *J. Leukoc. Biol.* **2008**, *83*, 536–545. [CrossRef] [PubMed]
40. De Caterina, R.; Libby, P.; Peng, H.B.; Thannickal, V.J.; Rajavashisth, T.B.; Gimbrone, J.M.A.; Shin, W.S.; Liao, J.K. Nitric Oxide Decreases Cytokine-induced Endothelial Activation. *J. Clin. Investig.* **1995**, *96*, 60–68. [CrossRef] [PubMed]
41. Zhang, W.J.; Stocker, R.; McCall, M.R.; Forte, T.M.; Frei, B. Lack of inhibitory effect of HDL on TNFalpha-induced adhesion molecule expression in human aortic endothelial cells. *Atherosclerosis* **2002**, *165*, 241–249. [CrossRef]
42. Tsou, J.K.; Gower, R.M.; Ting, H.J.; Schaff, U.Y.; Insana, M.F.; Passerini, A.G.; Simon, S.I. Spatial regulation of inflammation by human aortic endothelial cells in a linear gradient of shear stress. *Microcirculation* **2008**, *15*, 311–323. [PubMed]
43. Pu, F.R.; Williams, R.L.; Markkula, T.K.; Hunt, J.A. Expression of leukocyte-endothelial cell adhesion molecules on monocyte adhesion to human endothelial cells on plasma treated PET and PTFE in vitro. *Biomaterials* **2002**, *23*, 4705–4718. [CrossRef]
44. van der Zijpp, Y.J.T.; Poot, A.A.; Feijen, J. ICAM-1 and VCAM-1 expression by endothelial cells grown on fibronectin-coated TCPS and PS. *J. Biomed. Mater. Res. A* **2003**, *65*, 51–59. [CrossRef] [PubMed]

45. Litwin, M.; Clark, K.; Noack, L.; Furze, J.; Berndt, M.; Albelda, S.; Vadas, M.; Gamble, J. Novel Cytokine-independent Induction of Endothelial Adhesion Molecules Regulated by Platelet-Endothelial Cell Adhesion Molecule (CD31). *J. Cell Biol.* **1997**, *139*, 219–228. [CrossRef] [PubMed]
46. Luo, J.; Paranya, G.; Bischoff, J. Noninflammatory Expression of E-Selectin Is Regulated by Cell Growth. *Blood* **1999**, *93*, 3785–3791. [PubMed]
47. Martens, C.L.; Cwirla, S.E.; Lee, R.Y.W.; Whitehorn, E.; Chen, E.Y.F.; Bakker, A.; Martin, E.L.; Wagstrom, C.; Gopalan, P.; Smith, C.W.; et al. Peptides Which Bind to E-selectin and Block Neutrophil Adhesion. *J. Biol. Chem.* **1995**, *270*, 21129–21136. [CrossRef] [PubMed]
48. Goh, C.S.; Milburn, D.; Gerstein, M. Conformational changes associated with protein-protein interactions. *Curr. Opin. Struct. Biol.* **2004**, *14*, 104–109. [CrossRef] [PubMed]
49. Keskin, O. Binding induced conformational changes of proteins correlate with their intrinsic fluctuations: A case study of antibodies. *BMC Struct. Biol.* **2007**, *7*, 31. [CrossRef] [PubMed]
50. Cooke, R.M.; Hale, R.S.; Lister, S.G.; Shah, G.; Weir, M.P. The Conformation of the Sialyl Lewis X Ligand Changes upon Binding to E-Selectin. *Biochemistry* **1994**, *33*, 10591–10596. [PubMed]
51. Preston, R.C.; Jakob, R.P.; Binder, F.P.; Sager, C.P.; Ernst, B.; Maier, T. E-selectin ligand complexes adopt an extended high-affinity conformation. *J. Mol. Cell Biol.* **2016**, *8*, 62–72. [CrossRef] [PubMed]
52. Diaz, J.A.; Obi, A.T.; Myers, D.D., Jr.; Wrobleski, S.K.; Henke, P.K.; Mackman, N.; Wakefield, T.W. Critical review of mouse models of venous thrombosis. *Arterioscler. Thromb. Vasc. Biol.* **2012**, *32*, 556–562. [CrossRef] [PubMed]
53. Myers, D.D., Jr.; Rectenwald, J.E.; Bedard, P.W.; Kaila, N.; Shaw, G.D.; Schaub, R.G.; Farris, D.M.; Hawley, A.E.; Wrobleski, S.K.; Henke, P.K.; Wakefield, T.W. Decreased venous thrombosis with an oral inhibitor of P selectin. *J. Vasc. Surg.* **2005**, *42*, 329–336. [CrossRef] [PubMed]
54. Dhahri, M.; Mansour, M.B.; Bertholon, I.; Ollivier, V.; Boughattas, N.A.; Hassine, M.; Jandrot-Perrus, M.; Chaubet, F.; Maaroufi, R.M. Anticoagulant activity of a dermatan sulfate from the skin of the shark Scyliorhinus canicula. *Blood Coagul. Fibrinolysis* **2010**, *21*, 547–557. [CrossRef] [PubMed]
55. Duan, J.; Kasper, D.L. Oxidative depolymerization of polysaccharides by reactive oxygen/nitrogen species. *Glycobiology* **2011**, *21*, 401–409. [CrossRef] [PubMed]
56. van Golen, R.F.; Reiniers, M.J.; Vrisekoop, N.; Zuurbier, C.J.; Olthof, P.B.; van Rheenen, J.; van Gulik, T.M.; Parsons, B.J.; Heger, M. The mechanisms and physiological relevance of glycocalyx degradation in hepatic ischemia/reperfusion injury. *Antioxid. Redox Signal.* **2014**, *21*, 1098–1118. [CrossRef] [PubMed]
57. Zhang, J.; Nakayama, J.; Ohyama, C.; Suzuki, M.; Suzuki, A.; Fukuda, M.; Fukuda, M.N. Sialyl Lewis X-dependent Lung Colonization of B16 Melanoma Cells through a Selectin-like Endothelial Receptor Distinct from E- or P-Selectin. *Cancer Res.* **2002**, *62*, 4194–4198. [PubMed]
58. Damen, F.W.; Adelsperger, A.R.; Wilson, K.E.; Goergen, C.J. Comparison of Traditional and Integrated Digital Anesthetic Vaporizers. *J. Am. Assoc. Lab. Anim. Sci.* **2015**, *54*, 756–762. [PubMed]
59. Phillips, E.H.; Yrineo, A.A.; Schroeder, H.D.; Wilson, K.E.; Cheng, J.X.; Goergen, C.J. Morphological and Biomechanical Differences in the Elastase and AngII apoE$^{-/-}$ Rodent Models of Abdominal Aortic Aneurysms. *Biomed. Res. Int.* **2015**, *2015*, 413189. [CrossRef] [PubMed]
60. Phillips, E.H.; Di Achille, P.; Bersi, M.R.; Humphrey, J.D.; Goergen, C.J. Multi-Modality Imaging Enables Detailed Hemodynamic Simulations in Dissecting Aneurysms in Mice. *IEEE Trans Med Imaging* **2017**. [CrossRef] [PubMed]

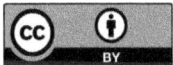

pharmaceuticals

MDPI

Article

Glycosaminoglycan Binding and Non-Endocytic Membrane Translocation of Cell-Permeable Octaarginine Monitored by Real-Time In-Cell NMR Spectroscopy

Yuki Takechi-Haraya [1,†], Kenzo Aki [1], Yumi Tohyama [1], Yuichi Harano [1], Toru Kawakami [2], Hiroyuki Saito [3] and Emiko Okamura [1,*]

1   Faculty of Pharmaceutical Sciences, Himeji Dokkyo University, 7-2-1 Kamiohno, Himeji 670-8524, Japan; haraya@nihs.go.jp (Y.T.-H.); aki@gm.himeji-du.ac.jp (K.A.); ytohyama@himeji-du.ac.jp (Y.T.); harano@gm.himeji-du.ac.jp (Y.H.)
2   Institute for Protein Research, Osaka University, 3-2 Yamadaoka, Suita, Osaka 565-0871, Japan; kawa@protein.osaka-u.ac.jp
3   Department of Biophysical Chemistry, Kyoto Pharmaceutical University, 5 Nakauchi-cho, Misasagi, Yamashina-ku, Kyoto 607-8414, Japan; hsaito@mb.kyoto-phu.ac.jp
*   Correspondence: emiko@himeji-du.ac.jp; Tel.: +81-79-223-6847
†   Present address: Division of Drugs, National Institute of Health Sciences, 1-18-1 Kamiyoga, Setagaya-ku, Tokyo 158-8501, Japan.

Academic Editor: Barbara Mulloy
Received: 16 February 2017; Accepted: 12 April 2017; Published: 15 April 2017

Abstract: Glycosaminoglycans (GAGs), which are covalently-linked membrane proteins at the cell surface have recently been suggested to involve in not only endocytic cellular uptake but also non-endocytic direct cell membrane translocation of arginine-rich cell-penetrating peptides (CPPs). However, in-situ comprehensive observation and the quantitative analysis of the direct membrane translocation processes are challenging, and the mechanism therefore remains still unresolved. In this work, real-time in-cell NMR spectroscopy was applied to investigate the direct membrane translocation of octaarginine (R8) into living cells. By introducing 4-trifluoromethyl-L-phenylalanine to the N terminus of R8, the non-endocytic membrane translocation of ^{19}F-labeled R8 (^{19}F-R8) into a human myeloid leukemia cell line was observed at 4 °C with a time resolution in the order of minutes. ^{19}F NMR successfully detected real-time R8 translocation: the binding to anionic GAGs at the cell surface, followed by the penetration into the cell membrane, and the entry into cytosol across the membrane. The NMR concentration analysis enabled quantification of how much of R8 was staying in the respective translocation processes with time in situ. Taken together, our in-cell NMR results provide the physicochemical rationale for spontaneous penetration of CPPs in cell membranes.

Keywords: glycosaminoglycan; heparin; cell penetrating peptide; octaarginine; non-endocytic membrane translocation; in-cell nuclear magnetic resonance spectroscopy

1. Introduction

Drug delivery using cell-penetrating peptides (CPPs) is one of the most powerful strategies to resolve the poor cell membrane permeability of new bioactive molecules such as oligonucleotides, plasmids, peptides and proteins for therapeutic pharmaceuticals [1]. Arginine- or lysine-rich CPPs can deliver such cargoes into cells in vitro and in vivo [2–4]. Although the endocytic pathway has been thought to be significant [5], more than 90% of the delivered cargo become biologically inactive because of lysosomal degradation [6]. CPPs also traverse cell membrane via the non-endocytic pathway at high concentrations, > ~5–10 μM [7,8]. This process is often named as direct membrane translocation or transduction. The mechanism is essentially a physicochemical, energy-independent process in which no receptors are required [9]. Although the direct membrane translocation is an alternative to endocytosis in order to avoid the lysosomal degradation, how cationic CPPs traverse hydrophobic cell membranes is still controversial [10].

As a first step of membrane translocation, cationic CPPs are thought to interact with negatively charged, sulfated glycosaminoglycans (GAGs) such as heparan sulfate and chondroitin sulfate which are covalently linked to membrane proteins at the cell surface [11–14]. The GAG clustering is induced via the electrostatic interaction with CPP, followed by the actin rearrangement that leads to endocytosis [15,16]. On the other hand, the GAG clustering also triggers the direct membrane translocation of CPPs at high CPP concentrations (> 5 μM) [17]. Although CPPs bind to and translocate into GAG-deficient cells and enzymatically GAG-removed cells [12,13,18,19], we have recently reported that the efficiency of the direct membrane translocation of arginine-rich CPPs is correlated with the favorable enthalpy of binding to heparin, of which the binding could be derived from formation of multidentate hydrogen bonding of the arginine residue with sulfate group of heparin [20]. In addition, the previous study has demonstrated that the direct membrane translocation of arginine-rich peptides including octaarginine (R8) is markedly reduced by the chlorate treatment, which prevents sulfation of both heparan sulfate and chondroitin sulfate chains [20]. Based on these facts, the non-endocytic membrane translocation of arginine-rich CPPs would follow three distinct steps: (1) binding to sulfated GAGs at the cell surface; (2) translocation into cells over potential barrier of the hydrophobic cell membrane; and (3) diffusion through the cytosol. However, in situ comprehensive observation and quantitative analysis of the non-endocytic membrane translocation processes are challenging, and the mechanism therefore remains still unsolved [10].

So far, almost all membrane translocation studies have relied upon the fluorescent labeling of CPPs or delivered cargo. Despite the high sensitivity, fluorophores are likely to strengthen the interaction of CPPs with lipid membrane [16,21], induce photodamage of lipid bilayer membranes [22], facilitate the uptake into the cell [23], modify the cellular distribution of the CPP [24,25], and change the structural flexibility and conformation of CPP [26]. Recently, an innovative MALDI TOF-MS quantification was reported by using biotin–avidin interaction [27–29]. Although the biotinylated CPP at as low as a femtomole scale has been quantified after the incubation with cells, the method has not been able to catch the real-time processes of CPP's translocation into cells. Recently- developed real-time NMR spectroscopy [30] is a potential technique for the observation of biologically-relevant functions in a natural manner.

In this work, the real-time solution NMR method is applied to natural living cells to investigate the mechanism for non-endocytic membrane translocation of cell-permeable octaarginine (R8). By introducing 4-trifluoromethyl-L-phenylalanine (4CF$_3$-Phe) to the N terminus of R8, the direct membrane translocation of ^{19}F-labeled R8 (^{19}F-R8) into a human myeloid leukemia cell line (HL60) is observed by ^{19}F NMR with a time resolution at a minute scale. ^{19}F NMR is advantageous because it is sensitive and no background is present in the cell. The small size, large chemical shift range, and 100% natural isotope abundance of the ^{19}F nucleus have made the use of ^{19}F-labeled peptides and proteins an attractive method for biologically-relevant NMR studies [31,32]. Labeling of R8 with 4CF$_3$-Phe is found to be an effective method to detect peptide uptake to cells with minimal perturbation [23]. In addition, ^{19}F NMR spectroscopy enables us to make a quantitative (concentration) analysis relevant to the molecular dynamics of biological interest without perturbing the system [33–36]. Here we observe the direct membrane translocation of ^{19}F-R8 at 4 °C, the temperature low enough to assure no endocytic pathway of the cellular uptake [37]. The method can detect the successive processes of ^{19}F-R8 translocation: (1) ^{19}F-R8 binds to GAG at the cell surface; (2) penetrates into the cell membrane; and (3) finally enters the cytosol through the membrane. In addition, ^{19}F NMR concentration analysis quantifies how much of ^{19}F-R8 is in the processes (1)–(3) with time. The information is valuable because the analysis of time-resolved drug transport has been limited to the uptake of a small drug-like ion via the *Escherichia coli* membrane by using second harmonic generation [38]. We also confirm the ^{19}F-R8 uptake to the cytosol of HL60 cells using cell fractionation after equilibrium was attained in the real-time NMR measurement. Finally, the most plausible mechanism of the non-endocytic ^{19}F-R8 entry into the cell is discussed.

2. Results

2.1. Real-Time In-Cell ^{19}F NMR Spectra

To capture the real-time process of non-endocytic membrane translocation of ^{19}F-R8, the solution ^{19}F NMR measurement was performed at 4 °C with a time resolution at a minute scale. In order to confirm no contribution of endocytosis at 4 °C, the comparative measurement was also performed at 37 °C. Figure 1a,b shows the real-time ^{19}F NMR spectra of ^{19}F-R8 before (0 min) and after the addition to HL60 cells at 4 and 37 °C, respectively. At 4 °C (Figure 1a), a signal is observed at −62.20 ppm, that is assignable to the F nuclei of $4CF_3$-Phe at the N terminus of R8. The assignment is confirmed by Figure S1 where signals of $4CF_3$-Phe at −62 ppm and trifluoroacetate (TFA) counter anions at −76 ppm are present with an intensity ratio ($4CF_3$-Phe/TFA) of 1:8. At 37 °C, the ^{19}F-R8 signal was shifted to −61.66 ppm (Figure 1b). In addition, a new peak was observed at −61.84 ppm after 10 min, and gradually increased with time. The increase of the peak at −61.84 ppm was coupled with a gradual decrease in the original signal at −61.66 ppm. The appearance of a new peak with the disappearance of the original one is due to the presence of cells because such kind of signal changes is not observed in the absence of cells at 37 °C (spectra not shown). Thus the new peak observed at 37 °C is thought to be the result of endocytosis involving peptide degradation [39]. Since such kind of spectral change is not found in Figure 1a, it is reasonable to consider that no endocytosis occurs at 4 °C. The absence of endocytosis at 4 °C is also consistent with the previous results of cell-penetrating peptides [8,9].

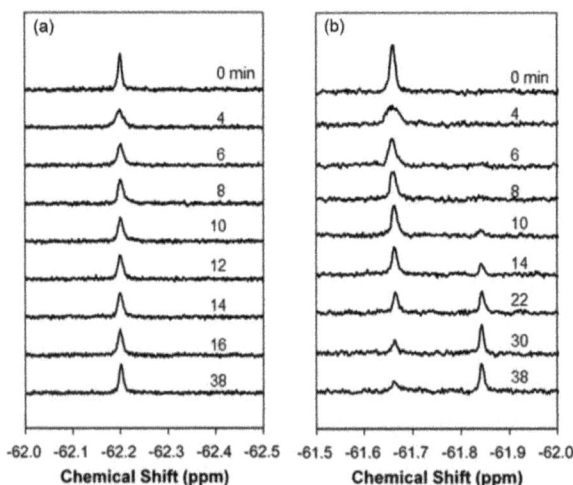

Figure 1. Real-time ^{19}F NMR spectra of ^{19}F-labeled R8 (^{19}F-R8) after addition to HL60 cells at (a) 4 and (b) 37 °C. The number attached to each spectrum indicates the passage of time before (0 min) and after the addition to cells (in min unit). The ^{19}F-R8 concentrations and pH values are (a) 80 μM at pH 7.4 and (b) 150 μM at pH 7.3, respectively. At 37 °C (b), a new peak is observed at −61.84 ppm after 10 min, and gradually increased with time. The increase of the peak at −61.84 ppm is coupled with a gradual decrease in the original signal of ^{19}F-R8 at −61.66 ppm. Notice that such kind of signal change is not observed at 4 °C (a).

Figure 2a shows an expansion of the real-time ^{19}F NMR spectra of ^{19}F-R8 at 4 °C in PBS (0 min) and 4, 6, 8, 10, 12, 14 and 16 min after the addition to HL60 cells. In comparison to the spectrum in PBS (0 min), the signal is broadened due to the appearance of new component (red arrow) at the low magnetic field within the first 4 min after ^{19}F-R8 was incubated with cells. We call it state I. After 6 min, the signal comes back to the high field and becomes sharper (state II). This is because the low field component gradually decreases in intensity during the period from 4 to 6 min. After 8 min, however, the peak top of the signal slightly moves to the lower field again (state III). No further change is observed in the ^{19}F-R8 signal after 10 min and later, indicating that the system reaches an equilibrium state.

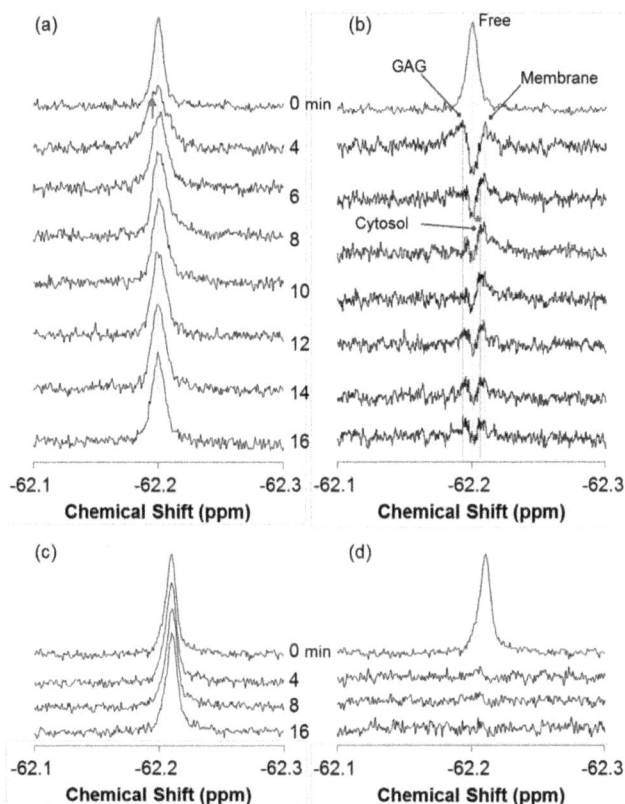

Figure 2. Real-time in-cell ^{19}F NMR spectra of ^{19}F-R8 and ^{19}F-T6 at 4 °C. (**a**) An expansion of the typical ^{19}F NMR spectra of 80 μM ^{19}F-R8 (Figure 1a) in PBS (0 min), and 4, 6, 8, 10, 12, 14 and 16 min after the addition to HL60 cells at 4 °C. The peak top of ^{19}F-R8 in the absence of cells (0 min) is designated by blue dotted line. The red arrow indicates a new component observed at the first step after addition to cells. (**b**) The difference spectra obtained by subtracting the spectrum of ^{19}F-R8 in PBS (0 min) from the respective spectra of Figure 2a in the presence of HL60 cells. Note that the top spectrum (Free) in Figure 2b is the ^{19}F NMR spectrum of ^{19}F-R8 in PBS (0 min). Four components of ^{19}F-R8 in cell outside (Free), bound to glycosaminoglycan (GAG), bound to cell membrane (Membrane), and in cytosol (Cytosol, *) are designated by the dotted lines in blue, black, green, and red, respectively. For comparison, the real-time in-cell ^{19}F NMR (**c**) and the difference spectra (**d**) of 100 μM ^{19}F-T6 in PBS (0 min), and at 4, 8, and 16 min after the addition to HL60 cells are also shown. The upper spectrum in (**d**) represents ^{19}F-T6 in PBS (0 min).

As mentioned above, the time-dependent spectral changes in Figure 2a imply that at least three different states I-III of ^{19}F-R8 are present after the addition to HL60 cells. We repeated in-cell NMR measurement three times, and confirmed such states every time of the measurement. To distinguish states I, II, and III clearly, it is convenient to see the difference spectrum. The difference spectrum analysis is useful in the present study because the integral intensity of ^{19}F-R8 is conserved all the time (see Supplementary Materials Figure S2); notice that no degradation of ^{19}F-R8 is induced at 4 °C by the presence of HL60 cells. By subtracting the spectrum of ^{19}F-R8 in PBS (0 min) from each spectrum after 4, 6, 8, 10, 12, 14 and 16 min with cells, we can obtain the difference spectra as illustrated in Figure 2b.

The time course of the difference spectra shows that probably three components of ^{19}F-R8 are present after ^{19}F-R8 is added to HL cells, in addition to the free component at −62.20 ppm. At first, two peaks are observed at −62.19 and −62.21 ppm after 4 min. These peaks can be assigned to ^{19}F-R8 bound to GAG (GAG in Figure 2b) and ^{19}F-R8 that interacts with the cell membrane (Membrane). Details of the assignment will be described later. Then, the third peak appears at −62.205 ppm after 6 min and increases in intensity after 8 min; see asterisk in Figure 2b. This peak can be assigned to ^{19}F-R8 in cytosol (Cytosol) after passing through the membrane.

It is noted that the peak assignments are reasonable in view of the following results of ^{19}F NMR and isothermal titration calorimetry (ITC). The first is that the NMR chemical shift of ^{19}F-R8 moves toward the low magnetic field as compared to ^{19}F-R8 in PBS when ^{19}F-R8 is mixed with heparin; see Figure 3a. Because heparin is frequently used as a model of GAG [40–45], it is reasonable to assign the broad component at −62.19 ppm to ^{19}F-R8 that is bound to GAG. According to the fact that NMR signal intensity is reduced by slower rotational movement of a molecule related to short transverse relaxation time, it should be noted that the rotational dynamics of ^{19}F-R8 are restricted due to the tighter binding to heparin, as previously discussed [20]. The high affinity of R8 for heparin is confirmed by the ITC result in Figure 4 that leads the association constant 1.3×10^8 M^{-1}, and the binding free energy, −10.9 kcal/mol at 25 °C, as listed in Table 1. The binding nature of R8 is largely derived from the electrostatic interaction between arginine residues and anionic sulfate/carboxyl groups of heparin [20]. The binding stoichiometry (molar ratio of peptide/heparin = ~11) corresponds approximately to the ratio for the charge neutralization (the heparin molecule used possesses an average of 80 anionic charges, whereas there are 8 cationic charges of octaarginine). The assignment also corresponds well with the previous consensus that R8 at first comes contact with GAG at the cell surface by the electrostatic interaction [46]. The second is that the ^{19}F NMR signal moves to a high magnetic field where ^{19}F-R8 interacts with cell membrane, in contrast to the electrostatic ^{19}F-R8 binding to GAG. As illustrated in Figure 3b, it is confirmed that the ^{19}F-R8 signal shifts to a high field after the binding to large unilamellar vesicle (LUV) composed of egg phosphatidylcholine (EPC) and egg phosphatidylglycerol (EPG) as model cell membrane. The result is consistent with the observation that the chemical shift of the ^{19}F NMR signal moves to the higher magnetic field when ^{19}F molecules are in a hydrophobic environment [23,47,48]. Similar to the case of heparin binding, the NMR signal intensity of ^{19}F-R8 is also reduced due to the binding to EPC/EPG LUV. The presence of energetically-favorable interaction between R8 and EPC-EPG membrane is also demonstrated by the ITC result in Figure 5 that gives the association constant, 1.5×10^6 M^{-1} and the binding free energy, −8.4 kcal/mol at 25 °C (Table 1). The binding stoichiometry (molar ratio of lipid/peptide = ~100) is close to the ratio for charge neutralization, that is, the molar ratio of EPG in the outer leaflet of the LUVs to the positively charged residues of octaarginine is ~1. Thus we can consider that the most plausible assignment of the peak at −62.21 ppm is ^{19}F-R8 in the cell membrane. Finally, it is reasonable to assign the third peak at −62.205 ppm (*) as ^{19}F-R8 in cytosol, because the peak comes back to the lower magnetic field due to rather hydrophilic cytosol environment as compared to the cell membrane. The presence of ^{19}F-R8 in cytosol is also confirmed by cell fractionation, the details of which will be described later.

Table 1. Thermodynamic parameters for the interaction of R8 with heparin or egg phosphatidylcholine (EPC)/egg phosphatidylglycerol (EPG) large unilamellar vesicles (LUVs) obtained from isothermal titration calorimetry (ITC).

	Binding Stoichiometry (n)	K (M^{-1})	$\Delta G°$ (kcal/mol)	$\Delta H°$ (kcal/mol)	$T\Delta S°$ (kcal/mol)
Heparin	R8/heparin = 11 ± 1.1	$(1.3 \pm 0.22) \times 10^8$	−10.9 ± 0.10	−9.6 ± 0.53	1.3 ± 0.54
EPC/EPG LUV	lipid/R8 = 100 ± 10	$(1.5 \pm 0.25) \times 10^6$	−8.4 ± 0.10	−6.3 ± 0.10	2.1 ± 0.10

For original ITC data, see Figures 4 and 5.

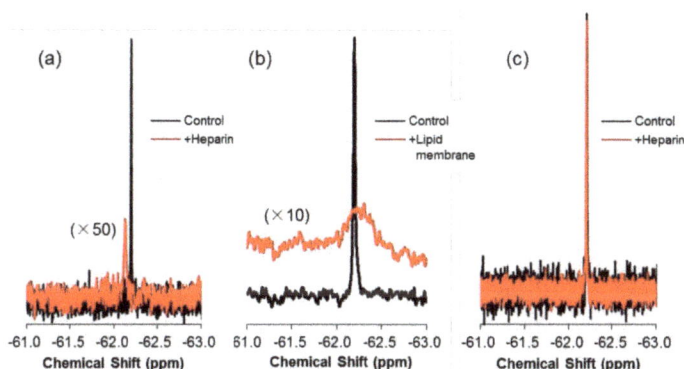

Figure 3. ^{19}F NMR spectra of ^{19}F-R8 in the presence of heparin and lipid membrane. ^{19}F NMR spectra of 80 μM ^{19}F-R8 in the presence (red) and absence (black) of (**a**) 80 μM heparin and (**b**) a 40-mM EPC/EPG bilayer membrane at 4 °C (pH 7.4). The spectra of 100 μM ^{19}F-T6 in the presence of 200 μM of heparin is also shown in (**c**) for comparison.

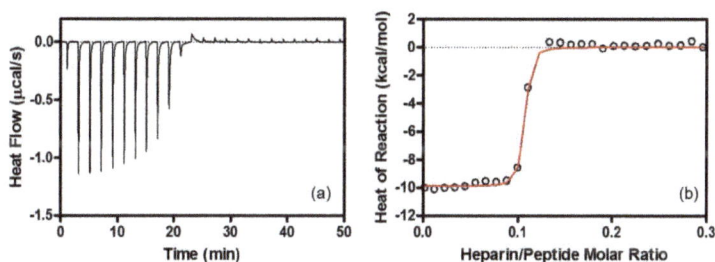

Figure 4. ITC associated with the interaction between R8 and heparin. (**a**) ITC for heparin (100 μM) injection into R8 (45 μM) at 25 °C. Each peak in heat flow chart corresponds to the injection of 1.0 μL aliquots of heparin. (**b**) Heat reactions (integrated from the calorimetric trace, and corrected for the dilution control) plotted as a function of heparin/peptide molar ratio. The solid line is the best fit to the experimental data. Buffer: 10 mM Tris-HCl buffer containing 15 mM NaCl at pH 7.4. The calculated parameters are listed in Table 1.

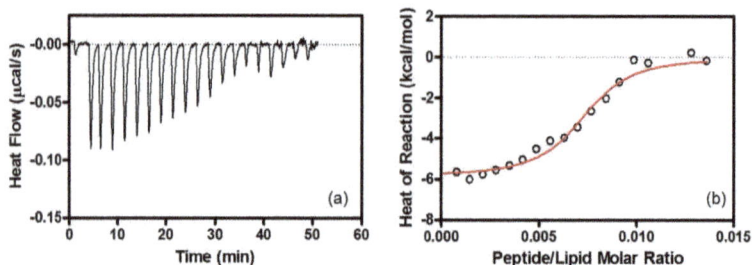

Figure 5. ITC associated with the interaction between R8 and lipid membrane. (**a**) ITC for R8 (51 µM) injection into EPC/EPG LUV (500 µM) at 25 °C. Each peak in heat flow chart corresponds to the injection of 2.0-µL aliquots of R8. (**b**) Heat reaction (integrated from the calorimetric trace, and corrected for the dilution control) plotted as a function of peptide/lipid molar ratio. The solid line is the best fit to the experimental data. Buffer: 10 mM Tris-HCl buffer containing 15 mM NaCl at pH 7.4. The calculated parameters are listed in Table 1.

Based on the assignment of the ^{19}F NMR spectra in Figure 2, here we propose a hypothesis about the most probable mechanism of non-endocytic membrane translocation of ^{19}F-R8 to HL60 cells as the following: (1) ^{19}F-R8 first binds to GAG (state I); (2) penetrates into cell membrane (state II); and (3) finally enters the cytosol (state III). In Figure 2b, the three components of ^{19}F-R8 bound to GAG, ^{19}F-R8 in membrane, and in cytosol are demonstrated by the dotted lines in black, green, and red, respectively, together with the free component (Free) in blue. It is found that the signal of ^{19}F-R8 bound to GAG and that in membrane already appear 4 min after the addition to cells. The GAG signal quickly decays with time and almost disappears after 6 min. Meanwhile, the membrane signal decays slowly as compared to GAG. Then, the signal in cytosol (Cytosol) is identified at 6 min, a few minutes after GAG and Membrane peaks are observed. The Cytosol signal is gradually increased with time and almost unchanged after 10 min, to confirm the equilibrium state of the translocation of ^{19}F-R8 to HL cells. The observed minute-ordered direct membrane translocation of ^{19}F-labeled octaarginine is consistent with our previous study that has confirmed the cell penetration of fluorescently-labeled octaarginine within at least 30 min [20]. There have also been reported that the fluorescently-labeled R8 and biotin-labeled nonaarginine penetrate into cells after about 5 min at 4 °C [7,8].

To verify the reliability of the analysis, a membrane-impermeable human lens αA-crystallin fragment, called ^{19}F-T6 (TV-(4CF$_3$-Phe)-DSGISEVR), was added to HL60 cells, and the spectra were compared. As ^{19}F-T6 includes two acidic and one cationic amino acids, the negative net charge is held under physiological conditions. The interaction between ^{19}F-T6 and negatively charged GAG is, therefore, not expected at the cell surface. In fact, as shown in Figure 2c,d, no changes were found in the ^{19}F NMR spectrum nor the difference spectrum of ^{19}F-T6 even 16 min after the addition to cells. The situation is a sharp contrast to ^{19}F-R8 where the equilibrium has been already attained for the membrane translocation process. The spectrum of ^{19}F-T6 was not changed even after 46 min (data not shown). The result demonstrates that no interaction occurs between ^{19}F-T6 and HL60 cells. This is also supported by the fact that the spectra of ^{19}F-T6 are not altered after it is added to heparin (Figure 3c), indicating no binding of ^{19}F-T6 to negatively charged GAG on the cell surface.

2.2. Quantitative Analysis of Direct Membrane Translocation

So far, no reports about in-situ quantity of CPPs in cells have been available. Here, by using the integral signal intensities of the real-time ^{19}F NMR difference spectra (Figure 2b), the quantities of four ^{19}F-R8 components, Free, GAG, Membrane, and Cytosol can be evaluated as a function of time. Detailed procedures are described in Appendix A. Figure 6 quantifies how the concentration of each ^{19}F-R8 component varied after the addition to HL60 cells. The amount of free ^{19}F-R8 gradually decreased for the first 5 min. This corresponds to the uptake of free ^{19}F-R8 to HL60 cells via the binding to GAG. At least 65 μM (81%) of ^{19}F-R8 was, however, remaining in a free state after the equilibrium was attained (at 16 min). The amount of ^{19}F-R8 bound to GAG, at first, increased but decreased to less than 5 μM within a short period of 4–6 min. This quick decrease is thought to be due to the transfer of ^{19}F-R8 to the membrane from the cell surface. In fact, the amount of ^{19}F-R8 in the membrane was gradually increased to 9 μM at 6 min, and then slightly decreased. The decrease in ^{19}F-R8 in membrane suggests that the peptide was delivered to cytosol after passing through the membrane. Actually, the transfer of ^{19}F-R8 to cytosol was first observed at around 5 min, followed by the increase up to about 6 μM.

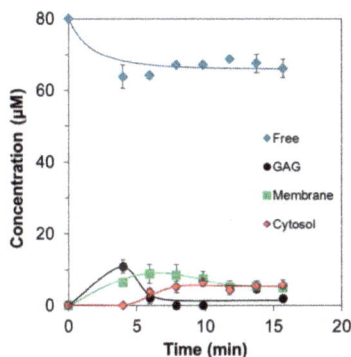

Figure 6. Real-time changes of ^{19}F-R8 concentrations in HL60 cells. The ^{19}F-R8 concentrations in outside (blue), bound to GAG (black), bound to membrane (green), and in cytosol (red) of HL60 cells at 4 °C are shown as a function of time. Each symbol represents the experimental value from the NMR signal intensity. Solid lines represent a visual guide.

It should be noted that the movement of ^{19}F-R8 from cytosol to the membrane occurs as frequently as the entry into cytosol because the concentrations of ^{19}F-R8 in membrane and in cytosol at the equilibrium state after 16 min are found to be equal within the experimental error. The relatively low concentrations are both reasonable from the fact that cell membranes impose a hydrophobic barrier on highly cationic R8 [49,50].

2.3. ^{19}F-R8 Distribution under Equilibrium

In the previous sections, we succeeded in comprehensive observation and quantitative analysis of the non-endocytic translocation of ^{19}F-R8 to the cell inside. To confirm that ^{19}F-R8 is actually transferred to cytosol across the cell membrane, the final distribution of ^{19}F-R8 was evaluated by cell fractionation after equilibrium was attained in real-time NMR measurements. Membrane solubilization and centrifugation techniques were combined in accordance with Scheme 1. First, we examined how much of ^{19}F-R8 was finally bound to cells. In Figure 7a, the ^{19}F NMR spectra of ^{19}F-R8 in the supernatant **I** is compared with total ^{19}F-R8 as a control at 4 °C. The ^{19}F NMR signal intensity of the supernatant **I** corresponds to ^{19}F-R8 that is still in a free (unbound) state under equilibrium. It is found that 77% of ^{19}F-R8 was in a free state. The value is consistent with the result of the real-time in-cell NMR measurement showing about 65 μM (81%) of ^{19}F-R8 is remaining in a free state after the equilibrium is attained (Figure 6). Next, to confirm that ^{19}F-R8 is actually bound to HL60 cell, the cell pellet **I** was solubilized by lysis buffer containing 1% Triton X-100. After the centrifugation, the supernatant **II** was subject to ^{19}F NMR measurement at 4 °C. The spectrum is shown in Figure 7b as Lysate, and 13% of the initial ^{19}F-R8 was detected.

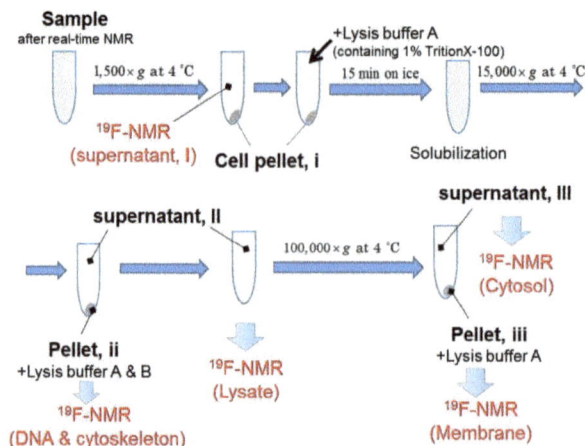

Scheme 1. Procedures of cell fractionation after real-time NMR measurement.

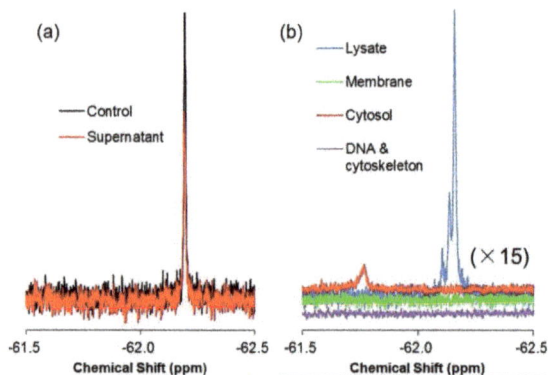

Figure 7. Final distribution of ^{19}F-R8 in HL60 cells. (**a**) ^{19}F NMR spectra of ^{19}F-R8 in PBS (control) and the supernatant I after real-time in-cell ^{19}F NMR measurement at 4 °C. The spectra were obtained at 4 °C, pH 7.4. (**b**) ^{19}F NMR spectra of ^{19}F-R8 fractions separated by solubilization and centrifugation in accordance with Scheme 1. All spectra were observed at 4 °C and pH 7.5. The signal of cytosol fraction is shifted as a result of the interaction with concentrated lysis buffer components, because supernatant III, containing lysis buffer A, was lyophilized and dissolved in large amount of lysis buffer again.

It is considered that three components of ^{19}F-R8 are contained in the Lysate. They include ^{19}F-R8 bound to GAG or cell membrane, and ^{19}F-R8 in cytosol. We separated these components as the supernatant **III** and the pellet **III** by centrifuging the Lysate at 100,000× *g*. Supernatant **III** consists of ^{19}F-R8 in cytosol, and pellet **III** contains ^{19}F-R8 bound to GAG or cell membrane (referred as Membrane); see Scheme 1. The ^{19}F NMR spectrum of the supernatant **III** at 4 °C shows that the signal of ^{19}F-R8 is observed in the cytosol fraction; see the red line in Figure 7b. The result is valuable because the ^{19}F-R8 entry into cytosol through HL60 cell membranes is actually demonstrated. This is a contrast to the absence of TFA peak in the Lysate fraction (Figure S3), indicating that the counter TFA ions of ^{19}F-R8 remain outside cells after the real-time in-cell ^{19}F NMR measurement. On the other hand, the ^{19}F-R8 in the membrane fraction is found to be within the experimental error at an equilibrium state. Although undesirable loss of peptide may be induced by the extensive solubilization and centrifugation for cell fractionation, almost no appearance of the membrane fraction is probably due to the signal broadening, as seen in spectra of ^{19}F-R8 bound to GAG or EPC/EPG LUV (Figure 3a,b). It should be noted that the observed chemical shift of NMR signal in this system is too complicated to understand. For example, the cell solubilization exposes ^{19}F-R8 to numerous molecules derived from cells. Also, the cytosol fraction was obtained by lyophilization of 50 mL lysis buffer A. This leads to the increased concentrations of components (Triton X-100, Tris-HCl, EDTA, NaCl in lysis buffer A) in the final sample to be measured. The condition of the solvent such as ionic strength and pH affects the chemical shift of ^{19}F-R8 NMR signal. Thus the integral NMR intensity is useful for the steady state NMR spectra because it is basically proportional to the nuclear concentration [51].

As ^{19}F-R8 is cationic, it is possible that ^{19}F-R8 is finally bound to DNA in the nucleus of HL60 cells. We explored whether ^{19}F-R8 was bound to DNA or cytoskeleton by solubilizing pellet **II** in accordance with Scheme 1. As shown in Figure 7b, the ^{19}F NMR signal of ^{19}F-R8 in the DNA and cytoskeleton was not yet detectable. Although further investigation is required, this may be due to the fact that the binding of ^{19}F-R8 to cellular component is too tight to be solubilized. In such case, the intensity of the NMR signal is underestimated by the signal broadening, similar to the case of membrane fraction.

3. Discussion

In the present study, we successfully observed the real-time processes of the direct membrane translocation of ^{19}F-R8 into HL60 cells without any perturbation of the system. Based on the results, we can discuss the plausible mechanism as illustrated in Figure 8.

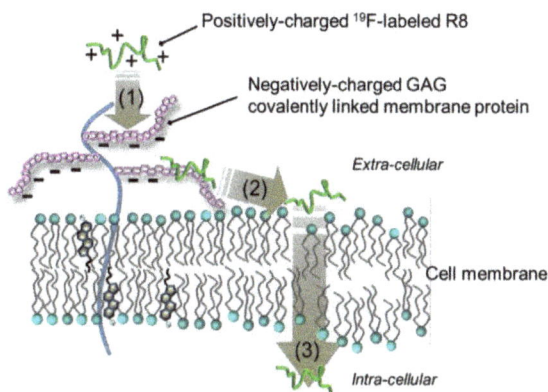

Figure 8. A plausible mechanism for non-endocytic, energy-independent translocation of ^{19}F-R8 into cells. The mechanism involves (1) binding of ^{19}F-R8 to GAG at the cell surface, followed by (2) the transfer to the cell membrane and (3) the entry into cytosol.

As a first step of the entry into cells, cationic ^{19}F-R8 electrostatically binds to negatively charged GAGs at the cell surface. Consistent with this, the same conclusion has been reached that arginine-rich CPPs such as R8 at first bind to GAGs at the cell surface [20,46]. Considering the fact that the fraction of acidic charged phospholipids in biological plasma membranes is only about 10%–20%, and that the lipids are predominantly distributed to inner leaflet of the membrane [52], it seems that ^{19}F-R8 bound to GAGs remains outside cells. However, contrary to the expectation, quantitative NMR analysis demonstrated the entry of cationic ^{19}F-R8 into hydrophobic cell membrane after binding to GAGs (Figures 2b and 6). One possibility is that the charge neutralization of polyarginine with GAGs would lead to insoluble peptide-GAG complexes [14,17,41], which is likely to be energetically unstable since GAGs are covalently immobilized to membrane protein at the water-abundant cell surface [53,54]. As a result, ^{19}F-R8 bound to GAG is likely to dissociate from GAGs to water or rapidly transfer to cell membrane. Indeed, it was reported that the cationic ^{19}F-R8 bound to the amphipathic sulfate compounds favorably partitions into octanol phase as cell membrane model via hydrophobic interactions [55,56]. In addition, bidentate hydrogen bonding between guanidino group of arginine and lipid phosphate makes the arginine-rich peptides stable in a hydrophobic environment [57–59]. Taken together, our results suggest that the charge neutralization of arginine-rich peptides by the presence of negatively charged GAG accelerates the peptide entry into the hydrophobic membrane inside.

Afterwards, ^{19}F-R8 is transferred to the cytosol. In order to enter the inside of cells, ^{19}F-R8 should pass through the hydrophobic cell membrane. Because ^{19}F-R8 is inherently hydrophilic, it is hard to enter the hydrophobic lipid bilayer.

One possibility to compensate this difficulty is to utilize the lipid movement in the vertical direction to the membrane surface. It is expected that the entry of ^{19}F-R8 into the cell is enhanced by synchronization with the vertical fluctuation of the membrane lipid. In fact, such movement, called protrusion, has been observed in the cell-sized lipid bilayer vesicle [60]. In this sense, the lipid protrusion motion is considered as one of the key factors for the direct membrane translocation of CPPs. This is especially the case under physiological conditions at 37 °C. At 4 °C, however, the direct translocation probability of ^{19}F-R8 is low due to impaired membrane fluidity. The protrusion is inhibited at low temperatures even in the fluid phase [60]. Recently, it has been reported that the most plausible mechanism for the direct membrane translocation of arginine-rich peptides is a transient pore formation, in which the peptides induce membrane perturbation so that it can easily pass through the membrane [56,61–65]. The lifetime of the toroidal pore is thought to be short enough to guarantee no cytotoxicity [66–68]. The trypan blue staining after the NMR measurement showed that ^{19}F-R8 did not lower cell viability, being consistent with the transient pore formation model.

In conclusion, the present in-cell NMR study is the first report to comprehensively observe and quantitatively analyze the direct translocation processes of cell penetrating ^{19}F-R8 in situ. Based on the results, a new insight into the mechanism for the entry of cationic ^{19}F-R8 into hydrophobic membrane after binding to negatively charged GAGs was obtained. The present study shows a potential for elucidating direct membrane translocation mechanism of CPPs with minimal perturbation.

4. Materials and Methods

4.1. Materials

The ^{19}F-labeled octaarginine (^{19}F-R8: (4CF$_3$-Phe)-RRRRRRRR) was synthesized manually by solid phase synthesis method using Fmoc chemistry. The amino and carboxyl termini of the peptide were acetylated and amidated, respectively. A fragment peptide, called ^{19}F-T6 (TV-(4CF$_3$-Phe)-DSGISEVR), from human lens αA-crystallin [69] was used as a negative control and synthesized by Fmoc solid-phase chemistry using an automated solid-phase synthesizer (PSSM-8; Shimadzu, Kyoto, Japan). The purity of each peptide was confirmed to be > 95% by reversed-phase high-performance liquid chromatography and MALDI-TOF mass spectrometry. Heparin sodium salt (from porcine intestinal mucosa; average molecular weight, 18,000 Da) was purchased from SIGMA (St. Louis, MO, USA). Egg phosphatidylcholine (EPC, > 96% pure) and egg phosphatidylglycerol (EPG, > 95% pure) were obtained from the NOF CORPORATION (Tokyo, Japan). All other reagents were of special grade and used without further purification.

4.2. Cell Culture

A human leukemia cell line HL60 was maintained in RPMI 1640 medium, supplemented with 8% heat-inactivated fetal calf serum (FCS), 100 U/mL penicillin and 100 µg/mL streptomycin in 5% CO$_2$ humidified air at 37 °C.

4.3. Preparation of Large Unilamellar Vesicle (LUV)

EPC/EPG LUV was prepared by using an extrusion method previously reported [70]. Briefly, EPC and EPG were dissolved in chloroform at a molar ratio of PC/PG = 4/1 in a round-bottomed flask and dried with a rotary evaporator to create a thin and homogeneous lipid film. The lipid film was vortexed in Tris-HCl buffer (pH 7.4) containing 15 mM NaCl to obtain vesicle suspension. The resultant suspension was subjected to five cycles of freeze–thawing and was then passed through a Mini-extruder equipped with two stacked 0.1-μm polycarbonate filters (Avanti Polar Lipids, Alabaster, AL, USA). The concentration of phospholipids was determined by the Bartlett method [71].

4.4. Real-Time In-Cell ^{19}F NMR Measurement

One-dimensional in-cell ^{19}F NMR measurements were carried out at 376.2 MHz by using a JEOL ECA400 NMR spectrometer equipped with a superconducting magnet of 9.4 T. A multinuclear probe (JEOL, NM40T10A/AT) for a 10-mm diameter tube was used. Detailed procedures of the measurement are described elsewhere [23]. Briefly, HL60 cells (the final concentration, 1×10^7 cells/mL) were suspended in phosphate-buffered saline (PBS, pH 7.4) at 4 °C and put into a NMR tube. In order to confirm no contribution of energy-dependent endocytosis at 4 °C, the comparative measurement was also performed at 37 °C. To avoid cellular toxicity, the amount of D_2O used for the signal lock was decreased to 10%. The sample was gently rotated to prevent the sedimentation of the cells. Field-gradient shimming was applied before the addition of the peptide, to quickly attain the spectral resolution. The measurements started immediately after the thermal equilibrium was attained, 1.5 min after the addition of the ^{19}F-labeled peptides. The final concentrations of ^{19}F-R8 and ^{19}F-T6 were 80 μM and 100 μM, respectively, and these were high enough to observe non-endocytic translocation [7,10,26]. Free induction decays (FIDs) were accumulated at 16 time/2-min intervals. For ^{19}F-R8, the in-cell ^{19}F NMR measurement was repeated three times. The spectra were processed by the JEOL DELTA software. Chemical shift of the ^{19}F NMR signal was obtained by referring to the absorption frequency of the trifluoroacetic acid in the solvent. Cell viability, assessed by the trypan blue staining after the NMR measurement at 4 °C, was 92% ± 1% for ^{19}F-R8 and 94% ± 1% for ^{19}F-T6 with respect to the control value, 94% ± 2%. At 37 °C, the viability was 92% ± 2% and 95% ± 3% in the presence and absence of ^{19}F-R8, respectively.

4.5. Steady State ^{19}F NMR Measurement

The amount of ^{19}F-R8 finally delivered to the cytosol was quantified by ^{19}F NMR under equilibrium in combination with the cell fractionation using membrane solubilization and centrifugation. The cell fractionation procedures are summarized in Scheme 1. After the real-time ^{19}F NMR measurement, 4 mL of the sample were centrifuged at 1500× *g* for 5 min at 4 °C. Pellet I was washed twice with 4 mL of PBS and centrifuged again. Then the 8 mL of supernatant I was collected and subject to ^{19}F NMR measurement at 4 °C, to quantify free ^{19}F-R8. Next, 4 mL of lysis buffer A (1% Triton X-100, 50 mM Tris-HCl, 50 mM EDTA, 150 mM NaCl, 10% D_2O) was added to pellet **I**, and left for 15 min on ice to complete the cell membrane solubilization. The solution was centrifuged at 15,000× *g* for 15 min at 4 °C, to separate pellet **II** and supernatant **II**. Then, supernatant **II** was collected and subjected to ^{19}F NMR measurement at 4 °C (called Lysate). After measurement, 50 mL of lysis buffer A was added and centrifuged at 100,000× *g* for 3 h at 4 °C. Pellet **III** contains cell membrane and supernatant **III** corresponded to the cytosol fraction [72]. Pellet **III** was resuspended in 4 mL of lysis buffer A and subjected to ^{19}F NMR measurement at 4 °C (called Membrane). On the other hand, supernatant **III** was lyophilized and resuspended in 4 mL of lysis buffer A, and subjected to ^{19}F NMR measurement at 4 °C (Cytosol). Pellet **II** was incubated in 1 mL of lysis buffer A containing 0.5 M NaCl for 15 min on ice, and added to 3 mL of lysis buffer B (0.05% SDS, 0.5% deoxycholic acid, 50 mM Tris-HCl, 5 mM EDTA, 150 mM NaCl, 10% D_2O, pH 7.5). Then the solubilized fractions were subjected to ^{19}F NMR measurement at 4 °C (DNA and cytoskeleton). In each experiment, the FIDs were accumulated 10,000–60,000 times to attain a high signal to noise ratio.

4.6. Isothermal Titration Calorimetry (ITC)

ITC measurements were carried out on an iTC200 system (MicroCal) at 25 °C in 10 mM Tris-HCl buffer at pH 7.4. Peptide solution was placed in the reaction cell, and titrated with aliquots of heparin, or EPC/EPG LUV. The ITC injections were repeated automatically at 25 °C under 1000 rpm stirring. The heats of reaction were corrected for dilution control. Thermodynamic parameters were determined by non-linear least-square fitting of the data using the single site binding model in program Origin for ITC version 7 (MicroCal) with the stoichiometry (n), the enthalpy of the reaction ($\Delta H°$), and the association constant (K) [45,73,74]. The Gibbs free energy $\Delta G°$ and entropy $\Delta S°$ for binding of R8 to heparin or EPC/EPG LUV were obtained by the following equations:

$$\Delta G° = -RT\ln K \tag{1}$$

and

$$T\Delta S° = \Delta H° - \Delta G° \tag{2}$$

where T is the absolute temperature.

Supplementary Materials: The following are available online at http://www.mdpi.com/1424-8247/10/2/42/s1, Figure S1: ^{19}F NMR spectrum of ^{19}F-R8 solution, Figure S2: Time course of ^{19}F NMR signal intensity of ^{19}F-R8 after addition to HL60 cells, Figure S3: Final distribution of trifluoroacetate counterions of ^{19}F-R8.

Acknowledgments: This work was partly supported by Grants-in-Aid for Scientific Research 24550035 and 15K05401 from Japan Society for the Promotion of Science, Hyogo Science and Technology Association Research Grant 25073 and performed under the Cooperative Research Program of Institute for Protein Research, Osaka University.

Author Contributions: Y.T.-H., Y.T. and E.O. conceived and designed the experiments; Y.T.-H., K.A., Y.T., T.K. and E.O. performed the experiments; Y.T.-H., K.A., Y.H. and E.O. analyzed the data; Y.T., T.K., H.S. and E.O. contributed reagents/materials/analysis tools; Y.T.-H. and E.O. wrote the paper.

Conflicts of Interest: The authors declare no conflict of interest.

Appendix A

Concentration Analysis

Cell peptide concentrations inside and outside were estimated by using the signal intensities of real-time ^{19}F NMR difference spectra in Figure 2b. Figure A1 illustrates how peptide concentrations were determined from the ^{19}F NMR spectra. As compared to the control signal at −62.20 ppm (a), one negative and two positive peaks are found in this case, with respect to the baseline in the difference spectrum (b). The negative peak corresponds to the decreased fraction of free (unbound) peptide because the peak minimum at −62.20 ppm is similar to the control (a). The positive peaks at −62.19 and −62.21 ppm can be assigned to ^{19}F-R8 bound to GAG and cell membrane; see Results for peak assignment.

The concentration of these three components can be evaluated from the signal intensities by integrating the respective peak areas. For example, the fraction of the decrease in free ^{19}F-R8 component, shaded blue area in the spectrum (b), is estimated as 16.3% with respect to the control, 100% (a). Thus, the free component remaining in cell outside is calculated as 83.7%. Similarly, the increase in the fraction bound to GAG (in gray) and membrane (in green) is estimated as 11.4 and 6.6%. Since the total ^{19}F-R8 concentration is 80 µM, the concentrations of free, bound to GAG, and membrane components are calculated to be 67, 9, and 5 µM, respectively.

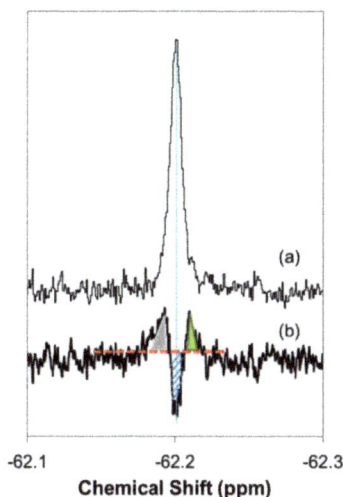

Chemical Shift (ppm)

Figure A1. Illustration of the signal intensity estimation in the ^{19}F NMR difference spectrum. The spectrum (**a**) shows an ^{19}F-R8 signal in PBS (control), and (**b**) is an example of an NMR difference spectrum obtained by subtracting (**a**) from the ^{19}F-R8 spectrum 4 min after the peptide was added to cells. The baseline in the difference spectrum is designated by a broken red line. In (**b**), one negative peak at −62.20 ppm and two positive peaks at −62.19 and −62.21 ppm are found. The negative signal (in blue, shaded) is assigned to ^{19}F-R8 in a free (unbound) state, and positive ones correspond to ^{19}F-R8 bound to GAG (in gray) and cell membrane (in green). The negative peak at −62.20 ppm means the decrease in free peptide. The concentration of these three components can be evaluated from the signal intensities by integrating the respective peak areas (see text).

References

1. Trabulo, S.; Cardoso, A.L.; Mano, M.; de Lima, M.C.P. Cell-penetrating peptides-mechanisms of cellular uptake and generation of delivery systems. *Pharmaceuticals* **2010**, *3*, 961–993. [CrossRef] [PubMed]
2. Keller, A.A.; Mussbach, F.; Breitling, R.; Hemmerich, P.; Schaefer, B.; Lorkowski, S.; Reissmann, S. Relationships between cargo, cell penetrating peptides and cell type for uptake of non-covalent complexes into live cells. *Pharmaceuticals* **2013**, *6*, 184–203. [CrossRef] [PubMed]
3. Howl, J.; Matou-Nasri, S.; West, D.C.; Farquhar, M.; Slaninová, J.; Östenson, C.G.; Zorko, M.; Östlund, P.; Kumar, S.; Langel, Ü.; et al. Bioportide: An emergent concept of bioactive cell-penetrating peptides. *Cell. Mol. Life Sci.* **2012**, *69*, 2951–2966. [CrossRef] [PubMed]
4. Liu, B.R.; Lin, M.D.; Chiang, H.J.; Lee, H.; Revon, B. Arginine-rich cell-penetrating peptides deliver gene into living human cells. *Gene* **2012**, *505*, 37–45. [CrossRef] [PubMed]
5. Jones, A.T.; Sayers, E.J. Cell entry of cell penetrating peptides and tales of tails wagging dogs. *J. Control. Release* **2012**, *161*, 582–591. [CrossRef] [PubMed]
6. Bechara, C.C.; Sagan, S. Cell-penetrating peptides: 20 years later, where do we stand? *FEBS Lett.* **2013**, *587*, 1693–1702. [CrossRef] [PubMed]
7. Kosuge, M.; Takeuchi, T.; Nakase, I.; Jones, A.T.; Futaki, S. Cellular internalization and distribution of arginine-rich peptides as a function of extracellular peptide concentration, serum, and plasma membrane associated proteoglycans. *Bioconjug. Chem.* **2008**, *19*, 656–664. [CrossRef] [PubMed]
8. Jiao, C.Y.; Delaroche, D.; Burlina, F.; Alves, I.D.; Chassaing, G.; Sagan, S. Translocation and Endocytosis for Cell-Penetrating Peptide Internalization. *J. Biol. Chem.* **2009**, *284*, 33957–33965. [CrossRef] [PubMed]
9. Watkins, C.L.; Schmaljohann, D.; Futaki, S.; Jones, A.T. Low concentration thresholds of plasma membranes for rapid energy-independent translocation of a cell-penetrating peptide. *Biochem. J.* **2009**, *420*, 179–189. [CrossRef] [PubMed]

10. Broc, R. The uptake of arginine-rich cell-penetrating peptides: Putting the puzzle together. *Bioconjug. Chem.* **2014**, *25*, 863–868. [CrossRef] [PubMed]
11. Ziegler, A. Thermodynamic studies and binding mechanisms of cell-penetrating peptides with lipids and glycosaminoglycans. *Adv. Drug Deliv. Rev.* **2008**, *60*, 580–597. [CrossRef] [PubMed]
12. Amand, H.L.; Rydberg, H.A.; Fornander, L.H.; Lincoln, P.; Nordén, B.; Esbjörner, E.K. Cell surface binding and uptake of arginine- and lysine-rich penetratin peptides in absence and presence of proteoglycans. *Biochim. Biophys. Acta Biomembr.* **2012**, *1818*, 2669–2678. [CrossRef] [PubMed]
13. Naik, R.J.; Chatterjee, A.; Ganguli, M. Different roles of cell surface and exogenous glycosaminoglycans in controlling gene delivery by arginine-rich peptides with varied distribution of arginines. *Biochim. Biophys. Acta Biomembr.* **2013**, *1828*, 1484–1493. [CrossRef] [PubMed]
14. Bechara, C.; Pallerla, M.; Zaltsman, Y.; Burlina, F.; Alves, I.D.; Lequin, O.; Sagan, S. Tryptophan within basic peptide sequences triggers glycosaminoglycan-dependent endocytosis. *FASEB J.* **2013**, *27*, 738–749. [CrossRef] [PubMed]
15. Nakase, I.; Niwa, M.; Takeuchi, T.; Sonomura, K.; Kawabata, N.; Koike, Y.; Takehashi, M.; Tanaka, S.; Ueda, K.; Simpson, J.C.; et al. Cellular uptake of arginine-rich peptides: Roles for macropinocytosis and actin rearrangement. *Mol. Ther.* **2004**, *10*, 1011–1022. [CrossRef] [PubMed]
16. Mishra, A.; Hwee, G.; Schmidt, N.W.; Sun, V.Z.; Rodriguez, A.R.; Tong, R.; Tang, L.; Lai, G.H.; Cheng, J.; Deming, T.J.; et al. Translocation of HIV TAT peptide and analogues induced by multiplexed membrane and cytoskeletal interactions. *Proc. Natl. Acad. Sci. USA* **2011**, *108*, 16883–16888. [CrossRef] [PubMed]
17. Ziegler, A.; Seelig, J. Contributions of glycosaminoglycan binding and clustering to the biological uptake of the nonamphipathic cell-penetrating peptide WR$_9$. *Biochemistry* **2011**, *50*, 4650–4664. [CrossRef] [PubMed]
18. Silhol, M.; Tyagi, M.; Giacca, M.; Lebleu, B.; Vivès, E. Different mechanisms for cellular internalization of the HIV-1 Tat-derived cell penetrating peptide and recombinant proteins fused to Tat. *Eur. J. Biochem.* **2002**, *269*, 494–501. [CrossRef] [PubMed]
19. Gump, J.M.; June, R.K.; Dowdy, S.F. Revised role of glycosaminoglycans in TAT protein transduction domain-mediated cellular transduction. *J. Biol. Chem.* **2010**, *285*, 1500–1507. [CrossRef] [PubMed]
20. Takechi-Haraya, Y.; Nadai, R.; Kimura, H.; Nishitsuji, K.; Uchimura, K.; Sakai-Kato, K.; Kawakami, K.; Shigenaga, A.; Kawakami, T.; Otaka, A.; et al. Enthalpy-driven interactions with sulfated glycosaminoglycans promote cell membrane penetration of arginine peptides. *Biochim. Biophys. Acta Biomembr.* **2016**, *1858*, 1339–1349. [CrossRef] [PubMed]
21. Hirose, H.; Takeuchi, T.; Osakada, H.; Pujals, S.; Katayama, S.; Nakase, I.; Kobayashi, S.; Haraguchi, T.; Futaki, S. Transient focal membrane deformation induced by arginine-rich peptides leads to their direct penetration into cells. *Mol. Ther.* **2012**, *20*, 984–993. [CrossRef] [PubMed]
22. Meerovich, I.; Muthukrishnan, N.; Johnson, G.A.; Erazo-Oliveras, A.; Pellois, J.P. Photodamage of lipid bilayers by irradiation of a fluorescently labeled cell-penetrating peptide. *Biochim. Biophys. Acta Gen. Subj.* **2014**, *1840*, 507–515. [CrossRef] [PubMed]
23. Okamura, E.; Ninomiya, K.; Futaki, S.; Nagai, Y.; Kimura, T.; Wakai, C.; Matubayasi, N.; Sugiura, Y.; Nakahara, M. Real-time in-cell ^{19}F NMR study on uptake of fluorescent and nonfluorescent ^{19}F-octaarginines into human jurkat cells. *Chem. Lett.* **2005**, *34*, 1064–1065. [CrossRef]
24. Szeto, H.H.; Schiller, P.W.; Zhao, K.; Luo, G. Fluorescent dyes alter intracellular targeting and function of cell-penetrating tetrapeptides. *FASEB J.* **2005**, *19*, 118–120. [CrossRef] [PubMed]
25. Puckett, C.A.; Barton, J.K. Fluorescein redirects a ruthenium-octaarginine conjugate to the nucleus. *J. Am. Chem. Soc.* **2009**, *131*, 8738–8739. [CrossRef] [PubMed]
26. Bertrand, J.R.; Malvy, C.; Auguste, T.; Tóth, G.K.; Kiss-Ivánkovits, O.; Illyés, E.; Hollósi, M.; Bottka, S.; Laczkó, I. Synthesis and studies on cell-penetrating peptides. *Bioconjug. Chem.* **2009**, *20*, 1307–1314. [CrossRef] [PubMed]
27. Aubry, S.; Aussedat, B.; Delaroche, D.; Jiao, C.Y.; Bolbach, G.; Lavielle, S.; Chassaing, G.; Sagan, S.; Burlina, F. MALDI-TOF mass spectrometry: A powerful tool to study the internalization of cell-penetrating peptides. *Biochim. Biophys. Acta Biomembr.* **2010**, *1798*, 2182–2189. [CrossRef] [PubMed]
28. Lécorché, P.; Walrant, A.; Burlina, F.; Dutot, L.; Sagan, S.; Mallet, J.; Desbat, B.; Chassaing, G.; Alves, I.D.; Lavielle, S. Cellular uptake and biophysical properties of galactose and/or tryptophan containing cell-penetrating peptides. *Biochim. Biophys. Acta Biomembr.* **2012**, *1818*, 448–457. [CrossRef] [PubMed]

29. Walrant, A.; Matheron, L.; Cribier, S.; Chaignepain, S.; Jobin, M.L.; Sagan, S.; Alves, I.D. Direct translocation of cell penetrating peptides in liposomes: A combined mass spectrometry quantification and fluorescence detection study. *Anal. Biochem.* **2013**, *438*, 1–10. [CrossRef] [PubMed]

30. Aki, K.; Okamura, E. D-β-aspartyl residue exhibiting uncommon high resistance to spontaneous peptide bond cleavage. *Sci. Rep.* **2016**, *6*, 21594. [CrossRef] [PubMed]

31. Cobb, S.L.; Murphy, C.D. ^{19}F NMR applications in chemical biology. *J. Fluor. Chem.* **2009**, *130*, 132–143. [CrossRef]

32. Kitevski-LeBlanc, J.L.; Prosser, R.S. Current applications of ^{19}F NMR to studies of protein structure and dynamics. *Prog. Nucl. Magn. Reson. Spectrosc.* **2012**, *62*, 1–33. [CrossRef] [PubMed]

33. Serber, B.Z.; Corsini, L.; Durst, F.; Serber, Z.; Dötsch, V. In-cell NMR spectroscopy. *Methods Enzymol.* **2005**, *394*, 17–41. [PubMed]

34. Suzuki, Y.; Brender, J.J.R.; Hartman, K.; Ramamoorthy, A.; Marsh, E.N.G. Alternative pathways of human islet amyloid polypeptide aggregation distinguished by 19F NMR-detected kinetics of monomer consumption. *Biochemistry* **2012**, *51*, 8154–8162. [CrossRef] [PubMed]

35. Shi, P.; Li, D.; Chen, H.; Xiong, Y.; Wang, Y.; Tian, C. In situ ^{19}F NMR studies of an *E. coli* membrane protein. *Protein Sci.* **2012**, *21*, 596–600. [CrossRef] [PubMed]

36. Kitevski-Leblanc, J.L.; Hoang, J.; Thach, W.; Larda, S.T.; Prosser, R.S. ^{19}F NMR studies of a desolvated near-native protein folding intermediate. *Biochemistry* **2013**, *52*, 5780–5789. [CrossRef] [PubMed]

37. De la Vega, M.; Marin, M.; Kondo, N.; Miyauchi, K.; Kim, Y.; Epand, R.F.; Emapnd, R.M.; Melikyan, G.B.; de la Vega, M. Inhibition of HIV-1 endocytosis allows lipid mixing at the plasma membrane, but not complete fusion. *Retrovirology* **2011**, *8*, 99. [CrossRef] [PubMed]

38. Zeng, J.; Eckenrode, H.M.; Dounce, S.M.; Dai, H. Time-resolved molecular transport across living cell membranes. *Biophys. J.* **2013**, *104*, 139–145. [CrossRef] [PubMed]

39. Palm, C.; Jayamanne, M.; Kjellander, M.; Hällbrink, M. Peptide degradation is a critical determinant for cell-penetrating peptide uptake. *Biochim. Biophys. Acta Biomembr.* **2007**, *1768*, 1769–1776. [CrossRef] [PubMed]

40. Capila, I.; VanderNoot, V.A.; Mealy, T.R.; Seaton, B.A.; Linhardt, R.J. Interaction of heparin with annexin V. *FEBS Lett.* **1999**, *446*, 327–330. [CrossRef]

41. Ziegler, A.; Seelig, J. Interaction of the protein transduction domain of HIV-1 TAT with heparan sulfate: Binding mechanism and thermodynamic parameters. *Biophys. J.* **2004**, *86*, 254–263. [CrossRef]

42. Futamura, M.; Dhanasekaran, P.; Handa, T.; Phillips, M.C.; Lund-Katz, S.; Saito, H. Two-step mechanism of binding of apolipoprotein E to heparin: Implications for the kinetics of apolipoprotein E-heparan sulfate proteoglycan complex formation on cell surfaces. *J. Biol. Chem.* **2005**, *280*, 5414–5422. [CrossRef] [PubMed]

43. Blaum, B.S.; Deakin, J.A.; Johansson, C.M.; Herbert, A.P.; Barlow, P.N.; Lyon, M.; Uhrín, D. Lysine and arginine side chains in glycosaminoglycan-protein complexes investigated by NMR, cross-linking, and mass spectrometry: A case study of the factor H-heparin interaction. *J. Am. Chem. Soc.* **2010**, *132*, 6374–6381. [CrossRef] [PubMed]

44. Noborn, F.; Callaghan, P.O.; Hermansson, E.; Zhang, X.; Ancsin, J.B.; Damas, A.M.; Dacklin, I.; O'Callaghan, P.; Presto, J.; Johansson, J.; et al. Heparan sulfate/heparin promotes transthyretin fibrillization through selective binding to a basic motif in the protein. *Proc. Natl. Acad. Sci. USA* **2011**, *108*, 5584–5589. [CrossRef] [PubMed]

45. Solomon, J.P.; Bourgault, S.; Powers, E.T.; Kelly, J.W. Heparin binds 8 kDa gelsolin cross-β-sheet oligomers and accelerates amyloidogenesis by hastening fibril extension. *Biochemistry* **2011**, *50*, 2486–2498. [CrossRef] [PubMed]

46. Gonçalves, E.; Kitas, E.; Seelig, J. Binding of oligoarginine to membrane lipids and heparan sulfate: Structural and thermodynamic characterization of a cell-penetrating peptide. *Biochemistry* **2005**, *44*, 2692–2702. [CrossRef] [PubMed]

47. Okamura, E.; Yoshii, N. Drug binding and mobility relating to the thermal fluctuation in fluid lipid membranes. *J. Chem. Phys.* **2008**, *129*, 215102. [CrossRef] [PubMed]

48. Lopes, S.; Simeonova, M.; Gameiro, P.; Rangel, M.; Ivanova, G. Interaction of 5-fluorouracil loaded nanoparticles with 1,2-dimyristoyl-sn-glycero-3-phosphocholine liposomes used as a cellular membrane model. *J. Phys. Chem. B* **2012**, *116*, 667–675. [CrossRef] [PubMed]

49. Esbjörner, E.K.; Lincoln, P.; Nordén, B. Counterion-mediated membrane penetration: Cationic cell-penetrating peptides overcome Born energy barrier by ion-pairing with phospholipids. *Biochim. Biophys. Acta Biomembr.* **2007**, *1768*, 1550–1558. [CrossRef] [PubMed]

50. Vorobyov, I.; Allen, T.W. On the role of anionic lipids in charged protein interactions with membranes. *Biochim. Biophys. Acta Biomembr.* **2011**, *1808*, 1673–1683. [CrossRef] [PubMed]

51. Wider, G.; Dreier, L. Measuring protein concentrations by NMR spectroscopy. *J. Am. Chem. Soc.* **2006**, *128*, 2571–2576. [CrossRef] [PubMed]

52. Deleu, M.; Crowet, J.M.; Nasir, M.N.; Lins, L. Complementary biophysical tools to investigate lipid specificity in the interaction between bioactive molecules and the plasma membrane: A review. *Biochim. Biophys. Acta Biomembr.* **2014**, *1838*, 3171–3190. [CrossRef] [PubMed]

53. Belting, M. Heparan sulfate proteoglycan as a plasma membrane carrier. *Trends Biochem. Sci.* **2003**, *28*, 145–151. [CrossRef]

54. Sarrazin, S.; Lamanna, W.C.; Esko, J.D. Heparan sulfate proteoglycans. *Cold Spring Harb. Perspect. Biol.* **2011**, *3*, 1–33. [CrossRef] [PubMed]

55. Perret, F.; Nishihara, M.; Takeuchi, T.; Futaki, S.; Lazar, A.N.; Coleman, A.W.; Sakai, N.; Matile, S. Anionic fullerenes, calixarenes, coronenes, and pyrenes as activators of oligo/polyarginines in model membranes and live cells. *J. Am. Chem. Soc.* **2005**, *127*, 1114–1115. [CrossRef] [PubMed]

56. Herce, H.D.; Garcia, A.E.; Cardoso, M.C. Fundamental molecular mechanism for the cellular uptake of guanidinium-rich molecules. *J. Am. Chem. Soc.* **2014**, *136*, 17459–17467. [CrossRef] [PubMed]

57. Rothbard, J.B.; Jessop, T.C.; Wender, P.A. Adaptive translocation: The role of hydrogen bonding and membrane potential in the uptake of guanidinium-rich transporters into cells. *Adv. Drug Deliv. Rev.* **2005**, *57*, 495–504. [CrossRef] [PubMed]

58. Tang, M.; Waring, A.J.; Hong, M. Phosphate-mediated arginine insertion into lipid membranes and pore formation by a cationic membrane peptide from solid-state NMR. *J. Am. Chem. Soc.* **2007**, *129*, 11438–11446. [CrossRef] [PubMed]

59. Su, Y.; Waring, A.J.; Ruchala, P.; Hong, M. Membrane-bound dynamic structure of an arginine-rich cell-penetrating peptide, the protein transduction domain of HIV TAT, from solid-state NMR. *Biochemistry* **2010**, *49*, 6009–6020. [CrossRef] [PubMed]

60. Takechi, Y.; Saito, H.; Okamura, E. Slow tumbling but large protrusion of phospholipids in the cell sized giant vesicle. *Chem. Phys. Lett.* **2013**, *570*, 136–140. [CrossRef]

61. Bobone, S.; Piazzon, A.; Orioni, B.; Pedersen, J.Z.; Nan, Y.H.; Hahm, K.S.; Shin, S.Y.; Stella, L. The thin line between cell-penetrating and antimicrobial peptides: The case of Pep-1 and Pep-1-K. *J. Pept. Sci.* **2011**, *17*, 335–341. [CrossRef] [PubMed]

62. Henriques, S.; Melo, M.; Castanho, M. Cell-penetrating peptides and antimicrobial peptides: How different are they? *Biochem. J.* **2006**, *7*, 1–7. [CrossRef] [PubMed]

63. Herce, H.D.; Garcia, A.E. Molecular dynamics simulations suggest a mechanism for translocation of the HIV-1 TAT peptide across lipid membranes. *Proc. Natl. Acad. Sci. USA* **2007**, *104*, 20805–20810. [CrossRef] [PubMed]

64. Clark, K.S.; Svetlovics, J.; McKeown, A.N.; Huskins, L.; Almeida, P.F. What determines the activity of antimicrobial and cytolytic peptides in model membranes. *Biochemistry* **2011**, *50*, 7919–7932. [CrossRef] [PubMed]

65. Last, N.B.; Schlamadinger, D.E.; Miranker, A.D. A common landscape for membrane-active peptides. *Protein Sci.* **2013**, *22*, 1–13. [CrossRef] [PubMed]

66. El-Andaloussi, S.; Järver, P.; Johansson, H.J.; Langel, U. Cargo-dependent cytotoxicity and delivery efficacy of cell-penetrating peptides: A comparative study. *Biochem. J.* **2007**, *407*, 285–292. [CrossRef] [PubMed]

67. Sawant, R.R.; Patel, N.R.; Torchilin, V.P. Therapeutic delivery using cell-penetrating peptides. *Eur. J. Nanomed.* **2013**, *5*, 141–158. [CrossRef]

68. Jo, J.; Hong, S.; Choi, W.Y.; Lee, D.R. Cell-penetrating peptide (CPP)-conjugated proteins is an efficient tool for manipulation of human mesenchymal stromal cells. *Sci. Rep.* **2014**, *4*, 4378. [CrossRef] [PubMed]

69. Aki, K.; Fujii, N. Kinetics of isomerization and inversion of aspartate 58 of αA-crystallin peptide mimics under physiological conditions. *PLoS ONE* **2013**, *8*, e58515. [CrossRef] [PubMed]

70. Takechi, Y.; Yoshii, H.; Tanaka, M.; Kawakami, T.; Aimoto, S.; Saito, H. Physicochemical mechanism for the enhanced ability of lipid membrane penetration of polyarginine. *Langmuir* **2011**, *27*, 7099–7107. [CrossRef] [PubMed]
71. Bartlett, G.R. Phosphorus assay in column chromatography. *J. Biol. Chem.* **1959**, *234*, 466–468. [PubMed]
72. Tohyama, Y.; Yanagi, S.; Sada, K.; Yamamura, H. Translocation of p72syk to the cytoskeleton in thrombin-stimulated platelets. *J. Biol. Chem.* **1994**, *269*, 32796–32799. [PubMed]
73. Ziegler, A.; Seelig, J. High affinity of the cell-penetrating peptide HIV-1 Tat-PTD for DNA. *Biochemistry* **2007**, *46*, 8138–8145. [CrossRef] [PubMed]
74. Ziegler, A.; Seelig, J. Binding and Clustering of Glycosaminoglycans: A Common Property of Mono- and Multivalent Cell-Penetrating Compounds. *Biophys. J.* **2008**, *94*, 2142–2149. [CrossRef] [PubMed]

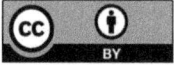

pharmaceuticals

MDPI

Review

The Good the Bad and the Ugly of Glycosaminoglycans in Tissue Engineering Applications

Bethanie I. Ayerst [1], Catherine L.R. Merry [2] and Anthony J. Day [1,*]

[1] Wellcome Trust Centre for Cell-Matrix Research, Division of Cell-Matrix Biology & Regenerative Medicine, School of Biology, Faculty of Biology, Medicine & Health, The University of Manchester, Manchester Academic Health Science Centre, Manchester M13 9PL, UK; bethayerst@me.com
[2] Stem Cell Glycobiology Group, Wolfson Centre for Stem Cells, Tissue Engineering & Modelling (STEM), Centre for Biomolecular Sciences, University of Nottingham, University Park, Nottingham NG7 2RD, UK; Cathy.Merry@nottingham.ac.uk
* Correspondence: Anthony.day@manchester.ac.uk; Tel.: +44-161-275-1495

Academic Editor: Jean Jacques Vanden Eynde
Received: 4 May 2017; Accepted: 6 June 2017; Published: 13 June 2017

Abstract: High sulfation, low cost, and the status of heparin as an already FDA- and EMA- approved product, mean that its inclusion in tissue engineering (TE) strategies is becoming increasingly popular. However, the use of heparin may represent a naïve approach. This is because tissue formation is a highly orchestrated process, involving the temporal expression of numerous growth factors and complex signaling networks. While heparin may enhance the retention and activity of certain growth factors under particular conditions, its binding 'promiscuity' means that it may also inhibit other factors that, for example, play an important role in tissue maintenance and repair. Within this review we focus on articular cartilage, highlighting the complexities and highly regulated processes that are involved in its formation, and the challenges that exist in trying to effectively engineer this tissue. Here we discuss the opportunities that glycosaminoglycans (GAGs) may provide in advancing this important area of regenerative medicine, placing emphasis on the need to move away from the common use of heparin, and instead focus research towards the utility of specific GAG preparations that are able to modulate the activity of growth factors in a more controlled and defined manner, with less off-target effects.

Keywords: glycosaminoglycans; heparin; heparan sulfate; cartilage; mesenchymal stem cells; tissue engineering; growth factors; growth differentiation factor 5; GDF5

1. Introduction

Tissue Engineering (TE) is a multidisciplinary research area involving combinations of biomaterials, differentiating cells, and bioactive factors to produce functional tissues and organs. Articular cartilage has limited ability to regenerate, and has therefore become a key target for TE strategies. However, despite sustained efforts, most techniques to date have failed to generate a truly biomimetic articular cartilage. Here we review the biology behind this highly structured tissue, the challenges that have been faced in trying to engineer cartilage, and the advancements that are currently being made within this field. In particular, we highlight the exciting potential that incorporating GAGs into cartilage TE strategies may provide, as well as the limitations and drawbacks that they may introduce if not used in a controlled manner.

2. Articular Cartilage

Articular (hyaline) cartilage is a predominantly alymphatic, aneural, and avascular tissue, consisting of chondrocytes, which make up only 1–5% of its total volume, embedded within an extensive extracellular matrix (ECM) (as reviewed [1–3]). Being widely dispersed, chondrocytes are responsible for the synthesis, maintenance and turnover of the ECM, in response to signals from growth factors, cytokines, adipokines, inflammatory mediators and matrix fragments (see [4]). Type II collagen and the proteoglycan (PG) aggrecan, play the most important structural roles in the ECM of cartilage, together forming a hydrodynamic, tensile meshwork, with a high compressive strength [2,5]. Given these properties, the tissue plays a vital role in load-bearing joints, and provides an almost frictionless surface to articulating bones [6]. The ECM of articular cartilage is also highly structured and organised, and can be divided into four spatially distinct regions, namely the superficial, middle, deep, and calcified zones (see [6–8]). As shown in Figure 1, each zone is characterised by unique ECM compositions, mechanical properties and cellular organisation. Studies have demonstrated that even small changes in the ECM of articular cartilage can lead to disruption in its mechanical properties, highlighting that structural organisation and continual remodelling of ECM molecules by chondrocytes is crucial to the proper functioning of the tissue [9,10].

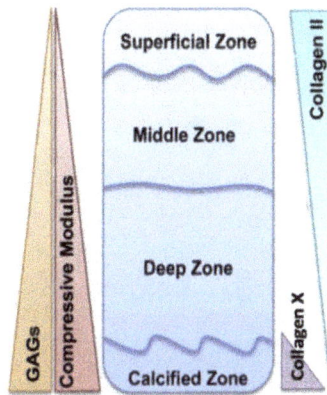

Figure 1. Schematic demonstrating the layered structure of articular cartilage. The transition from the superficial to the calcified zone is characterised by an increase in GAG content and compressive strength, but a decrease in collagen II. Collagen X is usually only found in the calcified zone of healthy articular cartilage. Figure adapted from [8,11]. Figure not to scale.

2.1. Formation

In many respects, our understanding of the mechanisms involved in the formation, organisation and maintenance of articular cartilage remain unclear and challenging [12]. Much of the progress that has been made to date has come from research into the formation of the axial and appendicular skeletons, which is initiated by limb bud development, through the highly regulated process of endochondral ossification [13–19]. This process begins early during embryogenesis with the aggregation and condensation of mesenchymal stem/stromal cells (MSCs) derived from the mesoderm germ layer. MSCs within these condensations then proliferate, increasing the cell density within the condensate, before undergoing differentiation into prechondrogenic cells that form a cartilage template/anlagen. At this stage the prechondrogenic cells are then thought to either further differentiate into chondrocytes that produce large amounts of ECM and form permanent hyaline cartilage, or into proliferating chondrocytes that form the growth plate and eventually undergo hypertrophy [19] (Figure 2A).

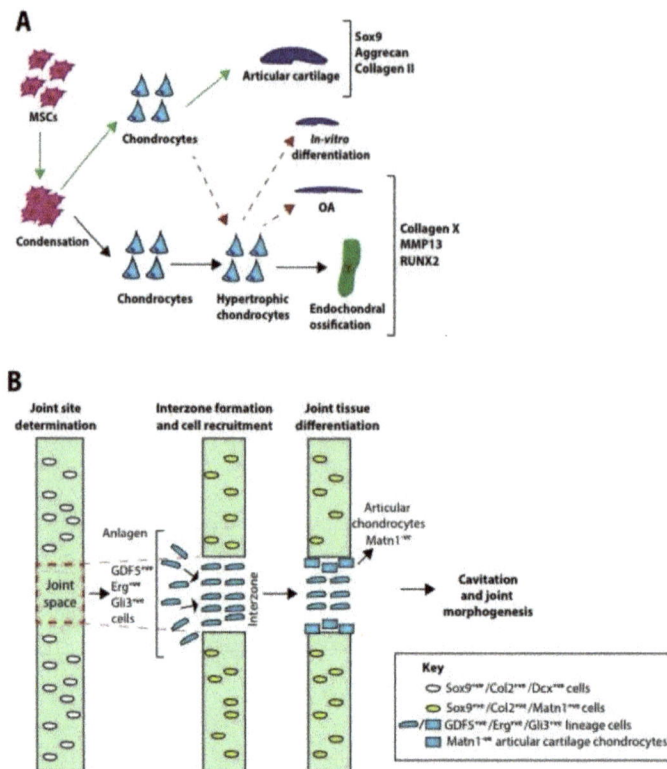

Figure 2. Articular cartilage formation. (**A**) Chondrogenesis is initiated during limb bud development with the condensation of MSCs. These progenitors then differentiate into chondrocytes that go on to form permanent articular cartilage, or into chondrocytes that eventually undergo hypertrophy and endochondral ossification. The complex spatiotemporal cues required to maintain chondrocytes in a permanent articular cartilage-like phenotype are not yet fully understood, and as such, the majority of regeneration strategies currently result in the formation of hypertrophic rather than hyaline-like tissue; (**B**) Articular cartilage is thought to originate from a distinct population of MSCs during limb joint formation; GDF5/Erg/Gli3 expressing cells within the joint space define the initial interzone MSC population, and this population becomes sandwiched between the two cartilage anlagen, while anlagen bound chondrocytes turn on expression of Matn1. GDF5/Erg/Gli3 expressing cells adjacent to their respective cartilaginous anlagen, but which have never expressed Matn1, then go on to differentiate into articular chondrocytes. (**A**) adapted from [20]; (**B**) adapted from [12]. Abbreviations: Dcx, doublecortin; OA, osteoarthritis.

Accumulating evidence suggests that permanent hyaline cartilage originates from a distinct population of MSCs, referred to as interzone cells (see [12,21]). These cells are found sandwiched between cartilage anlagen and are characterised by expression of genes such as erythroblast transformation-specific-related gene (Erg), growth differentiation factor 5 (GDF5), and GLI family zinc finger 3 (Gli3) [22–24] (see Figure 2B). Cell lineage tracing experiments have shown that as interzone cavitation and joint capsule formation occurs, articular cartilage and other synovial joint components are originated specifically from this interzone population of cells [24–26]. Notably, Hyde et al. [26], have shown that, unlike the remainder of chondrocytes in the cartilage anlagen, articular chondrocytes are derived from a specific group of chondrocytes, which have never expressed matrilin-1 (Matn1). In contrast, pre-chondrocytes found at secondary ossification sites at the edge of cartilage entities are instead transient in nature, proliferating and increasing in size before undergoing hypertrophy and contributing to bone growth [22]. Hypertrophic chondrocytes exit the cell cycle, secrete a distinct ECM rich in collagen X, and can be characterised by the expression of terminal markers of hypertrophic differentiation such as runt-related transcription factor 2 (Runx2), matrix metalloprotease 13 (MMP13), Indian hedgehog (Ihh), and collagen X [27–31]. Mineralization and blood vessel formation are also hallmarks of the phenotype [32]. Until recently, it was thought that the hypertrophic chondrocytes eventually undergo apoptosis allowing the infiltration of osteoblasts and bone formation, however, new evidence suggests some hypertrophic chondrocytes can survive the transition and become osteogenic cells [33]. Although evidence suggests that articular chondrocytes have a distinct embryonic origin from those that form the growth plate, under pathological conditions such as osteoarthritis (OA), chondrocyte hypertrophy is reactivated leading to calcification and outgrowths of bone, indicating that permanent articular chondrocytes can also acquire features of a more transient phenotype [34,35]. Chondrocyte hypertrophy is also a common outcome of in vitro and in vivo cartilage TE/regeneration strategies [30,36–41]. TE strategies must therefore focus on creating 'permanent' cartilage, which is able to maintain its structure and function throughout life and withstand hypertrophic differentiation [42] (see Figure 2A). A clearer understanding of the mechanisms and factors that trigger and suppress entry into the hypertrophic differentiation pathway will therefore be key to the success of future approaches.

2.2. Disease and Trauma

The low cell density and avascular nature of articular cartilage means that the tissue has limited potential for regeneration and repair following injury [3,43]. Instead, when a traumatic lesion, or degenerative disease occurs, the defect is filled with fibrous tissue, which is often unable to withstand the compressive and shear forces which act upon the joint, leading to cartilage breakdown, pain and immobility (as reviewed [3,43]). Cartilage damage can occur as a result of traumatic injuries such as ligament tears, impact, joint dislocation, infection and inflammation. While biomechanical loading is necessary for articular cartilage homeostasis, abnormal, or altered loading is associated with inflammation, metabolic imbalances and joint instability (see [44]). Damage can also occur gradually as the result of degenerative joint diseases such as OA, characterised by pain, structural changes, gradual loss of articular cartilage, and eventual direct bone-bone contact and joint destruction [45]. In OA it is still unclear whether it is the chondrocytes that drive cartilage pathology, or whether they are just responding to the disease process from elsewhere in the joint [46]; the balance between these processes may differ between patients and disease subgroups. OA is an epidemic problem and a major cause of decreased quality of life in adults [47]. It is estimated that one third of people over the age of 45 have sought treatment for OA in the UK [48], and this number is expected to rise in line with the ageing population and increasing obesity problem [49]. Therefore, there is a great need for the development of new approaches to prevent and treat cartilage damage.

2.3. Current Therapies

While knee-replacement surgery is becoming an increasingly common procedure, with around 97,000 replacements carried out each year in the UK alone [50], treatment of cartilage injury at an earlier stage to postpone or avoid total joint replacement would be preferable. Current treatments used in the clinic for cartilage damage include mosaicplasty, autologous chondrocyte implantation (ACI), and microfracture, each of which have shown various degrees of success, but which prove typically unsatisfactory in the long term [51,52]. For example, in the case of mosaicplasty, damaged cartilage is replaced with cartilage plugs (allo- or auto-grafts), which are poor at integrating with the host tissue, and in the case of allografts, have the potential for disease transmission [53]. ACI was first described in 1994, and involves the use of autologous chondrocytes, which are isolated from an uninjured area of the knee, expanded, and injected into the area of the defect [54]. The procedure has since been adapted to include the use of collagen/hyaluronan (HA) scaffolds (matrix-induced ACI

(MACI)), allowing for improved cell attachment and outcomes [55,56]. However, numerous limitations bedevil ACI/MACI outcomes, including donor site morbidity, the amount of time taken to expand the cells ex vivo, the inability to treat large cartilage defects, expense, and patient disability for long periods of time before surgical implantation can take place [51,57]. In addition, adult chondrocytes are known to de-differentiate during the expansion process, losing their spherical morphology and ability to synthesize aggrecan and collagen II [58,59]. Following implantation, hypertrophic growth has also been associated with these grafts [60]. Chondrocytes of older patients also have age-related intrinsic changes, such as decreased mitotic activity and telomere length [61,62]. As already mentioned, it is also unclear whether degenerative diseases such as OA are an ageing disorder of the chondrocyte itself, or whether chondrocytes are simply responding to the disease process initiated elsewhere [46]. Ultimately, therapeutic options for articular cartilage repair remain insufficient, despite the increasing prevalence of cartilage disease. While the use of chondrocytes in ACI/MACI procedures has marked the first steps in repairing damaged cartilage, with an ageing population the need for a more reliable, efficient and durable method of cartilage repair is clear.

3. Mesenchymal Stem Cells

Stem cells have become an attractive alternative to the use of chondrocytes for cartilage TE strategies, due to their relative abundance, self-renewal, and multipotent or pluripotent capabilities, therefore avoiding many of the limitations of chondrocytes [63–65]. The best stem cell source for cartilage TE is yet to be identified, with MSCs, embryonic stem cells (ESCs) and induced pluripotent stem cells (iPSCs), all being considered due to their individual strengths and weaknesses (as reviewed [66]). Ease of isolation, differentiation potential, surface marker expression and cost are just some of the factors that must be considered. An obvious benefit of ESCs and iPSCs is their therapeutic flexibility and continuous self-renewal capabilities. However, the use of ESCs carries high ethical and political concerns, the possible need for immunosuppressants, and the issue of tumorigenicity [67–69]. iPSCs also carry a high risk of teratoma formation, show low reprogramming efficiencies, and have been found to retain the epigenetic memory of their somatic cell of origin [70–72]. While the use of ESCs and iPSCs may become particularly important for the regeneration of tissues that cannot be repaired by alternative cell types, their limitations have meant that human MSCs (hMSCs) have remained a particularly attractive cell source for cartilage (and other) TE strategies [73,74]. hMSCs are relatively easily available, can be extracted from multiple tissue sources in relatively large quantities with limited morbidity, are capable of self-renewal, lack tumorigenicity, are applicable to autologous transplantation procedures, and can differentiate into multiple cell lineages, including chondrocytes [75–77]. MSCs are also known to secrete soluble cytokines and growth factors in a paracrine fashion, which are thought to add to their therapeutic effects [78]. In addition, MSCs have been indicated to have stronger immunomodulatory properties compared to other stem cell sources, and have been shown to suppress T cell, B cell, dendritic cell and natural killer cell activity [75,79–82]. MSCs are therefore not only attractive for tissue regeneration via their multilineage differentiation potential, but also for treatment of autoimmune diseases such as rheumatoid arthritis (RA), and to help bypass graft-versus-host disease (GVHD) [83–86]. In addition, MSCs have the obvious benefit over ESCs and iPSCs for cartilage TE, that they are already committed to mesoderm lineages [87], and therefore require less in vitro programming.

hMSCs were first used in a clinical trial to treat full thickness cartilage defects in 2004 [88], and have since been included in an increasing number of clinical trials [89–92]. Generally, results suggest that hMSCs are a promising cell source for cartilage repair, but there is a general lack of comparative studies and systematic reviews, and much remains to be investigated and optimised (see [73]). Some of these issues have been outlined below.

3.1. Isolation and Characterisation of MSCs

Adult MSCs are derived from the mesoderm and reside in the adult body throughout life, generally decreasing in abundance with age [87,93,94]. MSCs were first isolated from bone marrow [95,96], but have since been extracted from numerous sources including, adipose tissue [97], skeletal muscle [65], the synovium [98], and the umbilical cord [99]. The inherent differences among the microenvironments of each of these stem cell populations means that although each share similar phenotypic and functional properties, differences in differentiation capacities, and surface marker expression do exist [100,101]. This review will focus on bone marrow-derived MSCs (BMMSCs), which are the most well characterised and commonly used adult stem cell source for cartilage TE [102]. However, it is important to note that synovial membrane derived MSCs (SMSCs) are also becoming an interesting alternative due to their proximity to articular cartilage and tissue-specific properties for connective tissue repair [103–105]. Adipose derived MSCs are also gaining increased interest due to their abundance (5% of nucleated cells versus 0.0001–0.01% for BMMSCs) and the ease with which they can be harvested [106,107].

BMMSCs are isolated from the mononuclear layer of the bone marrow and are characterised by their fibroblast-like morphology, proliferation to form loose colonies of spindle shaped cells, and ability to adhere to tissue culture plastic [108,109]. The cells are passaged when they reach 80–90% confluence, with serial passages and washes generally thought to remove any non-MSC types. However, it is important to note that the resulting cultures are still heterogeneous and this will be discussed in the following section.

Phenotypically, no specific markers for hMSCs have been identified to date. Instead characterisation is based upon a panel of positive and negative markers. Generally, it is considered that hBMMSCs are negative for the hematopoietic markers CD45, CD34, CD14 and CD11, as well as for the co-stimulatory markers CD80, CD86 and CD40, and the adhesion molecules CD31, CD18 and CD56 [80]. The cells are also characterised as being positive for CD105, CD73, CD44, CD90, CD71 and Stro-1, as well as for the adhesion molecules CD106, CD166, ICAM-1 and CD29. Importantly, MSC surface markers have been shown to vary between species, tissue sources, and methods of isolation and culture. For example, a study by De Ugarte et al. [110], noted differences in expression of the cell adhesion molecules CD49d, CD54, CD34, and CD106, between MSCs isolated from bone marrow and adipose tissue. This highlights the need for a more uniform characterisation of MSCs, as it is becoming increasingly difficult to compare and contrast findings between investigators who are likely to be looking at distinct/different cell populations. A further way to identify MSCs is through their multilineage potential to differentiate into adipocytes, chondrocytes and osteoblasts [111]. However, the plasticity of MSCs has also come under further investigation, as studies have shown that the cells are also capable of differentiating down the myogenic and neuronal lineages [112–115].

In 2006 the Mesenchymal and Tissue Stem Cell Committee of the International Society for Cellular Therapy (ISCT) decided to try and address the inconsistent use of defining characteristics, and lack of universally accepted requirements to define MSCs [111]. It was proposed that the minimal requirements to define hMSCs would be: (i) the ability to adhere to culture tissue plastic; (ii) to express CD105, CD73 and CD90; (iii) to lack expression of CD45, CD34, CD14 or CD11b, CD79α or CD19, and HLA-DR surface markers; (iv) and to differentiate into osteoblasts, adipocytes and chondrocytes. Although these guidelines have provided the first steps in streamlining the characterisation of hMSCs, further refinements are clearly required if their full therapeutic potential is to be met [116–120]. Ultimately, the ubiquitous term of 'MSCs' remains one of the most undefined and controversial areas in stem cell research. It has even been suggested that this terminology should be abandoned altogether, with the argument that 'MSCs' with identical differentiation capacities do not exist [121].

3.2. MSC Heterogeneity

The low frequency of MSCs within human tissue means that the cells require extensive ex vivo expansion before they can be used for in vitro/in vivo testing, or indeed for potential clinical application. However differences in isolation methods, culture conditions and media additives used between different laboratories means that variability in cell yield and the phenotype of the expanded cell products are inevitable [122,123]. As well as improved characterisation of MSCs, standardisation of the procedures used for their isolation and expansion should therefore also be a priority, so that comparisons between studies can be made more effectively. MSCs are known to display a high degree of heterogeneity, and outgrowth of certain subsets of cells driven by the differences in culture conditions is likely to promote or inhibit their differentiation potential [124]. A better understanding of how this is controlled, and which conditions promote the differentiation of MSCs into certain cell types, is clearly needed. In the case of cartilage, better understanding of what drives permanent articular-cartilage formation, rather than fibrocartilage or hypertrophic differentiation is of the upmost importance to their success in TE/regeneration strategies [125–127]. Torensma et al. [124] suggest that the leading cause of heterogeneity within MSC cultures is, unsurprisingly, the tissue source, followed by the culture methodology, and then individual donor variation. Remarkably, in the same study, it was also shown that expanded cells which were then frozen and distributed to different laboratories to be grown for one passage, also developed some heterogeneity; indicating that cell culture location also has an effect.

3.3. In Vitro Chondrogenic Differentiation of MSCs

The most common and established method for in vitro chondrogenic differentiation of BMMSCs is often referred to as pellet culture and was developed by Johnstone et al. [36] using rabbit BMMSCs. The group then went on to use the same technique with hBMMSCs [37]. Briefly the technique involves spinning 200,000 cells at 500 g in 15 mL polypropylene conical tubes to form spherical cell aggregates. The spheroids are cultured in defined, serum-free medium consisting of high glucose Dulbecco's Modified Eagle's Medium (DMEM) supplemented with transforming growth factor beta 1 (TGFβ1), ascorbate-2-phosphate, sodium selenite, transferrin, dexamethasone, insulin, and sodium pyruvate. The technique is highly reproducible, with cell aggregates being harvested at time points up to 28 days, and some groups adapting the protocol to use up to 500,000 cells per aggregate [59]. Mackay et al. [128] went on to show that the addition of TGFβ3 rather than TGFβ1 better supports chondrogenesis.

The simplicity of the pellet culture method means it has remained popular for examining the various signalling pathways and soluble factors involved in chondrogenic differentiation, as well as for disease modelling [129–131]. However, mass transport limitations mean that the pellet cultures are not made up of a homogenous population of cells, and ECM production is not as extensive as you would hope for in an articular cartilage-like tissue, especially towards the centre of constructs [132]. In addition, the spheroid geometry of the pellet culture does not match the structured organisation of cartilage in vivo [7,8].

Murdoch et al. [41], modified the pellet culture method, introducing a porous membrane as a support for the cells. The method uses the same media and supplements as mentioned above, but the cells (500,000) are seeded onto Transwell filters and spun in a 24-well plate at 200 g, creating a shallow multilayer of MSCs that are then able to grow and differentiate into a disc of cartilage-like tissue [41,59,133]. The Transwell culture method has been shown to lead to more rapid and efficient differentiation of MSCs, and the deposition of a more extensive cartilage-like ECM when compared to the pellet culture system [41]. In addition there is a more uniform differentiation of the MSCs with improved mass transport within the shallow and permeable disc geometry [59]. Recently, it has also been shown that the Transwell system allows for the production and assembly of organised and cross-linked collagen networks; helping to explain the robust, flexible nature of the constructs that are formed [133]. However, despite the clear improvements in this technique, many researchers are still using the pellet culture method, perhaps due to the difficulty in reproducing the Transwell method effectively.

These difficulties and limitations have meant that the use of scaffolds/biomaterials to improve the in vitro chondrogenic differentiation of MSCs has become a popular avenue of research, allowing for a better recapitulation of the in vivo environment and production of larger scale cartilaginous constructs that are more clinically relevant. Ultimately though, despite much progress over the last two decades, current methods for the in vitro chondrogenic differentiation of hMSCs are still a long way off reaching the clinic. Indeed, as far as we are aware, pre-differentiated MSCs have not yet been used in any clinical trials for cartilage repair. Perhaps the most pressing concern/limitation regarding the application of pre-differentiated hMSCs is that of chondrocyte hypertrophy, with most differentiation protocols resulting in the formation of chondrocytes with endochondral-like maturation properties rather than a true articular cartilage-like phenotype [36–38,41,134–137]. In contrast, the use of undifferentiated hMSCs for cartilage repair has progressed further, with around 50 clinical trials currently registered at https://www.clinicaltrial.gov/. Published results have generally been promising, and the use of allogenic umbilical cord MSCs have already been approved by the Korean FDA for OA treatment [92,126,138–144]. However, the use of these cells for cartilage formation is still in its infancy, and from the evidence that is available, protocols to improve the quality of the regenerated cartilage are still clearly required [88,126,145–147]. As such, there is an overriding necessity to better understand the mechanisms controlling permanent articular cartilage formation, alongside further evaluation of ongoing clinical trials, before these cells can be used to their fullest potential in the clinic. Whether the greatest success will be seen with the in vitro chondrogenic differentiation of hMSCs, in vivo delivery of undifferentiated cells, or with cell-free approaches that instead harness the body's own MSCs for repair, remains to be seen. However, what is clear is that the use of current in vitro models (such as the pellet culture) to screen potential bioactive factors (such as growth factors) and culture conditions, as well as investigation into biomaterials that can help support articular cartilage formation, should be a priority, and will be of the upmost importance for the improved development of both in vivo and in vitro regeneration strategies.

4. Growth Factors Involved in the Chondrogenic Differentiation of MSCs

The differentiation of MSCs into chondrocytes involves the activation and suppression of a number of signalling pathways and growth factors, with members of the TGFβ, fibroblast growth factor (FGF), and insulin-like growth factor (IGF) families, among others, having all been implicated in the process (as reviewed in Table 1). The TGFβ superfamily has been the most researched of all stimulating factors in the area of chondrogenesis, and is described in more detail in the sections below.

Table 1. Growth factors implemented in chondrogenesis and associated PGs/GAGs.

Molecule Family	Molecule	Proposed Function during Chondrogenesis	Reference	Associated PGs/GAGs	Reference
FGF [1]	FGF2	Enhances proliferation and chondrogenic potential during expansion.	[59,148–151]	Role of HSPGs in FGF-receptor binding has been extensively studied; HSPGs play an important role in FGF-receptor signalling by facilitating ligand-receptor oligomerisation.	[155–159]
		Negative effect on matrix deposition and differentiation.	[151–153]		
		Addition during expansion primes cells for hypertrophy.	[149,151]		
		Prolongs lifespan of MSCs.	[154]		
	FGF9	Increases matrix production early on, but then promotes matrix resorption and hypertrophy.	[152]	CS sulfation patterns have also been implicated in articular cartilage formation and expression has been co-localised with FGF2. Perlecan can only deliver FGF2 to its receptors after its CS chains have been removed.	[160–162]
		However, also reported to promote matrix production and delay terminal hypertrophy.	[151]		
	FGF18	Suppresses proliferation and promotes matrix production.	[151,164]	Exogenous HS can be used to improve hMSC expansion.	[163]
		Delays terminal hypertrophy.	[151]		

Table 1. *Cont.*

Molecule Family	Molecule	Proposed Function during Chondrogenesis	Reference	Associated PGs/GAGs	Reference
TGFβ	TGFβ1/3	Promotes chondrogenic differentiation of MSCs. Considered a main chondrogenic inducer of MSCs, however, leads to chondrocyte hypertrophy.	[36–39,41,75,128,165]	TGFβ1 but not TGFβ3 has been shown to bind to HS; effects of the interaction remain conflicting.	[166–169]
		TGFβ3 better supports chondrogenic differentiation than TGFβ1.		TGFβ binds to the small leucine rich PGs, decorin, biglycan and fibromodulin, but via their protein core; CS/DS chains interfere with this binding.	[170]
BMP	GDF5	Important role in joint formation and organisation of articular cartilage; GDF5 expressed in healthy pre-hypertrophic cartilage, but not as OA develops; GDF5 dominant negative mutation results in articular cartilage degeneration.	[23,171–175]	Heparin binding sequence predicted.	[182]
		Increases cartilaginous ECM production in vitro.	[176–179]		
		Supplementation with TGFβ3 shown to promote hypertrophy. However, a combinatorial study with TGFβ1, BMP2 and GDF5 suggest that it is the TGFβ actually promoting hypertrophy.	[180,181]		
	BMP2/4/6/7	Promotes chondrogenic differentiation of MSCs, especially when used in combination with TGFβ. BMP2/7 indicated as particularly useful for inducing chondrogenesis. However, most studies indicate that BMP supplementation also leads to hypertrophy.	[153,181,183–186]	Use of heparin/HS to potentiate the activity of BMPs has been widely studied; especially in the case of BMP2 for bone TE.	[187–195]
Wnt	Wnt3a, Wnt5a	Promotes chondrogenic differentiation. Inhibits hypertrophy. However, Wnt5a also reported to promote hypertrophy during early stages of differentiation.	[196–198] [199]	Glypican3 is strongly linked to the Wnt pathway; HS chains bind to Wnts with different affinities to fine-tune access to Wnt receptors; 6-O-desulfation of HS reduces ability of Glypican1 HS chains to bind Wnt, and therefore facilitates Wnt-receptor interaction.	[200–202]
	Wnt11	Promotes chondrogenic differentiation and hypertrophy.	[203]		
	Wnt4, Wnt8	Inhibits chondrogenic differentiation. Promotes hypertrophy.	[196,204]		
	Wnt9a	Inhibits chondrogenic differentiation. Inhibits hypertrophy.	[205]		
IGF	IGF1	When used in combination with TGFβ3 collagen I production is reduced. Promotes hypertrophic differentiation.	[183] [206]	Heparin/HS/DS stimulate the release of free and bioactive IGF1 from IGF binding proteins	[207]
PTHrP	PTHrP (1–34) isoform	Inhibits TGFβ induced hypertrophic differentiation.	[39,153,208,209]	PTHrP is activated by Ihh signalling (feedback loop). HS binds Ihh and negatively regulates signalling.	[210,211]

[1] FGF, fibroblast growth factor; HSPG, heparan sulfate proteoglycan; CS, chondroitin sulfate; DS, dermatan sulfate; TGFβ, transforming growth factor beta; BMP, bone morphogenetic protein; GDF, growth differentiation factor; Wnt, Wingless-type MMTV integration site; IGF, insulin like growth factor; PTHrP, parathyroid hormone-related peptide.

4.1. Transforming Growth Factor Beta (TGFβ) Superfamily

The TGFβ superfamily of secreted factors is made up of more than 30 members that can be phylogenetically split into two main groups, namely the TGFβ/Activin and the BMP/GDF sub-families [212,213]. Members of the family are synthesised as large precursor (inactive) molecules, which then undergo proteolytic cleavage following dimerisation, to yield active, mature dimers [214]. All mature monomers of the family share a conserved cysteine knot structure, formed from six characteristically spaced disulfide-bonded cysteines within the C-terminal region [215,216]. In addition, with the exception of GDF3 and GDF9, members of the family contain a seventh conserved cysteine residue, which is required for the covalent linking of the dimeric structures [217]. Upon secretion, the active mature dimers are then able to bind to their respective receptors to initiate downstream signalling, although a number of further regulatory mechanisms exist, such as the secreted antagonists Noggin and Chordin [218], and where ECM molecules such as heparan sulfate (HS) also play a role [169]. In addition, it has been shown for some TGFβ superfamily members (such as TGFβ1/2/3 and GDF8), that the mature ligand is secreted from cells in a large complex which includes the cleaved pro-region, known as the latency-associated protein (LAP) (see [213,219]). These complexes have also been shown to bind to latent TGFβ-binding proteins (LTBPs), which are structurally related to fibrillins and allow for ECM localisation [220]. The complexes remain inactive in the ECM, until the mature ligand is released from the complex by activators such as integrin receptors, proteases, or reactive oxygen species [220–225]; thereby adding another level of control to ligand activity.

As extensively reviewed [137,226–228], upon binding of a TGFβ superfamily member to its receptor, the formation of a heterodimeric serine/threonine kinase complex is induced, which is composed of a pair of high affinity type I and type II receptors (see Table 2 and Figure 3). In addition, there are a number of type III co-receptors, able to indirectly regulate signalling by binding to TGFβ ligands and modulating their subsequent binding to type I and type II receptors. The type II serine/threonine kinases are constitutively active, and upon ligand binding undergo a conformational change, which leads to the recruitment and phosphorylation of the appropriate type I receptors. Type I receptors then specifically recognise and phosphorylate receptor-regulated Smad proteins (R-Smads). In this regard, there are two classes of R-Smads: the TGFβ responsive Smads, which include Smad 2 and 3, and the BMP-responsive Smads that include Smad 1, 5, and 8. Upon activation, R-Smads form a complex with the common-partner Smad (Co-Smad; Smad 4), and translocate to the nucleus to regulate the transcription of a multitude of target genes. Inhibitory Smads (I-Smads; Smad6/7) can also inhibit the receptor activation of R-Smads by mediating the degradation of receptors and R-Smads. While Smad 7 inhibits all TGFβ superfamily members, Smad 6 is more specific towards the BMP subfamily [229].

Aside from canonical Smad-mediated TGFβ superfamily signalling, other signalling pathways, such as the mitogen activated-protein kinase (MAPK) pathways have also been implicated in the process (reviewed [230]). These non-Smad-mediated pathways can either be directly activated by TGFβ ligands, or can modulate the activity of TGFβ-induced Smad signalling, allowing for crosstalk and modification/fine-tuning of initial Smad-mediated signals.

Table 2. Components of the TGFβ Smad-dependent canonical signalling pathway.

Molecular Category	TGFβ Sub-Family Pathway [1]	BMP Sub-Family Pathway
Ligands	TGFβs, ActivinsGDF8/9/10/11, BMP3, Nodal	BMP2/4/5/6/7/8/9/10, GDF1/3/5/6/7, MIS
Type II receptors	TβRII, ActRIIA, ActRIIB	BMPRII, ActRIIA, ActRIIB
Type I receptors	ALK4, TβRI (ALK5), ALK7	ALK1/2, BMPR1A (ALK3), BMPR1B (ALK6)
R-Smad	Smad2/3	Smad1/5/8
Co-Smad	Smad4	Smad4
I-Smad	Smad7	Smad6/7

[1] Alternative protein names are listed in brackets. TβR, TGFβ receptor; MIS, muellerian inhibiting substance; BMPR, BMP receptor; ActR, activin receptor; ALK, activin receptor-like kinase. Table adapted from [226].

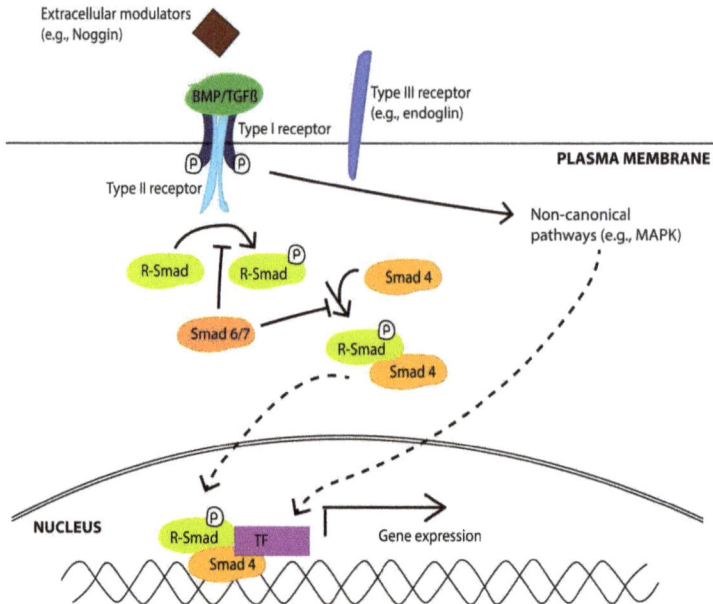

Figure 3. Schematic overview of TGFβ signalling. Binding of a TGFβ/BMP ligand to specific cell surface receptors induces the formation of a heteromeric type II/type I receptor complex. This binding is further regulated by type III receptors/co-receptors. Upon ligand binding, constitutively active type II receptors activate type I receptors. This then leads to the phosphorylation of R-Smads (Smad 2/3 for the TGFβ subfamily; Smad1/5/8 for the BMP subfamily). R-Smads then form heterodimeric complexes with Smad 4 (Co-Smad) and translocate to the nucleus, where they regulate gene expression through interaction with transcription factors (TFs). I-Smads (Smad 6/7) inhibit receptor activation of R-Smads. Besides the canonical Smad signalling pathway, non-Smad pathways, such as the MAPK pathways have also been implicated in TGFβ signalling. Figure adapted from [227].

4.1.1. TGFβ Subfamily

TGFβ is crucial for cartilage maintenance and integrity, as highlighted by mutations in these genes/proteins, which have been shown to lead to OA-like pathology [231,232]. Lack of TGFβ signalling is also reported in aged mice, and murine models of OA [233,234]. This has led to the majority of in vitro chondrogenic differentiation protocols including supplementation with either TGFβ1 or TGFβ3, of which TGFβ3 has been shown to support chondrogenesis more efficiently [36–41,59,75,128,133,165]. It has generally been considered that TGFβ is the only well-established inducer of chondrogenesis, leading to the deposition of a matrix rich in PG and collagen II. However, TGFβ-induced chondrogenic differentiation of MSCs is also clearly accompanied by the expression of unwanted hypertrophic markers such as collagen X and MMP13 [36,37,39,41,75,128,165]. In addition, the ectopic transplantation of TGFβ-differentiated MSCs into the subcutaneous pouches of severe combined immunodifficient (SCID) mice has been shown to result in matrix calcification and vascular invasion [38]. Human articular chondrocytes have also been shown to be directed towards hypertrophy when expanded in the presence of TGFβ1 [235]. Interestingly, it has been reported that MSCs differentiated in the presence of TGFβ1 had significantly less mineralisation than those cultured with TGFβ3 [236]. However, taken together, these drawbacks have indicated that further refinement of chondrogenic differentiation protocols are required; as such, researchers are now looking into the use of other/combinations of chondrogenic factors, which can induce the differentiation of MSCs into a permanent articular chondrocyte-like phenotype, and that can withstand hypertrophy. For example, it has been indicated that PTHrP may be able to suppress the hypertrophic effects of TGFβ treatment, without affecting the deposition of a cartilaginous matrix [39,153,208,209]. The use of a wide range of BMP subfamily members are also being increasingly investigated (see Section 4.1.2). Importantly, mutations which lead to elevated TGFβ activity have also been associated with increased bone mass and ossification [237,238], and TGFβ supplementation has been shown to stimulate osteophyte formation in the murine knee joint [239]. This therefore highlights that TGFβ activity is not limited to the articular cartilage tissue of synovial joints, and may well help explain why TGFβ stimulation also leads to chondrocyte hypertrophy and mineralisation (i.e., if MSCs are not first primed towards the articular cartilage pathway). The medium formulations (including growth factors) that are currently used for inducing chondrogenic differentiation of MSCs are potentially overly simplistic, since the formation of permanent articular cartilage is likely to be dependent upon the cross-talk from multiple signalling pathways [20,240]. Investigation into the effects of other chondrogenic factors has therefore become vital.

4.1.2. BMP Subfamily

The unsatisfactory results from in vitro chondrogenic protocols using TGFβ supplementation has led to the extensive investigation of the BMP subfamily of the TGFβ superfamily [153,183–186,241–243]. BMPs have been shown to play a number of essential roles in endochondral ossification, and are important for chondrocyte proliferation and differentiation, helping to maintain the expression of the chondrogenic transcription factor Sox9 [244,245]. Dual knockdown of BMP2 and BMP4 in mice has been shown to lead to abnormalities in chondrogenic condensations, and severe disorganisation of chondrocytes within the growth plate [246,247]. BMP7 is also thought to play a particularly important role in articular cartilage maintenance, with intra-articular injections of the ligand being shown to delay cartilage degradation in mice [248]. In vitro studies have demonstrated that BMPs (predominantly BMP2/4/6/7) can also induce the chondrogenic differentiation of MSCs, and that the use of BMPs in combination with TGFβ is more effective at inducing chondrogenesis than TGFβ treatment alone [183–186,241,242]; however, the majority of these protocols have also led to extensive hypertrophic differentiation. In contrast, Weiss et al. [153] have suggested that BMP2/4/6/7 and IGF1 were individually not sufficient to induce chondrogenesis of MSCs and that instead TGFβ was also required. Again, when these growth factors were used in combination with TGFβ, collagen X expression was still observed. Caron et al. [186] also looked at the effects of both BMP2 and BMP7 in combination with TGFβ3, and found that while BMP2 promoted chondrocyte hypertrophy, BMP7 inhibited this terminal differentiation. Handorf and Li [243], have looked at varying growth factor requirements throughout the differentiation protocol, evaluating if MSCs may have differing requirements depending on their stage of differentiation. While sequential administration of TGFβ1 and BMP7 did not enhance chondrogenesis to a greater extent than treatment with both growth factors at every feed, the hypertrophic phenotype was significantly reduced; but, while these results were promising, additional reductions in hypertrophy were still thought to be required. This therefore further highlights that examination of factors that can repress hypertrophy, or prime MSCs early on towards a phenotypically stable articular cartilage state, is of profound importance. The identification of such a factor, and its use in combination/sequence with other TGFβ and BMP treatments may be key to generating a permanent hyaline cartilage tissue.

4.1.2.1. GDF5

GDF5, also known as BMP14 or cartilage derived morphogenetic protein 1 (CDMP1), is a particularly interesting member of the BMP subfamily. It is synthesised as a 501 amino acid preprotein (UNIPROT accession number: P43026) [249]. Upon cleavage of the signal sequence (27 residues), the proregion (70 kDa) is proteolytically removed, leaving a 13.5 kDa (120 amino acid) monomer, which will then go on to form a disulfide linked homodimer, or a heterodimer with another TGFβ superfamily member [250–252]. GDF5 is well established as playing a critical role in joint development and maintenance [23,171–173,253–256]. Its importance was first highlighted in mice carrying the brachypodism (bp) mutation, which results in changes to the length and number of bones in the limbs, and was found to be the result of mutations in the GDF5 gene [253]; GDF5 was also shown to be highly expressed in the joint interzone, and that mice lacking both GDF5 and GDF6 have further wide spread joint defects and skeletal growth retardation [257,258]; highlighting its importance in the formation of synovial joints. Importantly, GDF5 has also been shown to be required for proper joint formation and homeostasis in humans, and is predominantly expressed in areas of cartilage formation during embryonic development [171,259–263]. Loss of function mutations in the human GDF5 gene have been shown to result in a number of chondrodysplasias such as Grebe and Hunter-Thompson syndromes [259,263], and a single nucleotide polymorphism in the 5′UTR of human GDF5 has also been linked to OA susceptibility [261]. In contrast, overexpression of GDF5 has been shown to enhance chondrogenesis, increase the length and width of bones, and lead to joint fusions [260,262].

Despite the clear importance of GDF5 for skeletal formation, its use for chondrogenic in vitro differentiation protocols and regeneration strategies has been somewhat under-researched compared to other TGFβ superfamily members. However, previous work comparing the effects of TGFβ1 and GDF5 in fetal hMSCs via histological staining, has demonstrated that while TGFβ1 was more stimulatory in terms of GAG production, the combination of both TGFβ1 and GDF5 was synergistic [264]. In contrast, Feng et al. [176] indicated that compared to TGFβ1 (10 ng/mL), GDF5 (100 ng/mL) had a much greater effect on the chondrogenic differentiation of adipose derived rat MSCs, although collagen X levels appeared similar in both TGFβ and GDF5 treated pellets. Interestingly, MSCs transfected with GDF5 and implanted into full thickness articular cartilage defects in the knee joints of rabbits have shown promising results; demonstrating superior repair of hyaline cartilage compared to MSC implantation alone [265]. In addition, most crucially, Zhang et al. [177], have reported that GDF5 (100 ng/mL) inhibited hBMMSCs from expressing collagen X, while promoting the deposition of a cartilage-like matrix. Although their results were not compared to the more commonly used TGFβ, this study has sparked interest in GDF5 as a target for cartilage TE/repair strategies.

This is exemplified by our own recent work, showing that GDF5 can induce the chondrogenic differentiation of hMSCs, while overcoming the hurdle of hypertrophy [266]. In contrast to TGFβ1, we found that GDF5 induced aggrecan and Sox9 expression (both markers associated with chondrogenesis and ECM production [267]), without increasing the expression of collagen X (the major marker of chondrocyte hypertrophy [268]); see Figure 4A–C [266]. Our data suggests that GDF5 could be used to generate a clinically useful cartilage matrix with a high PG content, while maintaining the chondrocytes in a mature articular cartilage phenotype. As well as building on the results of Zhang et al. [177], our research [266] also complements several other studies published over the past few years [175,179,181,269]. For example, work in an OA rat model has demonstrated that GDF5 is expressed in healthy pre-hypertrophic cartilage, but is not evident as OA develops [175]. A further study with human chondrocytes has also shown that GDF5 stimulation promoted the expression of aggrecan, while inhibiting collagen X expression [179]. Consistent with what we observed, Murphy et al. [181] demonstrated that collagen X expression was significantly increased in the presence of TGFβ1 but not GDF5, i.e., in 7-day hMSC-derived chondrocyte pellets. However, our results are in contrast to another recent study suggesting that GDF5 can promote the hypertrophy of hMSC-derived chondrocyte pellets [180]. This work, however, looked at the effect of GDF5 in combination with TGFβ3, and not in isolation. We have demonstrated that GDF5 alone does not increase collagen X expression, and that the combination of GDF5 and TGFβ1 is no more potent at inducing collagen X than TGFβ1 treatment alone [266].

Thus, overall, there is increasing evidence supporting the potential use of GDF5 in cartilage TE strategies, especially when this growth factor is supplied to hMSCs in the absence of TGFβ. Future studies to look at the expression of a wider repertoire of genes involved in chondrogenesis, as well as additional biochemical assays (for example to quantify PG content) would help to further determine the effects of GDF5 on the chondrogenic differentiation of hMSCs. A recent study in human umbilical cord perivascular stem cell-derived chondrocyte pellets demonstrated that GDF5 enhanced proliferation, but had no effect on the expression of chondrogenic-related genes [270], therefore indicating that the effect of GDF5 may be specific to the source of stem/stromal cells.

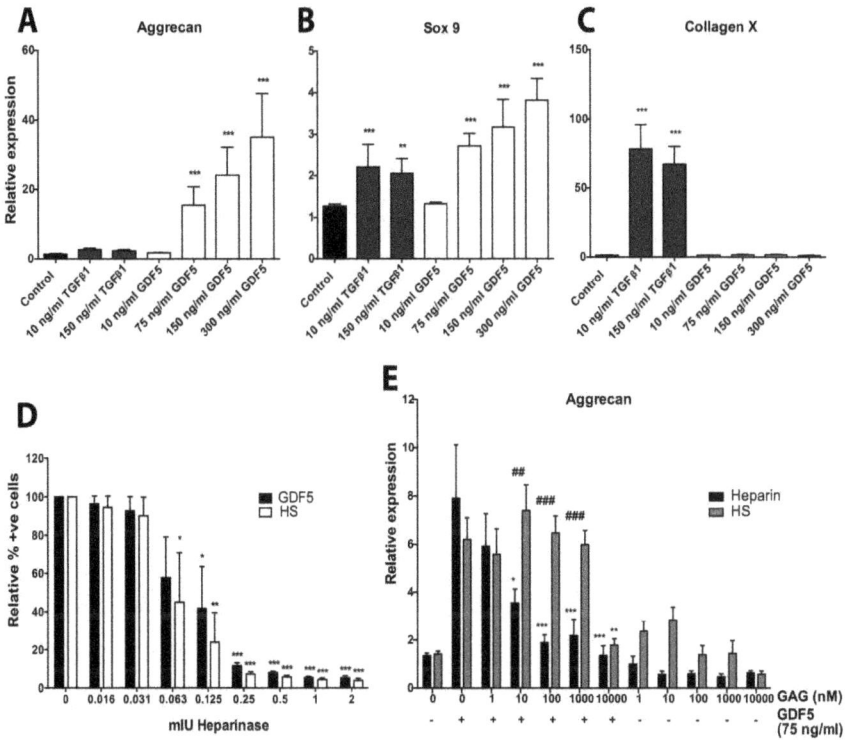

Figure 4. GDF5 promotes the chondrogenic differentiation of hMSCs without inducing hypertrophy, and its activity is modulated by GAGs. GDF5 promotes the expression of aggrecan (**A**) and Sox 9 (**B**), both markers associated with chondrogenesis and ECM production, in hMSC-derived chondrogenic pellets, but importantly, does this without inducing collagen X expression; (**C**), a marker of chondrocyte hypertrophy. The removal of endogenous HSPGs (HS) from the cell surface (by using heparinase) is positively correlated with the reduced level of GDF5 able to bind to the cell surface; (**D**), Exogenous heparin, but not equivalent doses of HS, inhibit GDF5-induced chondrogenic differentiation of hMSCs as monitored by aggrecan expression (**E**), * $p < 0.05$, ** $p < 0.01$, *** $p < 0.001$ versus no addition control; ## $p < 0.01$, ### $p < 0.001$, comparing heparin and HS of same dose (see [266] for full experimental details).

Importantly, the supplementation of hMSCs with GDF5 rather than TGFβ1/3 may provide an effective way to achieve the aim of forming hyaline rather than hypertrophic chondrocytes from hMSCs, and strongly suggests that a transition to using GDF5 in hMSC-based cartilage engineering strategies could help to overcome this long-standing hurdle [266]. However, hMSC heterogeneity [271], along with the inability of being able to form a scalable tissue, need to be overcome if successful clinical implementation is to be achieved. A more robust quality control of cell preparations, that can better predict clinical outcomes, and/or allow for the purification of subpopulations of cells with improved chondrogenic potential, is therefore of the upmost importance (see [272]). The difficulties surrounding the use of hMSCs, has also meant that researchers are now looking into alternative solutions to cell therapy. Conventionally the strategy would be to deliver expanded hMSCs (undifferentiated or differentiated) to the repair site, but recent work has led to the opinion that the beneficial effects of hMSCs (or other stem cells) for tissue regeneration are not only due to cell restoration (and engraftment), but can also be attributed to the trophic factors that hMSCs release (see reviews [273,274]). As a result, research is now being directed into the identification and delivery of paracrine factors to the injury site, which can then modulate the environment and evoke a repair response from the resident cells [275–279]. These cell free approaches to tissue regeneration are exciting; e.g., overcoming the issues of cell sourcing, expansion and differentiation, as well as the strict regulatory issues that surround cell therapy. However, they come with other challenges, including the effective and safe delivery and/or controlled release of the bioactive factors [277,280]. These issues, which are relevant to both cell-free and cell-based regeneration strategies, will be explored in further detail within the following sections.

5. Glycosaminoglycans

As well as the difficulties in identifying the correct growth factors (and combinations thereof) to target for cartilage TE/regeneration strategies, the inherent instability of these proteins has also hampered their potential use. Growth factors are known to be susceptible to proteolytic degradation, are rapidly cleared from the injury site, and demonstrate burst release pharmkinetics [281–283]. Together these factors have largely meant that supraphysiological quantities are required to get anywhere near the desired outcome, resulting in economically unsustainable costs for clinical translation [284–287]. In addition, the safety of growth factors is still under debate due to the increasing number that are being identified as proto-oncogenic, and this worry is only heightened by the high doses that are currently required [288–291]. The use of carriers that can reduce the quantity of exogenous growth factors required, through their localisation, protection or enhancement, or indeed that could harness endogenously produced growth factors, would therefore be ideal. Research into the use of GAGs for these approaches is proving particularly promising, and presents an attractive therapeutic opportunity for TE strategies [163,195,292–295].

In animal cells there are an estimated 10^5–10^6 copies of HS and chondroitin sulfate (CS) on the cell surface, which range from ~40–160 nm in length; these GAGs are present at mg/mL concentrations in the ECM, highlighting their abundance and importance. Moreover, solution structure studies of sulfated GAGs have indicated that the oligosaccharides are highly dynamic, with a high degree of conformational plasticity (although forming stiffened random coils), allowing them to interact with a diverse number of proteins, and adding to the complexity of the interactions [296]. All GAGs, with the exception of HA (and heparin, once it has been secreted by mast cells), exist as PGs by attaching to serine residues on core proteins [297]; alternatively, keratan sulfate (KS) can be N-linked. PGs are produced by virtually all mammalian cells and can be found on the cell surface, within the ECM, or stored in secretory granules [298]. PGs can include only one GAG chain (e.g., decorin), or can have over 100 GAG chains, as is the case for aggrecan, the most predominant PG in cartilage [299,300]. Aggrecan consists of around 100 CS and 30 KS GAG chains extending from a large protein core of approximately 250 kDa [301]. In addition, this PG forms large aggregates (size, 1–4 μm), with hundreds of aggrecan molecules non-covalently bound on a single HA chain, where the interaction is stabilised by cartilage link protein [302]. The biomechanical properties of cartilage are largely due to the high negative charge provided by associated GAG chains, and the large size of the biopolymer, which is held in place by collagen networks. These factors render the PG immobile and unable to redistribute itself, allowing the matrix to become water swollen (Gibbs-Donnan effect), resistant to deformation, and able to resist compressive force [303]. The highly sulfated GAG chains of aggrecan are also responsible for sequestering and modulating the accessibility of molecules, such as growth factors, which bind via positively charged amino acid residues [304]. Other PGs expressed in cartilage include glypican, cell surface syndecans and the large HSPG perlecan [162,305–307]. Via its HS chains, perlecan has strong affinity for collagen VI, and can bind to fibronectin and laminin, via both its HS chains and core protein [308]. Through these interactions perlecan has been shown to play an important role in sequestering FGF2 and softening the ECM within the immediate vicinity of the chondrocytes (the pericellular matrix (PCM)), providing an environment suitable for mechanotransduction [161,308].

The physiological and pathological functions of PGs are vast; e.g., helping to define tissue form, and dynamically modulate function and remodelling during health and disease [309,310]. The specific functions of GAGs/PGs include ligand binding/immobilisation/retention, promotion of ligand/receptor interactions, protection of ligands from proteolysis, and facilitation of cell-cell and cell-matrix interactions [156,311–320]; all of which can have a profound effect on cellular activity. The variable lengths and sulfation patterns of GAG chains on PGs, makes them the most structurally complex and information dense molecules found in nature [309]. Importantly, the intrinsic heterogeneity of sulfated GAGs allows for diverse patterning and multifunctionality, and as such the understanding of how these 'sugar codes' control tissue development and homeostasis is of huge therapeutic interest [321–324]. This is particularly apparent in the case of heparin/HS, where the huge degree of versatility has opened up the concept of 'heparanomics', seeking to better understand how HS structures interact with proteins to modulate biological activity [325,326]. It has been estimated that over 1×10^6 structurally different sequences are possible from a just a short HS octasaccharide; emphasising the point that these molecules could potentially accommodate an enormous number of protein-binding epitopes [327]. Research aimed at enabling a better understanding of this complexity and its functional consequences is ongoing [328–330], and it is ultimately hoped that this will allow for improved modulation of cellular activity and thus, TE/regeneration strategies.

Role of GAGs in Stem Cell Differentiation and Development

The extensive work of Merry and colleagues has highlighted the importance of HS and HSPGs in stem cell differentiation and embryonic development [331–335]. For example, the neural differentiation of mouse ESCs (mESCs) expressing green fluorescent protein (GFP) under the control of the neural marker Sox1, has been used to show that, compared to undifferentiated mESCs where HS sulfation was low, GFP-expressing neural progenitor cells demonstrated increased levels of both N- and O-sulfation, as supported by high levels of HS biosynthesis enzymes such as NDST4 and 3OST [331]. Variations in sulfation patterns between mESCs and neural progenitor cells were also confirmed using epitope specific antibodies, which show preferential binding to specific patterns of sulfation in the HS chain [331]. The group also demonstrated that the phage-display antibody RB4EA-12, which specifically binds to 6-O sulfated structures, had significantly increased expression in the Sox1-GFP expressing neural progenitors compared to the undifferentiated mESCs. Further to this, EXT1$^{-/-}$ mESCs (that are unable to form an HS polymer) placed in neural media were unable to differentiate, unless supplemented with soluble heparin. It was also shown that exogenously added GAGs, of particular sulfation patterns, concentrations, and chain lengths were also able to support the neural differentiation of wild type mESCs [334].

Taking a similar approach, the Merry group have also characterised changes in HS expression during differentiation of mESCs down the mesoderm/hematopoietic lineage, using a cell line where GFP is under the control of the Bry gene (which is expressed in mesoderm but not in ESCs), alongside a panel of HS sequence specific antibodies [332]. Of particular significance was the antibody HS4C3 which was specifically expressed within the emerging Bry$^+$ population, but that disappeared from the cell surface as cells differentiated into mature hematopoietic cells. In vivo findings also demonstrated that HS4C3 binding sequences were restricted to the mesoderm during gastrulation. The rapid turnover of the HS4C3 HS binding sequences at the cell surface during different stages of differentiation indicates how highly regulated and important HS sulfation patterns are during development, allowing different growth factors to bind at specific spatio-temporal locations to instigate specific signalling pathways. Understanding the details of HS sequences that are involved in the formation of various tissues, will therefore lead to a better understanding of how stem cell differentiation and development is regulated and controlled. In a subsequent study, EXT1$^{-/-}$ mESCs were only able to differentiate into hematopoietic lineages with the addition of heparin [333]. In contrast (and in contrast to the previously discussed work in the neural differentiation system), the addition of chemically N- or O-desulfated heparin oligosaccharides, or heparin chains shorter than 18 saccharides, were unable to restore differentiation. Together these results highlight the widespread importance of HS in embryonic tissue development. While the low sulfation patterns seen in mESCs help to keep the cells in a pluripotent, undifferentiated state, dynamic changes in the sulfation patterns of HS appear to be required for growth factor activity and stem cell differentiation.

Consistent with the findings above, Nairn et al., [336] examined transcripts encoding the glycosylation machinery during stem cell differentiation, and demonstrated clear correlations between transcripts and changes in glycan structures. In addition, with more particular reference to the importance of GAGs in cartilage development, bioimaging has been used to demonstrate changes in the staining intensity of CS and HS during the chondrogenic differentiation of ESCs [337]. In addition, homozygous mice lacking either exostosin 1 or 2 (EXT1/EXT2; responsible for the polymerisation of growing HS chains), fail to gastrulate, while heterozygous mutants are likely to develop hereditary multiple exotoses, characterised by abnormal cartilage differentiation, premature hypertrophy and bony outgrowths [338,339]. In addition, Stickens et al. [339] showed that all EXT2$^{+/-}$ mice display abnormalities in cartilage differentiation, with disorganisation of chondrocytes and premature hypertrophy in the cartilage. Similarly, conditional knockdown of EXT1 in limb bud mesenchyme also leads to dysregulation of BMP signalling and delayed chondrogenic differentiation [340]. Furthermore, HS chains on the PG perlecan within the growth plate have been shown to be involved in the binding of FGF2 to its receptors FGFR1–4, leading to the regulation of chondrocyte proliferation and bone growth [162]. Importantly, however, perlecan can only deliver FGF2 to its receptors following the removal of CS; thus the CS chains on perlecan allow for the sequestration of FGF2 within the PCM of cartilage tissue, while the HS chains help with its delivery to receptors [161,162]. FGF2 has also been demonstrated to be liberated from perlecan HS chains upon injury or mechanical compression [341]. In humans, a mutation in 3′-phosphoadenosine 5′-phosphosulfate synthase 1 (PAPSS1; a bi-functional enzyme with both ATP sulfurylase and adenosine 5′-phosphosulfate kinase activity), which introduces a premature stop codon and disrupts GAG sulfation, as well as other mutations that lead to disruption in sulfation patterns, have been shown to result in osteochondrodysplasias (disorders in the development of cartilage/bone) [342]. A study has also shown that there is significantly higher expression of the endosulfatases, Sulf1 and Sulf2, in OA versus normal articular cartilage, indicating that changes in 6-O sulfation patterns post biosynthesis can contribute to cartilage pathology [343]. In addition, Sulf1 and Sulf2 have been shown to modulate cartilage homeostasis via their differential effects on BMP and FGF signalling [344]. Together these studies indicate that cartilage is particularly sensitive to sulfation patterns within GAG sequences, with key signalling pathways being dependent upon particular domain structures and sulfation patterns being present; see Table 1. The predominant role of GAGs and PGs in the formation and maintenance of the ECM of articular cartilage, makes them particularly interesting as factors for improving cartilage TE strategies, and a better understanding and identification of GAG sequences involved in articular cartilage formation and disease is clearly required.

Exogenously added HS, and heparin have been shown to stimulate cartilage nodule formation and growth in chick limb bud mesenchyme micromass cultures [345]. In contrast, although HS treatment alone does not appear to have an effect on the in vitro chondrogenic differentiation of MSCs, addition in combination with TGFβ3 and BMP2 has been shown to potentiate chondrogenic activity, more so than growth factor treatment alone [346,347]. It has been suggested that this may be due to exogenous HS limiting the ability of ligands to bind to endogenous HSPGs that would usually prevent/regulate their binding to receptors [346]. Consistent with this, overexpression of syndecan-3, a major HSPG expressed during chondrogenesis, was shown to impair the ability of BMP2 to promote chondrogenic differentiation [346]. On the other hand, the inclusion of the HSPG perlecan in biomaterials has been shown to enhance cartilage TE strategies, prolonging the release of BMP2 [348]. Exogenous HS has also been shown to prolong TGFβ1-mediated signalling in hMSCs [169]. In addition, a recent study has also demonstrated that knockdown of perlecan inhibits the chondrogenic and adipogenic differentiation of SMSCs, but not osteogenic differentiation [349].

Ultimately, the ECM, and more specifically the PCM, which consists of the cell surface and immediate local ECM, plays a major role in maintaining homeostasis and directing cell behavior [350]. It provides a scaffold for cell attachment and spreading and helps provide the shape and mechanical properties of many tissues, including cartilage [304,351–354]. GAGs and PGs are key components of the PCM/ECM, keeping the matrix hydrated through their high negative charge, determining the compressive properties of the tissue, modulating morphogen gradients, and controlling the activity of ligands. A greater understanding of GAG structure within target tissues (the composition of which varies considerably with cell type and location), and how these are altered during development and disease, will therefore be of huge importance in the success of future TE strategies [355–357]. The elucidation of GAG structure/function relationships has lagged behind that of proteins and nucleic acids, largely because of limitations in the research methods available; e.g., GAGs cannot be amplified against a template, and as such cannot be sequenced in the same manner as DNA/RNA [297]. Adding to the challenge is their vast heterogeneity [321] and the high degree of sequence/conformational flexibility, likely underpinning the diversity and complexity of GAG-ligand interactions [296,328,358]. Despite these challenges, the persistence of the PG community has meant that much more advanced synthesis, modelling and sequencing tools are now becoming available (see [321,326,359–361]); in line with these developments, there is the hope that the full potential and full biological significance GAGs can soon be realised.

6. Biomaterials

A wide range of materials have been used for cartilage scaffold fabrication, including natural polymers such as collagen, fibrin and HA, as well as synthetic polymers such as polylactic acid (PLA) and polyglycolic acid (PGA), and self-assembling peptides (see [362]). Natural polymers have the obvious advantage of biological recognition, providing the cells with ECM molecules that can positively support cell function and adhesion [363–366]. Collagen, being a major component of the cartilage ECM, is a widely used natural polymer in cartilage TE, and is the most common scaffold to be incorporated into MACI procedures [55,60,367,368]. However, due to its abundance and versatility, collagen I (rather than type II) is usually used [369]. Collagen scaffolds have also been used in clinical trials immediately after microfracture treatment, although assessment of the benefit of this treatment still requires further analysis [370–372]. Multi-layered collagen scaffolds, which can more effectively mimic the zonal structure of articular cartilage, have also been recently examined in large animal models [373,374]. Histological analysis demonstrated that these scaffolds alone (i.e., cell-free) were able to initiate the formation of well-structured osteochondral tissue. Collagen I gels in combination with 2D micro patterning and single cell culture has also been used as a platform to investigate conditions that control chondrocyte de-differentiation [375]. This approach also offers a method from which niches for targeted differentiation of hMSCs could be investigated.

As well as collagen, HA and chitosan have also been extensively studied as natural polymers for cartilage TE/regeneration strategies. The HA-based scaffold, Hyalograft C, demonstrated promising results for the treatment of articular cartilage lesions, and like collagen, has also been used in MACI procedures [376,377]. However, results appeared less convincing for chronic lesions [378], and the product was recently discontinued failing EMA approval. More promisingly, a chitosan-based product, BST-CarGel, has been shown to result in better organised tissue repair compared to microfracture treatment alone [379], and further clinical evaluation will indeed be interesting to follow.

However, a number of concerns over the use of natural polymers, such as the feasibility of producing sufficient amounts of these materials for clinical applications, the degree of reproducibility, and assurance of pathogen removal, has led to a number of synthetic polymers being investigated as alternatives (as reviewed [380]). Synthetic polymers offer the benefits of processing flexibility and mass production, lack of immunological concerns, and greater control over degradation rates (see [381]).

Research involving synthetic polymers for cartilage TE is largely focused around degradable polyesters that have been FDA/EMA approved, such as PGA, PLA and their copolymer, poly (lactic-co-glycolic acid) (PLGA) (see [382,383]). PGA and PLA are degraded into glycolic acid and lactic acid respectively, both of which can be metabolised by the body and removed by natural pathways. A recent study has also indicated that the release of lactic acid from PLA scaffolds can be beneficial to chondrocyte ECM synthesis [384]. PLA contains a methyl side group within each monomer unit, which contributes to its hydrophobicity and slower degradation rate compared to PGA [385]. While the greater stability and high compressive strength of PLA may be beneficial to cartilage TE strategies [386], the hydrophobicity of the polymer limits cell attachment and viability [387]. In contrast to PLA, PGA is a rigid polymer with a high degree of crystallinity [385]; it is also hydrophilic and lacks methyl groups, which contributes to its higher degradation rate. The copolymer PLGA can therefore be used to tailor degradation rates and compressive strength, with altered ratios of PLA and PGA being used to fine-tune these properties. One study looked at the effects of PLGA composition on the cell adhesion and growth of bovine articular chondrocytes [388]; here non-woven PGA meshes were coated with varying quantities of PLA via solvent evaporation to give composites with PLA contents ranging from 0 to 68%. The compressive strength and degradation time was shown to increase with increasing PLA content, with those meshes containing 68% PLA lasting for 45 days with a compressive modulus of 20 kPa, while 0% PLA meshes degraded after just 5 days and had a compressive modulus of 1 kPa; however, the hydrophobic PLA was shown to decrease cell seeding efficiency, adhesion and proliferation. PLGA is also considered an expensive synthetic polymer and, as such, the relatively inexpensive polycaprolactone (PCL) is also being widely incorporated into many strategies [389–391]. This polymer has also been used to overcome the brittle properties of PLGA and its flexibility means that electrospun PCL nanofibrous sheets can be rolled or moulded over surfaces, e.g., of articular joints; making them excellent candidates for skeletal TE strategies [392]. However, like PLA, the downside of PCL lies in its hydrophobic nature and lack of cell surface recognition sites. Together the relative positive and negative attributes of synthetic polymers means that co-polymerisation of various combinations of both synthetic and natural polymers has become an active area of research [389,391,393–398].

6.1. Electrospun Scaffolds

As well as choice of polymer, scaffold form is also an important factor to consider. Electrospinning is a popular, simple, and cost-effective technique which allows for the production of both nano- and microfibrous polymer scaffolds (see [399]). Briefly, the technique involves dissolving a polymer in a suitable solvent and feeding it through a metal capillary with a high voltage applied, sending a jet of highly charged molecules in solution towards a collector of opposite charge [400]. As the jet travels, the solvent is evaporated, leaving a mesh of polymer fibers. The applied voltage, working distance, rotation rate, choice of solvent, polymer concentration, and flow rate, are all parameters that can be adjusted to generate scaffolds with different characteristics and fiber morphologies [401]. A number of groups have used electrospun scaffolds for cartilage TE purposes [398,402,403]. Sonomoto et al. [398] demonstrated that their PLGA electrospun nanofibrous scaffolds (a 50:50 ratio of PLA to PGA) could induce the differentiation of hMSCs into chondrocytes, without the addition of any cytokines. Wise et al. [402], have also compared orientated PCL electrospun scaffolds of approximately 500 nm and 3000 nm fiber diameter. The group demonstrated that hMSCs preferentially orientated along the direction of the fibers, and maintained their orientation during chondrogenic differentiation. The nanofibrous scaffolds (500 nm) were shown to enhance chondrogenic differentiation when compared to the microfibrous scaffolds (3000 nm), as indicated by type II collagen and aggrecan expression.

An issue of electrospinning is the inherently small pore sizes generated (typically < 10 μm), and the low thickness of fibers (typically ranging from 10 to 10,000 nm in diameter; limited by the slow rate of production), which together means that 2D membranes with poor cellular infiltration rather than true 3D scaffolds are often formed [404,405]. As such, techniques such as multilayering, or the incorporation of hydrogels are being investigated [395,406–409]. Indeed, the native ECM consists of a fibrous protein network infiltrated with PGs, and so inclusion of a hydrogel within electrospun fibers seems a natural step in creating an ECM-mimetic with good levels of hydration, cell infiltration and the potential for controlled release of bioactive factors. A technique involving the combination of electrospinning and electrospraying allows for the rapid fabrication of fiber/hydrogel hybrid scaffolds with improved and more uniform cell infiltration [407,409]. Chen et al. [395] have also recently designed a porous 3D scaffold using electrospun gelatin/PLA nanofibers crosslinked with HA. Chondrocytes cultured in the scaffolds remained viable, and histological staining demonstrated that the construct could enhance the repair of cartilage in vivo. In an alternative approach Coburn et al. [410] have developed a fiber-hydrogel composite, using a novel electrospinning technique, whereby the fibers are spun onto a water coagulation bath (rather than a solid surface). This allows for the formation of a rapid 3D fiber mesh with porosity suitable for hydrogel and cell infusion by means of simple mixing, and which is injectable and allows for homogenous tissue growth. They demonstrated that the density of the fibers within the constructs had an effect on tissue formation, with higher (40% dry weight) fiber density leading to greater MSC proliferation, while lower (10% dry weight) fiber density led to the greatest amount of matrix production following chondrogenesis. However, most characterisation of chondrogenesis in this study seems to have been on fiber-hydrogel composites made from stacking to form a 3D multilayered scaffold, rather than those made by the novel electrospinning technique. Compared to hydrogels alone, the stacked composites showed increased ECM production and greater response to mechanical stimulation, which resulted in a drastic increase in tissue production and near native levels of ECM (although ECM composition was not examined). Owing to the structured composition of articular cartilage, stacked composites, where each layer could be engineered to release different combinations of bioactive factors, may be more effective compared to one homogenous matrix. However, it should be noted that Coburn et al. [410] did not look at any markers of chondrocyte hypertrophy within their study.

6.2. Hydrogels

Hydrogels, water swollen hydrophilic polymers that are able to retain large quantities of water, are also popular for cartilage TE strategies, as they allow the formation of an effective 3D environment, can be processed in relatively mild conditions, and can be delivered in a minimally invasive manner (see [411,412]). The high water content of these gels creates a permeable matrix that can effectively mimic the 'softness' of cartilage, allowing for easy nutrient transfer, and which can signal to cells through both mechanical and chemical signals [411]. Given these properties, a wide range of both natural and synthetic hydrogels have been investigated for cartilage TE.

Examples of natural hydrogels frequently used for cartilage TE include fibrin and alginate. Ho et al. [413], compared the chondrogenic differentiation of BMMSCs seeded into fibrin hydrogels or fibrin-alginate composites. MSCs encapsulated within fibrin hydrogels showed increased mesenchymal condensation compared to fibrin-alginate constructs. The fibrin hydrogel encapsulated cells also showed increased chondrogenic differentiation with an increase in expression of collagen type II and aggrecan, and unlike the fibrin-alginate gels, did not appear to undergo hypertrophy. Interestingly though, alginate sulfate hydrogels have been shown to support a chondrocyte phenotype, and by combining alginate sulfate with nanocellulose it is possible to create a printable bioink, which could therefore allow for the spatial deposition of hydrogels with micrometer precision [414].

Nguyen et al. [7], have used different combinations of both synthetic and natural biopolymers to create hydrogels that can direct MSCs to differentiate and form ECM that is characteristic of the superficial, middle, or deep zones of articular cartilage (see Figure 1). For example, the combination of CS and MMP-sensitive peptides incorporated into polyethylene glycol (PEG) hydrogels reportedly led to high levels of type II collagen, low levels of PG expression, and a low compressive modulus characteristic of the superficial zone. In contrast, PEG-HA hydrogels induced low collagen II and high PG levels leading to a high compressive modulus more characteristic to that of the deep zone. In a further study they demonstrated that layer-by-layer organisation of these hydrogels to create a single 3D scaffold can stimulate MSCs to differentiate and form a multilayered ECM similar to that of native articular cartilage [8].

Although hydrogels clearly offer much promise, a common issue is the toxicity problems associated with their chemical crosslinking [415]. A number of groups have therefore been investigating self-assembling peptides, made up of alternating hydrophilic and hydrophobic amino acids, which spontaneously form nanofiber scaffold hydrogels in NaCl solutions [416,417]. These self-assembling peptide hydrogels have the advantages of traditional hydrogels, but also avoid the use of toxic cross-links, harmful degradation products, and undesired immunological responses, making them a very attractive option for TE strategies [416]. Zhou et al. have developed a novel self-assembling peptide hydrogel, which is based around the co-assembly of two aromatic peptide amphiphiles; i.e., a structural peptide, fluorenylmethoxycarbonyl-diphenylalanine (Fmoc-FF) and a functional Fmoc-coupled RGD peptide (arginine-glycine-aspartic acid) (Fmoc-RGD), which corresponds to the cell-binding domain of the common ECM component fibronectin [418]. These short di/tri-peptides were shown to lead to the formation of a simple, cost-effective and bioactive hydrogel, which could be formed at neutral pH and effectively support cell attachment and spreading [418,419]. In addition, the versatility of the hydrogel means that it could also be decorated with other bioactive peptides. Similarly, Saiani et al. [420] have formed simple FEFEFKFK self-assembling octapeptide gels, which can also allow for the addition of bioactive peptides. The gels have been shown to self-assemble into β-sheet structures which can promote the round morphology and ECM production of chondrocytes [421].

Another limitation of hydrogels is that although MSCs undergoing chondrogenesis appear to prefer the softer material of a hydrogel over fibrous scaffolds, hydrogels are limited in their mechanical properties and, thus, this may negatively affect their survival within a joint [410]. As such, the use of fiber/hydrogel composites (as discussed in Section 6.1) is perhaps more likely to succeed in cartilage TE applications. However, considerable variation in the stiffness of self-assembling peptide hydrogels can be achieved through modulating the assembly conditions [422].

6.3. GAG Incorporation and Application

As discussed above, synthetic polymers are becoming increasingly popular in TE strategies, due to their reproducibility, non-immunogenic properties, and ability for up-scaled production [381]. However, the bioinert properties of synthetic materials, means that they usually have to be enhanced with additives such as expensive growth factors and cytokines. A more cost effective method of promoting the biofunctionality of synthetic scaffolds is thought to be through the use of GAGs (as discussed in Section 5).

A number of groups have pioneered the incorporation of GAGs into synthetic polymers, in order to produce functionalised scaffolds that combine the advantages of both synthetic and natural polymeric materials [335,423,424]. The incorporation of GAGs into hydrogels has utilised both covalent and non-covalent conjugation, which allow for the tunable adjustment of matrix characteristics and release of bioactive factors [424]. Kim et al. [425] seeded MSCs into photocrosslinkable HA hydrogels and cultured them with varying levels and durations of TGFβ3. Results demonstrated that relatively short-term exposure (7 days) to a high level of TGFβ3 (100 ng/mL) was more effective at inducing and maintaining cartilage formation when compared to constant delivery of a lower dose (10 ng/mL) over a 9-week period. In agreement with this, Bhakta et al. [189], have reported that heparin containing hydrogels reduced the burst release of BMP2, and sustained its activity, however, it was the initial burst release of BMP2 that was found to be important for optimal bone formation. These results indicate that the controlled degradation of biphasic scaffolds might allow for both the initial release of a high dose of growth factor, followed by prolonged activity [426].

Compared to the incorporation of GAGs into hydrogels, their immobilisation onto surfaces such as electrospun fibrous scaffolds has proved a more difficult task. Typically GAGs are anchored via covalent immobilisation, however, this has been shown to restrict the conformation of the bound

GAGs and their functionality [395,427–429]; e.g., in some situations the oligosaccharides are required to be internalised with signalling receptors [430–432]. Mahoney et al. [433] have developed a method for the non-covalent immobilisation of heparin to surfaces, which involves the use of cold plasma polymerisation of allylamine (ppAm) and avoids the need for labelling or chemical modification of the GAGs. The ppAm coats the surface in positively charged amine groups ($-NH_2$) [434], thereby allowing for the subsequent immobilisation of negatively charged GAGs. Plasma polymerisation is an established technology involving a vessel containing the vapour of a monomer at low pressure and an energy source (see [435]). Generally, the lower the ratio of power to monomer input rate, the higher the retention of monomer functionality, and in addition substrate temperature and the location of the plasma discharge relative to the substrate have been shown to affect surface chemistry [436]. Heparin immobilised onto ppAm-coated microtiter plates was able to interact with the heparin-binding proteins tumour necrosis factor-stimulated gene-6 (TSG-6), complement factor H, and the chemokine interleukin 8, whereas no functional heparin was present on untreated plates [433]. The positive charge of the allylamine coating, and the fact that the binding of heparin to the surface was salt-strength dependent indicates that the binding is at least partly through an ionic interaction [433,437]. It was also demonstrated that the ppAm coating could be used to create heparin gradients, and as well as heparin, can also support the functional binding of a wide range of GAGs, including CS, HA, and DS, although differences existed in their protein-binding capabilities depending on the surface chemistry to which they were adsorbed [437,438]. Yang et al. [439] have also coated stainless steel with ppAm, in order to develop a heparinised surface with biological function. They found that the heparin-binding surface inhibited the ability of human umbilical artery smooth muscle cells to adhere and proliferate, while enhancing that of human umbilical vein endothelial cells. The heparinised surface was also shown to inhibit thrombosis and promote re-endothelialisation in vivo. Meade et al. [335] translated the cold plasma polymerisation technology onto 3D constructs, developing a novel electrospun scaffold functionalised with GAGs non-covalently attached to the fiber surface via a ppAm coating. Bound GAGs were shown to be biologically active, restoring the ability of $EXT1^{-/-}$ (HS-deficient) mESCs to differentiate down the neural lineage. Use of these scaffolds to investigate how GAGs can control the chondrogenic differentiation of hMSCs would therefore be interesting.

Whilst the incorporation of GAGs into biomaterials for improved TE strategies is not new, most attempts thus far have relied upon the use of poorly defined, heterogeneous, commercially available, preparations [188–190,192,194,335,395,426,428,439–441]. Although these strategies have generally proven effective, it is difficult to decipher specific structure-function relationships, and there is the worry that off-target effects may lead to sub-optimal or even detrimental effects [190,442–446]. In addition, the use of natural polymers, generally isolated from animal tissues, is a concern for clinical translation, not only due to the high levels of structural complexity, but also due to potential contamination. As recently as 2008, batches of heparin containing oversulfated CS, caused allergic-type reactions in patients and led to over 100 deaths, highlighting the need for a more controllable method of production [447]; this requirement has also recently been underlined by the identification of significant batch variation in commercially available preparations of HS used in research [448]. In an effort to purify more defined HS preparations, Cool and colleagues have successfully employed a peptide affinity isolation method [163,169,193,195,295]; this technique is suitable for scale-up to meet clinical demand, and has already been shown to be effective for potentiating the bioactivity and bioavailability of a number of growth factors. Further to this, the advancement of GAG modelling, sequencing and synthesis tools over the past decade (see [326,359–361]), has also meant that the feasibility of generating synthetic GAG mimetics is progressing rapidly (see [449]). Chemoenzymatic methods using bacterial glycosyltransferases and synthetic UDP monosaccharide donors can now allow for the rapid production of structurally defined HS oligosaccharides [450], where the expression of HS biosynthetic enzymes at high levels in *E. coli* is making the process amenable to scale-up [451]. In addition, a novel strategy, whereby the 6-hydroxyl group of synthetic UDP-GlcNAc or UDP-GlcNS nucleotides is substituted by an azido group, is facilitating the synthesis of GAG mimetics in excellent yields [452];

here the azido moiety is converted to a sulfate group, leading to the production of oligosaccharides with N-sulfates at both the 2- and 6- positions, allowing for close mimicry of natural N-sulfated, 6-O sulfated GlcN residues. Improved understanding of the substrate specificity of C5 epimerase activity has also meant that single product IdoA2S-GlcNS residues can now be irreversibly synthesised (i.e., rather than a mixture of GlcA and IdoA residues) [453]. These improved methods have meant that over 30 synthetic heparin oligosaccharides have now been generated [449]. Ultimately, our ability to uncover structure/function relationships in heparin/HS oligosaccharides is evolving rapidly, and with this, the incorporation of more defined and specific HS sequences into TE strategies, in a cost-effective manner, has now become a realistic goal.

7. The Problems Associated with Heparin

The high level of sulfation (and thus negative charge) carried by the GAG heparin, means that it is able to bind, stabilise, and modulate the activity of a wide range of growth factors (see [454]). In addition, the low cost, easy availability, and status of heparin as an already FDA- and EMA-approved product, has meant that researchers are harnessing its properties, preferentially over that of other GAGs (such as HS) to improve growth factor delivery [188,189,192,194,440]. Gaining particular prominence is the use of heparin-loaded delivery vehicles for skeletal TE, where biomaterials decorated with heparin have been extensively studied both in vitro and in vivo, for their ability to reduce the dosing requirements and improve the therapeutic potential of BMPs, such as BMP2 [188,189,194,455–460]. Most of these studies have shown very promising results, with heparin-loaded biomaterials improving BMP2 delivery, release, and osteogenic potential. It should be noted, however, that some inhibitory effects of heparin on TGFβ superfamily members (and other proteins) have been reported when high doses of the GAG are used [461,462]. In addition, in some cases the use of heparin-loaded biomaterials have proven ineffective in vivo [192] and the long-term side effects have not been tested. Adding to this, it has been shown in a rat ectopic model, that while collagen sponges soaked with BMP2 and heparin did result in more bone formation compared to sponges soaked with BMP2 alone, the use of an HS variant, rather than heparin, improved bone formation even further [190]. On this basis we hypothesised that while heparin may enhance the retention/activity of BMP2 (or other growth factors) under certain conditions, its binding 'promiscuity' means that it may also inhibit other factors that play a role in the repair process, leading to sub-optimal or even deleterious results [266].

In addition to the potential off-target effects from heparin-incorporated biomaterials, the long-term use of heparin as an anticoagulant has also resulted in a number of adverse clinical effects being reported, including thrombocytopenia, vascular reactions and osteoporosis [442–445]. Cool and colleagues, recently showed that heparin has donor-dependent effects on the stemness and multipotency of hMSCs, and alters a number of signalling pathways associated with hMSC growth and differentiation [446]. This raises a concern regarding the long-term use of heparin in the clinic and its suitability in skeletal (and other) TE strategies. Furthermore, the potential of GDF5 in cartilage TE strategies (see Section 4.1.2.1 above) lead us to investigate the interaction between GDF5 and heparin. We identified GDF5 as a novel heparin/HS-binding protein, and demonstrated that heparin (but not equivalent doses of HS) has a strong and clear inhibitory effect on the biological activity of GDF5, even at doses 10-fold lower than those that would be clinically administered (Figure 4E) [266]; e.g., for patients with venous thromboembolism, the dose of heparin is usually maintained at 0.3 to 0.7 U/mL [463], while 10 nM of heparin used in our study equates to around 0.03 to 0.04 U/mL. In addition, the inhibitory effect of heparin was seen across multiple hMSC donors and in the skeletal cell line ATDC5. Given the importance of GDF5 for skeletal development, our results might help explain the reported increased risk of developing osteoporosis following long-term heparin treatment [442,444], and the variable (and disappointing) results seen with heparin-loaded biomaterials for skeletal repair [190,192]. As illustrated in Figure 5, these data add further caution to the widespread use of unfractionated heparin, both in the clinic and research settings.

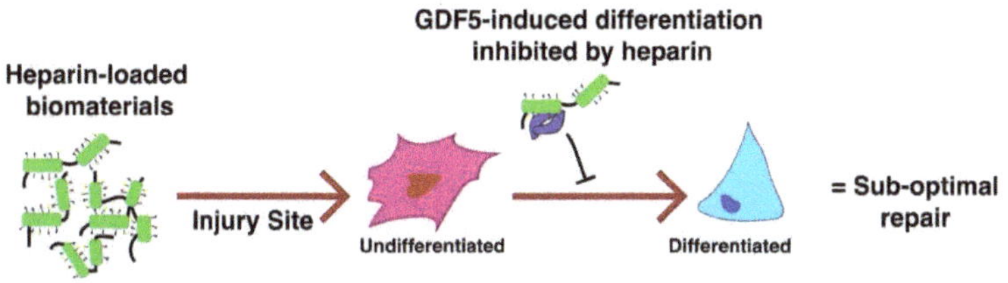

Figure 5. Urging caution over the use of heparin-loaded biomaterials for TE strategies. Heparin has an inhibitory effect on the activity of GDF5. As such, the incorporation of heparin-loaded biomaterials into skeletal TE strategies may have an inhibitory effect on GDF5, which is found naturally at the repair site and that may also be important to the repair process, leading to suboptimal or deleterious outcomes.

Importantly, the HS used in our study did not show the same inhibitory effect as heparin on GDF5 activity (Figure 4E), indicating that HS may be a more suitable, safe and effective alternative for incorporation into TE strategies and stem cell expansion/differentiation protocols. However, it is hard to generalise when HS is so heterogeneous/diverse, and additional studies with better-defined HS preparations will of course be necessary to investigate this further. It should also be noted, that the unfractionated HS preparation we used (from porcine intestinal mucosa) did not significantly promote the activity of GDF5 either. Again, given the sequence diversity of HS [309,328,330], we anticipate that it will be possible to identify HS variants that promote GDF5 activity while retaining other beneficial effects on chondrocyte function/phenotype [266]. Previous work by the Cool/Nurcombe group indicates that isolation of HS variants by their affinity for particular growth factors, enables the selection of saccharides markedly more potent at promoting growth factor activity compared to using unfractionated HS starting material, with its intrinsically high level of compositional heterogeneity [190,193,195,295]. Thus, there is the possibility to potentiate the activity of specific growth factors, to the same extent as heparin, while avoiding the adverse and off-target effects stemming from heparin's pleiotropic nature. Indeed, our work has revealed that the HS3 variant (selected through its affinity for BMP2 and shown to promote BMP2 activity [193,195]), did not inhibit GDF5 in the same manner as heparin [266]. Therefore, by using this particular HS preparation, there is the possibility of promoting BMP2 activity (as with heparin) without affecting the activity of GDF5, which would also be present at the injury site and be involved in the repair process [259,261,464]. This further highlights the therapeutic utility of developing selective HS variants, rather than using heparin. Interestingly, given that HS3 has a higher level of sulfation compared to unfractionated HS [193], and carries an overall charge more similar to heparin, it might have been expected to also inhibit GDF5 activity. However, this was not the case [266] and suggests that charge density is not the dominant feature in the interaction between GDF5 and heparin/HS, and that GAG structure and sequence may also play a role.

The clear inhibitory effects of exogenously added heparin on GDF5 activity, also led us to look at whether there was a requirement for endogenous HSPGs for GDF5 binding and localisation [266]. Previous studies have shown that overexpression of *Drosophila* HSPGs (i.e., division abnormally delayed (Dally) and Dally-like protein (Dlp)), result in enhanced *Drosophila* Decapentaplegic (Dpp) (an ortholog of vertebrate BMP2/4) signalling in the wing [465]. However, in HSPG deficient mutants, Dpp signalling is reduced [466]. These results therefore suggest a positive role for HSPGs in BMP signalling, perhaps by acting as a co-receptor for BMPs (as with FGF signalling [467,468]), or by modulating the bioavailability of BMPs at the cell surface. In favour of the latter hypothesis, our data [266] demonstrated that pericellular HSPGs play a key role in localising GDF5 to the cell surface, with a positive correlation between HSPG and GDF5 concentration being observed (Figure 4D). This is in good agreement with results reported for BMP2 [190,469], and further emphasises the importance of HSPGs in regulating the activity of many TGFβ superfamily members. These results then led us to hypothesise that the inhibitory effects of heparin on GDF5-induced activity may be due to the exogenous heparin out-competing the binding of pericellular HSPGs to GDF5; i.e., preventing GDF5 from localising to the cell surface and binding to its receptors to initiate downstream signalling/activity [266]. In agreement with this hypothesis, we were able to show that heparin (but not equivalent doses of HS) inhibited both GDF5 association to the cell surface, and GDF5-induced downstream Smad 1/5/8 signalling. Interestingly, we have recently observed that despite the lack of HS on the surface of HSPG-deficient CHO cells, and the decreased binding of GDF5 to these cells (compared to WT CHO), over a one hour time period, GDF5 signalling appeared similar in both cell lines (B.I. Ayerst, V. Nurcome, A.J. Day, C.L.R. Merry and S. Cool, *unpublished observations*). We therefore suggest that while HSPGs are important for capturing and improving the bioavailability of GDF5 at the cell surface, and perhaps protecting the growth factor from proteolytic degradation, unlike the FGF family of growth factors [467,468], HSPGs are not critical for the interaction between GDF5 and its receptor for downstream signalling.

Since the inhibitory effect of exogenous heparin on GDF5 activity cannot simply be explained by a lack of accumulation of GDF5 at the cell surface, we suggest that the high affinity of heparin for GDF5 may also more directly inhibit GDF5-receptor interaction [266]. In addition, heparin has also been shown to inhibit the activity of heparanases [470–472]. While treatment with heparanse has been shown to stimulate chondrogenesis in micromass cultures of mouse embryo limb mesenchymal cells, the heparanase antagonist SST0001 (a heparin molecule, modified so that it lacks anticoagulant activity) strongly inhibited chondrogenesis [473]. Heparanase was also found to be over expressed in chondrocytes from patients with hereditary multiple exostoses; a skeletal disorder resulting in the formation of benign cartilagenous tumours. In this sense, the inhibitory effect of heparin on GDF5-induced activity seen in our study may be three fold; firstly the high affinity of heparin for GDF5 may directly inhibit GDF5-receptor interactions; secondly, heparin may bind to GDF5, preventing it from associating with cell surface HS, and therefore limiting its bioavailability; thirdly heparin may inhibit the activity of heparanases, thereby preventing GDF5 from being released from cell surface HSPGs, which is required for its interaction with its receptors and the initiation of downstream signaling (Figure 6).

The pleiotropic nature and off-target effects of heparin render it, in our opinion, unsuitable for use in TE strategies [442–446]. Importantly, HS-based therapeutics may offer improved outcomes, with a more direct and targeted control of growth factor activity [357]. Indeed, a successful strategy for isolating HS fractions according to their affinity for specific growth factors has been developed [163,193,195,295]. The arrangement of sulfate groups within HS chains are thought to align with basic amino acids within the heparin-binding domain of target proteins [474]. As such, the synthesis of peptides based on heparin-binding domains of proteins, can allow for affinity-based HS purification and the isolation of variants with increased growth factor potency. The technology has already been used to isolate HS variants with increased affinity for BMP2, $VEGF_{165}$, and FGF2, which have all proved more efficacious than unfractionated HS for bone healing, angiogenesis, and stem cell expansion, respectively [163,193,195,295].

However, although successful in the cases above, limitations and challenges still exist in the widespread translation of this affinity purification platform. The use of linear heparin-binding peptide sequences is simplistic and not representative of the majority of heparin-protein interactions [158,169,475–478]. Ultimately, a major obstacle for the use of HS as a therapeutic lies in its vast heterogeneity, including (large) variations in its domain structure, sulfation level/pattern, and chain length [479]. On top of this, simple/effective methodologies for the sequencing of HS (and other GAG) chains are not yet available; thus, making it difficult to determine and interpret structure-function relationships [321]. In addition, the degree of specificity involved in protein-HS interactions is still very much open for discussion [159,328,330,480–482], adding doubt over how precisely protein-HS interactions can be controlled in vivo. Another important factor is that binding affinity does not always directly equate to activity, and broad recognition/specificity does not necessarily indicate insignificance [483,484]; further adding to the complexities of developing a standard and effective method for targeted HS therapeutics.

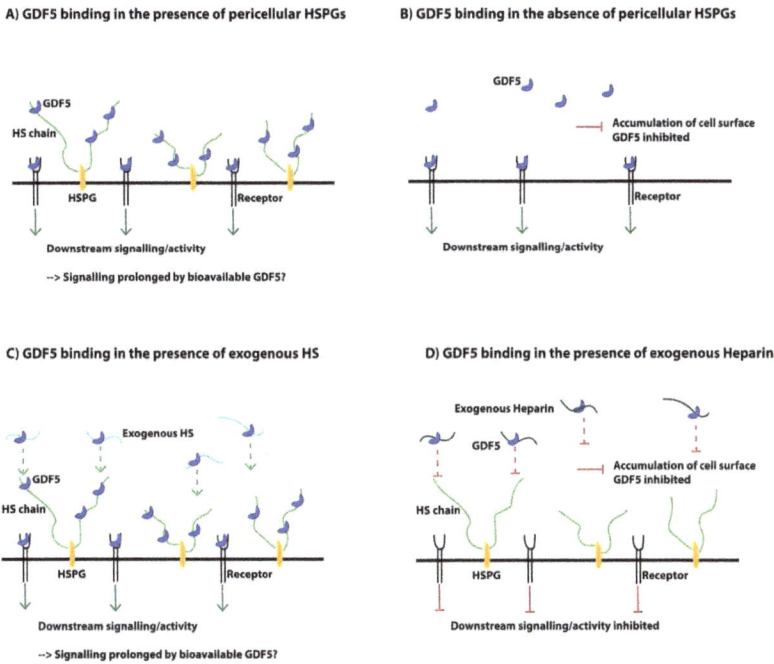

Figure 6. Proposed methods of regulation of GDF5 activity by cell surface HSPGs and exogenously added heparin/HS. GDF5 is captured by HSPGs and accumulates at the cell surface, where it is then available for prolonged receptor binding and activity (**A**). In the absence of HSPGs the accumulation of GDF5 at the cell surface does not occur; GDF5 is still able to bind to its receptors to initiate activity, but the free ligand may be more susceptible to proteolytic degradation, and as a result the duration of downstream signalling and activity may not be as prolonged as in the presence of HSPGs; (**B**). Exogenous HS is able to bind to GDF5, but the higher affinity of cell surface HSPGs and receptors for GDF5 binding, means that the interaction is only transient in nature; cell surface HSPGs and receptors out-compete exogenous HS for the GDF5 interaction and, as a result, similar levels of signalling are seen as in situation part A. However, if a specific high affinity HS is used (at a high enough concentration) then inhibition would be seen (**C**). The high affinity of heparin for GDF5 means that this GAG binds and out-competes cell-surface HSPGs and receptors for binding. Both the accumulation of GDF5 at the cell surface and downstream signalling is inhibited (**D**).

Early on, the discovery of the sequence required for antithrombin III (ATIII) binding indicated that protein-HS interactions may be governed by specific sequences encoded within the primary structure of HS [485]. ATIII requires a 3-O-sulfated pentasaccharide in order to bind HS; i.e., GlcNS/NAc(6S)-GlcA-GlcNS(3S±6S)-IdoA(±2S)-GlcNS(±6S). Removal of the 3-O sulfate reduces the pentasaccharide's affinity for ATIII by 17,000 fold [486]. However, since this finding, very few specific binding sequences have been identified, perhaps with the exception of FGF2 [155,487], and it has been suggested that the specificity of protein-HS interactions instead exists on many different levels; with some interactions being more specific than others [484]. The importance of sulfation patterning also exists at a chain level as well as at an individual saccharide level, where the distribution of sulfated domains within an HS chain can dictate binding specificity as well as (or in some cases, in preference over) the specific sulfation sequence within those domains [159,488,489]. In support of this, HS chains produced by biosynthetic mutant mice, lacking HS 2-O-sulfotransferase activity, were still able to support FGF2 activity despite lacking 2-O sulfation, apparently because they had compensatory increases in N- and 6-O sulfation that maintained the charge distribution along the HS chain [489]. While HS contains regions of both high and low sulfation, known as NS and NA domains, respectively, heparin can be seen as a hypersulfated version of HS, with virtually continuous sulfation along its chains, i.e., forming essentially one long NS domain [479,490]. The overall high level of sulfation in heparin may therefore mask selectivity, leading to its pleiotropic nature. It has been suggested that in the case of some heparin/HS-protein interactions little specificity exists, and that instead overall charge density is the predominant factor in determining binding [483,491].

It is therefore likely that the extent of HS-binding specificity varies among different proteins, and that overall charge density, sulfate patterning, and sequence specificity on HS chains can all play an important role. In addition, while electrostatic interactions between sulfate/carboxyl groups in the GAG chains and surface exposed positively charged arginine/lysine residues in the protein are undoubtedly important [492], evidence also suggests that non-ionic interactions, such as van der Waals forces, hydrogen bonding, and aromatic ring stacking, can also play a role [328,481,492–496]. Interestingly, a recent study has suggested that the presence of residues such as asparagine or glutamine can help to identify heparin/HS binding sites [496]; where these uncharged residues confer specificity on the interaction. If correct, this could revolutionise the identification of HS-protein binding sites, and thus facilitate the design of targeted HS-based therapeutics.

While experimental and modelling techniques are rapidly advancing, we are still only in the infancy of being able to fully characterise protein-GAG interactions. The high level of heterogeneity, conformational flexibility, and uncertainty over binding mechanisms has meant that it is hard to model and identify interactions in a high-throughput and effective manner. In addition, it appears that the level of specificity involved in protein-GAG interactions is not universal, and high affinity HS variants may not always lead to the desired outcome. As such, the development of targeted HS therapeutics may be a more complex task than first envisioned. However, the fact that a degree of specificity does seem to exist for certain proteins, means that the use of HS variants, rather than heparin, to more tightly control protein activity, is still an exciting and realistic prospect. The development of more advanced modelling and sequencing tools, along with the further refinement of biomaterials for the delivery and application of HS variants, will however first be required, before the full potential of HS glycotherapeutics can be realised.

8. Conclusions

The low cost, easy availability, high level of sulfation, and status of heparin as an already FDA- and EMA- approved product, has meant that it has largely been the GAG of choice for TE applications. While the use of heparin has generally proven effective, the long-term side effects of its incorporation into biomaterials has not been tested, and in some cases the use of heparin-loaded biomaterials have proven ineffective in vivo. While heparin may enhance the retention/activity of certain growth factors under certain conditions, its binding 'promiscuity' means that it may also inhibit other factors that play an important role in the repair process, leading to suboptimal or even deleterious effects. These concerns have been highlighted by our recent work, indicating that exogenous heparin has a strong inhibitory effect on the activity of growth differentiation factor 5 (GDF5), a growth factor which plays a critical role in cartilage/skeletal formation and homeostasis. This is particularly worrying, given the increasing incorporation of heparin into skeletal TE strategies. Overall, there is growing evidence cautioning the use of heparin both in the clinic and in TE applications, and emphasising the need to transition to using more specific GAGs (e.g., HS derivatives or synthetics), with better-defined structures and fewer off-target effects, if optimal therapy is to be achieved. Importantly, the advancement of GAG modelling, sequencing and synthesis tools over the past decade are starting to allow for this transition; enabling us to move away from the use of heterogenous undefined GAG preparations, and opening up more advanced opportunities for the use of GAGs in a more controlled and defined manner.

Acknowledgments: B.I.A acknowledges the receipt of a University of Manchester and A*STAR, Singapore, PhD Studentship and A*STAR Research Attachment Programme (ARAP) scholarship. AJD thanks Arthritis Research UK for its long-term support. We also acknowledge Prof. Barbara Mulloy from Imperial College London, for inviting us to contribute to this issue.

Author Contributions: B.I.A wrote the review, with the guidance, support and contribution of A.J.D and C.L.R.M.

Conflicts of Interest: The authors declare no conflict of interest.

References

1. Bhosale, M.A.; Richardson, J.B. Articular cartilage: Structure, injuries and review of management. *Br. Med. Bull.* **2008**, *87*, 77–95. [CrossRef] [PubMed]
2. Hardingham, T.E. Fell-Muir lecture: Cartilage 2010—The known unknowns. *Int. J. Exp. Pathol.* **2010**, *91*, 203–209. [CrossRef] [PubMed]
3. Correa, D.; Lietman, S.A. Articular cartilage repair: Current needs, methods and research directions. *Semin. Cell Dev. Bio.* **2016**, *62*, 67–77. [CrossRef] [PubMed]
4. Goldring, M.B. Chondrogenesis, chondrocyte differentiation, and articular cartilage metabolism in health and osteoarthritis. *Ther. Adv. Musculoskelet. Dis.* **2012**, *4*, 269–285. [CrossRef] [PubMed]
5. Schinagl, R.M.; Gurskis, D.; Chen, A.C.; Sah, R.L. Depth-dependent confined compression modulus of full-thickness bovine articular cartilage. *J. Orthop. Res.* **1997**, *15*, 499–506. [CrossRef] [PubMed]
6. Seror, J.; Zhu, L.; Goldberg, R.; Day, A.J.; Klein, J. Supramolecular synergy in the boundary lubrication of synovial joints. *Nat. Commun.* **2015**, *6*, 6497. [CrossRef] [PubMed]
7. Nguyen, L.H.; Kudva, A.K.; Guckert, N.L.; Linse, K.D.; Roy, K. Unique biomaterial compositions direct bone marrow stem cells into specific chondrocytic phenotypes corresponding to the various zones of articular cartilage. *Biomaterials* **2011**, *32*, 1327–1338. [CrossRef] [PubMed]
8. Nguyen, L.H.; Kudva, A.K.; Saxena, N.S.; Roy, K. Engineering articular cartilage with spatially-varying matrix composition and mechanical properties from a single stem cell population using a multi-layered hydrogel. *Biomaterials* **2011**, *32*, 6946–6952. [CrossRef] [PubMed]
9. Boschetti, F.; Peretti, G.M. Tensile and compressive properties of healthy and osteoarthritic human articular cartilage. *Biorheology* **2008**, *45*, 337–344. [PubMed]
10. Yang, N.; Meng, Q.J. Circadian Clocks in Articular Cartilage and Bone: A Compass in the Sea of Matrices. *J. Biol. Rhythm.* **2016**, *31*, 415–427. [CrossRef] [PubMed]
11. Shen, G. The role of type X collagen in facilitating and regulating endochondral ossification of articular cartilage. *Orthod. Craniofac. Res.* **2005**, *8*, 11–17. [CrossRef] [PubMed]
12. Decker, R.S.; Koyama, E.; Pacifici, M. Genesis and morphogenesis of limb synovial joints and articular cartilage. *Matrix Biol.* **2014**, *39*, 5–10. [CrossRef] [PubMed]
13. Mitrovic, D. Development of the diarthrodial joints in the rat embryo. *Am. J. Anat.* **1978**, *151*, 475–485. [CrossRef] [PubMed]
14. Hunziker, E.B. Growth plate structure and function. *Pathol. Immunopathol. Res.* **1988**, *7*, 9–13. [CrossRef] [PubMed]
15. Hall, B.K.; Miyake, T. The membranous skeleton: The role of cell condensations in vertebrate skeletogenesis. *Anat. Embryol. (Berl)* **1992**, *186*, 107–124. [CrossRef] [PubMed]
16. Kronenberg, H.M. Developmental regulation of the growth plate. *Nature* **2003**, *423*, 332–336. [CrossRef] [PubMed]
17. Long, F.; Ornitz, D.M. Development of the endochondral skeleton. *Cold Spring Harb. Perspect. Biol.* **2013**, *5*, a008334. [CrossRef] [PubMed]
18. Kozhemyakina, E.; Lassar, A.B.; Zelzer, E. A pathway to bone: Signaling molecules and transcription factors involved in chondrocyte development and maturation. *Development* **2015**, *142*, 817–831. [CrossRef] [PubMed]
19. Camarero-Espinosa, S.; Rothen-Rutishauser, B.; Foster, E.J.; Weder, C. Articular cartilage: From formation to tissue engineering. *Biomater. Sci.* **2016**, *4*, 734–767. [CrossRef] [PubMed]

20. Zhong, L.; Huang, X.; Karperien, M.; Post, J.N. The Regulatory Role of Signaling Crosstalk in Hypertrophy of MSCs and Human Articular Chondrocytes. *Int. J. Mol. Sci.* **2015**, *16*, 19225–19247. [CrossRef] [PubMed]

21. Iwamoto, M.; Ohta, Y.; Larmour, C.; Enomoto-Iwamoto, M. Toward regeneration of articular cartilage. *Birth Defects Res. C Embryo Today* **2013**, *99*, 192–202. [CrossRef] [PubMed]

22. Pacifici, M.; Koyama, E.; Shibukawa, Y.; Wu, C.; Tamamura, Y.; Enomoto-Iwamoto, M.; Iwamoto, M. Cellular and molecular mechanisms of synovial joint and articular cartilage formation. *Ann. N. Y. Acad. Sci.* **2006**, *1068*, 74–86. [CrossRef] [PubMed]

23. Iwamoto, M.; Tamamura, Y.; Koyama, E.; Komori, T.; Takeshita, N.; Williams, J.A.; Nakamura, T.; Enomoto-Iwamoto, M.; Pacifici, M. Transcription factor ERG and joint and articular cartilage formation during mouse limb and spine skeletogenesis. *Dev. Biol.* **2007**, *305*, 40–51. [CrossRef] [PubMed]

24. Koyama, E.; Shibukawa, Y.; Nagayama, M.; Sugito, H.; Young, B.; Yuasa, T.; Okabe, T.; Ochiai, T.; Kamiya, N.; Rountree, R.B.; et al. A distinct cohort of progenitor cells participates in synovial joint and articular cartilage formation during mouse limb skeletogenesis. *Dev. Biol.* **2008**, *316*, 62–73. [CrossRef] [PubMed]

25. Rountree, R.B.; Schoor, M.; Chen, H.; Marks, M.E.; Harley, V.; Mishina, Y.; Kingsley, D.M. BMP receptor signaling is required for postnatal maintenance of articular cartilage. *PLoS Biol.* **2004**, *2*, e355. [CrossRef] [PubMed]

26. Hyde, G.; Dover, S.; Aszodi, A.; Wallis, G.A.; Boot-Handford, R.P. Lineage tracing using matrilin-1 gene expression reveals that articular chondrocytes exist as the joint interzone forms. *Dev. Biol.* **2007**, *304*, 825–833. [CrossRef] [PubMed]

27. Von der Mark, K.; Kirsch, T.; Nerlich, A.; Kuss, A.; Weseloh, G.; Glückert, K.; Stöss, H. Type X collagen synthesis in human osteoarthritic cartilage. Indication of chondrocyte hypertrophy. *Arthritis Rheum.* **1992**, *35*, 806–811. [CrossRef] [PubMed]

28. St-Jacques, B.; Hammerschmidt, M.; McMahon, A.P. Indian hedgehog signaling regulates proliferation and differentiation of chondrocytes and is essential for bone formation. *Genes Dev.* **1999**, *13*, 2072–2086. [CrossRef] [PubMed]

29. Yoshida, C.A.; Yamamoto, H.; Fujita, T.; Furuichi, T.; Ito, K.; Inoue, K.; Yamana, K.; Zanma, A.; Takada, K.; Ito, Y.; Komori, T. Runx2 and Runx3 are essential for chondrocyte maturation, and Runx2 regulates limb growth through induction of Indian hedgehog. *Genes Dev.* **2004**, *18*, 952–963. [CrossRef] [PubMed]

30. Mueller, M.B.; Tuan, R.S. Functional characterization of hypertrophy in chondrogenesis of human mesenchymal stem cells. *Arthritis Rheum.* **2008**, *58*, 1377–1388. [CrossRef] [PubMed]

31. Shimizu, E.; Selvamurugan, N.; Westendorf, J.J.; Olson, E.N.; Partridge, N.C. HDAC4 represses matrix metalloproteinase-13 transcription in osteoblastic cells, and parathyroid hormone controls this repression. *J. Biol. Chem.* **2010**, *285*, 9616–9626. [CrossRef] [PubMed]

32. Davoli, M.A.; Lamplugh, L.; Beauchemin, A.; Chan, K.; Mordier, S.; Mort, J.S.; Murphy, G.; Docherty, A.J.; Leblond, C.P.; Lee, E.R. Enzymes active in the areas undergoing cartilage resorption during the development of the secondary ossification center in the tibiae of rats aged 0–21 days: II. Two proteinases, gelatinase B and collagenase-3, are implicated in the lysis of collagen fibrils. *Dev. Dyn.* **2001**, *222*, 71–88. [PubMed]

33. Yang, L.; Tsang, K.Y.; Tang, H.C.; Chan, D.; Cheah, K.S. Hypertrophic chondrocytes can become osteoblasts and osteocytes in endochondral bone formation. *Proc. Natl. Acad. Sci. USA* **2014**, *111*, 12097–12102. [CrossRef] [PubMed]

34. Drissi, H.; Zuscik, M.; Rosier, R.; O'Keefe, R. Transcriptional regulation of chondrocyte maturation: Potential involvement of transcription factors in OA pathogenesis. *Mol. Aspects Med.* **2005**, *26*, 169–179. [CrossRef] [PubMed]

35. Zhang, W.; Chen, J.; Zhang, S.; Ouyang, H.W. Inhibitory function of parathyroid hormone-related protein on chondrocyte hypertrophy: The implication for articular cartilage repair. *Arthritis Res. Ther.* **2012**, *14*, 221. [PubMed]

36. Johnstone, B.; Hering, T.M.; Caplan, A.I.; Goldberg, V.M.; Yoo, J.U. In vitro chondrogenesis of bone marrow-derived mesenchymal progenitor cells. *Exp. Cell Res.* **1998**, *238*, 265–272. [CrossRef] [PubMed]

37. Yoo, J.U.; Barthel, T.S.; Nishimura, K.; Solchaga, L.; Caplan, A.I.; Goldberg, V.M.; Johnstone, B. The chondrogenic potential of human bone-marrow-derived mesenchymal progenitor cells. *J. Bone Joint Surg. Am.* **1998**, *80*, 1745–1757. [CrossRef] [PubMed]

38. Pelttari, K.; Winter, A.; Steck, E.; Goetzke, K.; Hennig, T.; Ochs, B.G.; Aigner, T.; Richter, W. Premature induction of hypertrophy during in vitro chondrogenesis of human mesenchymal stem cells correlates with calcification and vascular invasion after ectopic transplantation in SCID mice. *Arthritis Rheum.* **2006**, *54*, 3254–3266. [CrossRef] [PubMed]
39. Kafienah, W.; Mistry, S.; Dickinson, S.C.; Sims, T.J.; Learmonth, I.; Hollander, A.P. Three-dimensional cartilage tissue engineering using adult stem cells from osteoarthritis patients. *Arthritis Rheum.* **2007**, *56*, 177–187. [CrossRef] [PubMed]
40. Kreuz, P.C.; Steinwachs, M.; Erggelet, C.; Krause, S.J.; Ossendorf, C.; Maier, D.; Ghanem, N.; Uhl, M.; Haag, M. Classification of graft hypertrophy after autologous chondrocyte implantation of full-thickness chondral defects in the knee. *Osteoarthr. Cartil.* **2007**, *15*, 1339–1347. [CrossRef] [PubMed]
41. Murdoch, A.D.; Grady, L.M.; Ablett, M.P.; Katopodi, T.; Meadows, R.S.; Hardingham, T.E. Chondrogenic differentiation of human bone marrow stem cells in transwell cultures: Generation of scaffold-free cartilage. *Stem. Cells* **2007**, *25*, 2786–2796. [CrossRef] [PubMed]
42. Chen, S.; Fu, P.; Cong, R.; Wu, H.; Pei, M. Strategies to minimize hypertrophy in cartilage engineering and regeneration. *Genes Dis.* **2015**, *2*, 76–95. [CrossRef] [PubMed]
43. Hunziker, E.B.; Lippuner, K.; Keel, M.J.; Shintani, N. An educational review of cartilage repair: Precepts & practice-myths & misconceptions-progress & prospects. *Osteoarthr. Cartil.* **2015**, *23*, 334–350. [PubMed]
44. Guilak, F. Biomechanical factors in osteoarthritis. *Best Pract. Res. Clin. Rheumatol.* **2011**, *25*, 815–823. [CrossRef] [PubMed]
45. Antony, B.; Jones, G.; Jin, X.; Ding, C. Do early life factors affect the development of knee osteoarthritis in later life: A narrative review. *Arthritis Res. Ther.* **2016**, *18*, 202. [CrossRef] [PubMed]
46. Fosang, A.J.; Beier, F. Emerging Frontiers in cartilage and chondrocyte biology. *Best Pract. Res. Clin. Rheumatol.* **2011**, *25*, 751–766. [CrossRef] [PubMed]
47. Xie, F.; Kovic, B.; Jin, X.; He, X.; Wang, M.; Silvestre, C. Economic and Humanistic Burden of Osteoarthritis: A Systematic Review of Large Sample Studies. *Pharmacoeconomics* **2016**, *34*, 1087–1100. [CrossRef] [PubMed]
48. *Osteoarthritis in General Practice*; Arthritis Research UK: Scotland, UK, 2013.
49. Cross, M.; Smith, E.; Hoy, D.; Nolte, S.; Ackerman, I.; Fransen, M.; Bridgett, L.; Williams, S.; Guillemin, F.; Hill, C.L.; et al. The global burden of hip and knee osteoarthritis: Estimates from the global burden of disease 2010 study. *Ann. Rheum. Dis.* **2014**, *73*, 1323–1330. [CrossRef] [PubMed]
50. Kulkarni, K.; Karssiens, T.; Kumar, V.; Pandit, H. Obesity and osteoarthritis. *Maturitas* **2016**, *89*, 22–28. [CrossRef] [PubMed]
51. Harris, J.D.; Siston, R.A.; Pan, X.; Flanigan, D.C. Autologous chondrocyte implantation: A systematic review. *J. Bone Joint Surg. Am.* **2010**, *92*, 2220–2233. [CrossRef] [PubMed]
52. Rodriguez-Merchan, E.C. Regeneration of articular cartilage of the knee. *Rheumatol. Int.* **2013**, *33*, 837–845. [CrossRef] [PubMed]
53. Tibesku, C.O.; Szuwart, T.; Kleffner, T.O.; Schlegel, P.M.; Jahn, U.R.; Van Aken, H.; Fuchs, S. Hyaline cartilage degenerates after autologous osteochondral transplantation. *J. Orthop. Res.* **2004**, *22*, 1210–1214. [CrossRef] [PubMed]
54. Brittberg, M.; Lindahl, A.; Nilsson, A.; Ohlsson, C.; Isaksson, O.; Peterson, L. Treatment of deep cartilage defects in the knee with autologous chondrocyte transplantation. *N. Engl. J. Med.* **1994**, *331*, 889–895. [CrossRef] [PubMed]
55. Marlovits, S.; Striessnig, G.; Kutscha-Lissberg, F.; Resinger, C.; Aldrian, S.M.; Vecsei, V.; Trattnig, S. Early postoperative adherence of matrix-induced autologous chondrocyte implantation for the treatment of full-thickness cartilage defects of the femoral condyle. *Knee Surg. Sports Traumatol. Arthrosc.* **2005**, *13*, 451–457. [CrossRef] [PubMed]
56. Gobbi, A.; Kon, E.; Berruto, M.; Francisco, R.; Filardo, G.; Marcacci, M. Patellofemoral full-thickness chondral defects treated with Hyalograft-C: A clinical, arthroscopic, and histologic review. *Am. J. Sports Med.* **2006**, *34*, 1763–1773. [CrossRef] [PubMed]
57. Wood, J.J.; Malek, M.A.; Frassica, F.J.; Polder, J.A.; Mohan, A.K.; Bloom, E.T.; Braun, M.M.; Cote, T.R. Autologous cultured chondrocytes: Adverse events reported to the United States Food and Drug Administration. *J. Bone Joint Surg. Am.* **2006**, *88*, 503–507. [CrossRef] [PubMed]
58. Benya, P.D.; Padilla, S.R.; Nimni, M.E. Independent regulation of collagen types by chondrocytes during the loss of differentiated function in culture. *Cell* **1978**, *15*, 1313–1321. [CrossRef]

59.	Tew, S.R.; Murdoch, A.D.; Rauchenberg, R.P.; Hardingham, T.E. Cellular methods in cartilage research: Primary human chondrocytes in culture and chondrogenesis in human bone marrow stem cells. *Methods* **2008**, *45*, 2–9. [CrossRef] [PubMed]
60.	Ebert, J.R.; Smith, A.; Fallon, M.; Butler, R.; Nairn, R.; Breidahl, W.; Wood, D.J. Incidence, degree, and development of graft hypertrophy 24 months after matrix-induced autologous chondrocyte implantation: Association with clinical outcomes. *Am. J. Sports Med.* **2015**, *43*, 2208–2215. [CrossRef] [PubMed]
61.	Martin, J.A.; Buckwalter, J.A. Telomere erosion and senescence in human articular cartilage chondrocytes. *J. Gerontol. A Biol. Sci. Med. Sci.* **2001**, *56*, B172–B179. [CrossRef] [PubMed]
62.	Kuszel, L.; Trzeciak, T.; Richter, M.; Czarny-Ratajczak, M. Osteoarthritis and telomere shortening. *J. Appl. Genet.* **2015**, *56*, 169–176. [CrossRef] [PubMed]
63.	Martin, G.R. Isolation of a pluripotent cell line from early mouse embryos cultured in medium conditioned by teratocarcinoma stem cells. *Proc. Natl. Acad. Sci. USA* **1981**, *78*, 7634–7638. [CrossRef] [PubMed]
64.	Williams, R.L.; Hilton, D.J.; Pease, S.; Willson, T.A.; Stewart, C.L.; Gearing, D.P.; Wagner, E.F.; Metcalf, D.; Nicola, N.A.; Gough, N.M. Myeloid leukaemia inhibitory factor maintains the developmental potential of embryonic stem cells. *Nature* **1988**, *336*, 684–687. [CrossRef] [PubMed]
65.	Williams, J.T.; Southerland, S.S.; Souza, J.; Calcutt, A.F.; Cartledge, R.G. Cells isolated from adult human skeletal muscle capable of differentiating into multiple mesodermal phenotypes. *Am. Surg.* **1999**, *65*, 22–26. [PubMed]
66.	Beane, O.S.; Darling, E.M. Isolation, characterization, and differentiation of stem cells for cartilage regeneration. *Ann. Biomed. Eng.* **2012**, *40*, 2079–2097. [CrossRef] [PubMed]
67.	Okita, K.; Ichisaka, T.; Yamanaka, S. Generation of germline-competent induced pluripotent stem cells. *Nature* **2007**, *448*, 313–317. [CrossRef] [PubMed]
68.	Shih, C.C.; Forman, S.J.; Chu, P.; Slovak, M. Human embryonic stem cells are prone to generate primitive, undifferentiated tumors in engrafted human fetal tissues in severe combined immunodeficient mice. *Stem. Cells Dev.* **2007**, *16*, 893–902. [CrossRef] [PubMed]
69.	Swijnenburg, R.J.; Schrepfer, S.; Govaert, J.A.; Cao, F.; Ransohoff, K.; Sheikh, A.Y.; Haddad, M.; Connolly, A.J.; Davis, M.M.; Robbins, R.C.; et al. Immunosuppressive therapy mitigates immunological rejection of human embryonic stem cell xenografts. *Proc. Natl. Acad. Sci. USA* **2008**, *105*, 12991–12996. [CrossRef] [PubMed]
70.	Gutierrez-Aranda, I.; Ramos-Mejia, V.; Bueno, C.; Munoz-Lopez, M.; Real, P.J.; Macia, A.; Sanchez, L.; Ligero, G.; Garcia-Parez, J.L.; Menendez, P. Human induced pluripotent stem cells develop teratoma more efficiently and faster than human embryonic stem cells regardless the site of injection. *Stem. Cells* **2010**, *28*, 1568–1570. [CrossRef] [PubMed]
71.	Polo, J.M.; Liu, S.; Figueroa, M.E.; Kulalert, W.; Eminli, S.; Tan, K.Y.; Apostolou, E.; Stadtfeld, M.; Li, Y.; Shioda, T.; et al. Cell type of origin influences the molecular and functional properties of mouse induced pluripotent stem cells. *Nat. Biotechnol.* **2010**, *28*, 848–855. [CrossRef] [PubMed]
72.	Ebrahimi, B. Reprogramming barriers and enhancers: Strategies to enhance the efficiency and kinetics of induced pluripotency. *Cell Regen. (Lond.)* **2015**, *4*, 10. [CrossRef] [PubMed]
73.	Vonk, L.A.; de Windt, T.S.; Slaper-Cortenbach, I.C.; Saris, D.B. Autologous, allogeneic, induced pluripotent stem cell or a combination stem cell therapy? Where are we headed in cartilage repair and why: A concise review. *Stem. Cell Res. Ther.* **2015**, *6*, 94. [CrossRef] [PubMed]
74.	Martin, I.; Ireland, H.; Baldomero, H.; Dominici, M.; Saris, D.B.; Passweg, J. The Survey on Cellular and Engineered Tissue Therapies in Europe in 2013. *Tissue Eng. Part A* **2016**, *22*, 5–16. [CrossRef] [PubMed]
75.	Pittenger, M.F.; Mackay, A.M.; Beck, S.C.; Jaiswal, R.K.; Douglas, R.; Mosca, J.D.; Moorman, M.A.; Simonetti, D.W.; Craig, S.; Marshak, D.R. Multilineage potential of adult human mesenchymal stem cells. *Science* **1999**, *284*, 143–147. [CrossRef] [PubMed]
76.	Jiang, Y.; Jahagirdar, B.N.; Reinhardt, R.L.; Schwartz, R.E.; Keene, C.D.; Ortiz-Gonzalez, X.R.; Reyes, M.; Lenvik, T.; Lund, T.; Blackstad, M.; et al. Pluripotency of mesenchymal stem cells derived from adult marrow. *Nature* **2002**, *418*, 41–49. [CrossRef] [PubMed]
77.	Ham, O.; Song, B.W.; Lee, S.Y.; Choi, E.; Cha, M.J.; Lee, C.Y.; Park, J.H.; Kim, I.K.; Chang, W.; Lim, S.; et al. The role of microRNA-23b in the differentiation of MSC into chondrocyte by targeting protein kinase A signaling. *Biomaterials* **2012**, *33*, 4500–4507. [CrossRef] [PubMed]

78. Monsel, A.; Zhu, Y.G.; Gennai, S.; Hao, Q.; Liu, J.; Lee, J.W. Cell-based therapy for acute organ injury: Preclinical evidence and ongoing clinical trials using mesenchymal stem cells. *Anesthesiology* **2014**, *121*, 1099–1121. [CrossRef] [PubMed]

79. Le Blanc, K.; Tammik, C.; Rosendahl, K.; Zetterberg, E.; Ringden, O. HLA expression and immunologic properties of differentiated and undifferentiated mesenchymal stem cells. *Exp. Hematol.* **2003**, *31*, 890–896. [CrossRef]

80. Chamberlain, G.; Fox, J.; Ashton, B.; Middleton, J. Concise review: Mesenchymal stem cells: Their phenotype, differentiation capacity, immunological features, and potential for homing. *Stem. Cells.* **2007**, *25*, 2739–2749. [CrossRef] [PubMed]

81. Uccelli, A.; Moretta, L.; Pistoia, V. Mesenchymal stem cells in health and disease. *Nat. Rev. Immunol.* **2008**, *8*, 726–736. [CrossRef] [PubMed]

82. Atoui, R.; Chiu, R.C. Mesenchymal stromal cells as universal donor cells. *Exp. Opin. Biol. Ther.* **2012**, *12*, 1293–1297. [CrossRef] [PubMed]

83. Le Blanc, K.; Rasmusson, I.; Sundberg, B.; Gotherstrom, C.; Hassan, M.; Uzunel, M.; Ringden, O. Treatment of severe acute graft-versus-host disease with third party haploidentical mesenchymal stem cells. *Lancet* **2004**, *363*, 1439–1441. [CrossRef]

84. Ra, J.C.; Kang, S.K.; Shin, I.S.; Park, H.G.; Joo, S.A.; Kim, J.G.; Kang, B.C.; Lee, Y.S.; Nakama, K.; Piao, M.; et al. Stem cell treatment for patients with autoimmune disease by systemic infusion of culture-expanded autologous adipose tissue derived mesenchymal stem cells. *J. Transl. Med.* **2011**, *9*, 181. [PubMed]

85. Wang, L.; Wang, L.; Cong, X.; Liu, G.; Zhou, J.; Bai, B.; Li, Y.; Bai, W.; Li, M.; Ji, H.; et al. Human umbilical cord mesenchymal stem cell therapy for patients with active rheumatoid arthritis: Safety and efficacy. *Stem. Cells Dev.* **2013**, *22*, 3192–3202. [CrossRef] [PubMed]

86. Wang, L.; Zhang, H.; Guan, L.; Zhao, S.; Gu, Z.; Wei, H.; Gao, Z.; Wang, F.; Yang, N.; Luo, L.; et al. Mesenchymal stem cells provide prophylaxis against acute graft-versus-host disease following allogeneic hematopoietic stem cell transplantation: A meta-analysis of animal models. *Oncotarget* **2016**, *7*, 61764–61774. [PubMed]

87. Dennis, J.E.; Charbord, P. Origin and differentiation of human and murine stroma. *Stem. Cells* **2002**, *20*, 205–214. [CrossRef] [PubMed]

88. Wakitani, S.; Mitsuoka, T.; Nakamura, N.; Toritsuka, Y.; Nakamura, Y.; Horibe, S. Autologous bone marrow stromal cell transplantation for repair of full-thickness articular cartilage defects in human patellae: Two case reports. *Cell Trans.* **2004**, *13*, 595–600. [CrossRef]

89. Giannini, S.; Buda, R.; Battaglia, M.; Cavallo, M.; Ruffilli, A.; Ramponi, L.; Pagliazzi, G.; Vannini, F. One-step repair in talar osteochondral lesions: 4-year clinical results and t2-mapping capability in outcome prediction. *Am. J. Sports Med.* **2013**, *41*, 511–518. [CrossRef] [PubMed]

90. Skowronski, J.; Rutka, M. Osteochondral lesions of the knee reconstructed with mesenchymal stem cells—Results. *Ortop. Traumatol. Rehabil.* **2013**, *15*, 195–204. [CrossRef] [PubMed]

91. Vega, A.; Martin-Ferrero, M.A.; Del Canto, F.; Alberca, M.; Garcia, V.; Munar, A.; Orozco, L.; Soler, R.; Fuertes, J.J.; Huguet, M.; et al. Treatment of Knee Osteoarthritis With Allogeneic Bone Marrow Mesenchymal Stem Cells: A Randomized Controlled Trial. *Transplantation* **2015**, *99*, 1681–1690. [CrossRef] [PubMed]

92. Soler, R.; Orozco, L.; Munar, A.; Huguet, M.; Lopez, R.; Vives, J.; Coll, R.; Codinach, M.; Garcia-Lopez, J. Final results of a phase I-II trial using ex vivo expanded autologous Mesenchymal Stromal Cells for the treatment of osteoarthritis of the knee confirming safety and suggesting cartilage regeneration. *Knee* **2016**, *23*, 647–654. [CrossRef] [PubMed]

93. Vodyanik, M.A.; Yu, J.; Zhang, X.; Tian, S.; Stewart, R.; Thomson, J.A.; Slukvin, I.I. A mesoderm-derived precursor for mesenchymal stem and endothelial cells. *Cell Stem. Cell* **2010**, *7*, 718–729. [CrossRef] [PubMed]

94. Alrefaei, G.I.; Ayuob, N.N.; Ali, S.S.; Al-Karim, S. Effects of maternal age on the expression of mesenchymal stem cell markers in the components of human umbilical cord. *Folia Histochem. Cytobiol.* **2015**, *53*, 259–271. [CrossRef] [PubMed]

95. Friedenstein, A.J.; Gorskaja, J.F.; Kulagina, N.N. Fibroblast precursors in normal and irradiated mouse hematopoietic organs. *Exp. Hematol.* **1976**, *4*, 267–274. [PubMed]

96. Caplan, A.I. Mesenchymal stem cells. *J. Orthop. Res.* **1991**, *9*, 641–650. [CrossRef] [PubMed]

97. Zuk, P.A.; Zhu, M.; Ashjian, P.; De Ugarte, D.A.; Huang, J.I.; Mizuno, H.; Alfonso, Z.C.; Fraser, J.K.; Benhaim, P.; Hedrick, M.H. Human adipose tissue is a source of multipotent stem cells. *Mol. Biol. Cell* **2002**, *13*, 4279–4295. [CrossRef] [PubMed]

98. De Bari, C.; Dell'Accio, F.; Tylzanowski, P.; Luyten, F.P. Multipotent mesenchymal stem cells from adult human synovial membrane. *Arthritis Rheum* **2001**, *44*, 1928–1942. [CrossRef]

99. Erices, A.; Conget, P.; Minguell, J.J. Mesenchymal progenitor cells in human umbilical cord blood. *Br. J. Haematol.* **2000**, *109*, 235–242. [CrossRef] [PubMed]

100. Arufe, M.C.; De la Fuente, A.; Fuentes-Boquete, I.; De Toro, F.J.; Blanco, F.J. Differentiation of synovial CD-105(+) human mesenchymal stem cells into chondrocyte-like cells through spheroid formation. *J. Cell Biochem.* **2009**, *108*, 145–155. [CrossRef] [PubMed]

101. Heo, J.S.; Choi, Y.; Kim, H.S.; Kim, H.O. Comparison of molecular profiles of human mesenchymal stem cells derived from bone marrow, umbilical cord blood, placenta and adipose tissue. *Int. J. Mol. Med.* **2016**, *37*, 115–125. [PubMed]

102. Nazempour, A.; Van Wie, B.J. Chondrocytes, Mesenchymal Stem Cells, and Their Combination in Articular Cartilage Regenerative Medicine. *Ann. Biomed. Eng.* **2016**, *44*, 1325–1354. [CrossRef] [PubMed]

103. Sakaguchi, Y.; Sekiya, I.; Yagishita, K.; Muneta, T. Comparison of human stem cells derived from various mesenchymal tissues: Superiority of synovium as a cell source. *Arthritis Rheum.* **2005**, *52*, 2521–2529. [CrossRef] [PubMed]

104. Koga, H.; Muneta, T.; Ju, Y.J.; Nagase, T.; Nimura, A.; Mochizuki, T.; Ichinose, S.; von der Mark, K.; Sekiya, I. Synovial stem cells are regionally specified according to local microenvironments after implantation for cartilage regeneration. *Stem. Cells* **2007**, *25*, 689–696. [CrossRef] [PubMed]

105. Jones, B.A.; Pei, M. Synovium-derived stem cells: A tissue-specific stem cell for cartilage engineering and regeneration. *Tissue Eng. Part B* **2012**, *18*, 301–311. [CrossRef] [PubMed]

106. Wu, L.; Cai, X.; Zhang, S.; Karperien, M.; Lin, Y. Regeneration of articular cartilage by adipose tissue derived mesenchymal stem cells: Perspectives from stem cell biology and molecular medicine. *J. Cell Physiol.* **2013**, *228*, 938–944. [CrossRef] [PubMed]

107. Perdisa, F.; Gostynska, N.; Roffi, A.; Filardo, G.; Marcacci, M.; Kon, E. Adipose-Derived Mesenchymal Stem Cells for the Treatment of Articular Cartilage: A Systematic Review on Preclinical and Clinical Evidence. *Stem. Cells Int.* **2015**, *2015*, 597652. [CrossRef] [PubMed]

108. Caterson, E.J.; Nesti, L.J.; Danielson, K.G.; Tuan, R.S. Human marrow-derived mesenchymal progenitor cells: Isolation, culture expansion, and analysis of differentiation. *Mol. Biotechnol.* **2002**, *20*, 245–256. [CrossRef]

109. Hung, S.C.; Chen, N.J.; Hsieh, S.L.; Li, H.; Ma, H.L.; Lo, W.H. Isolation and characterization of size-sieved stem cells from human bone marrow. *Stem. Cells* **2002**, *20*, 249–258. [CrossRef] [PubMed]

110. De Ugarte, D.A.; Alfonso, Z.; Zuk, P.A.; Elbarbary, A.; Zhu, M.; Ashjian, P.; Benhaim, P.; Hedrick, M.H.; Fraser, J.K. Differential expression of stem cell mobilization-associated molecules on multi-lineage cells from adipose tissue and bone marrow. *Immunol. Lett.* **2003**, *89*, 267–270. [CrossRef]

111. Dominici, M.; Le Blanc, K.; Mueller, I.; Slaper-Cortenbach, I.; Marini, F.; Krause, D.; Deans, R.; Keating, A.; Prockop, D.; Horwitz, E. Minimal criteria for defining multipotent mesenchymal stromal cells. The International Society for Cellular Therapy position statement. *Cytotherapy* **2006**, *8*, 315–317. [CrossRef] [PubMed]

112. Xie, X.J.; Wang, J.A.; Cao, J.; Zhang, X. Differentiation of bone marrow mesenchymal stem cells induced by myocardial medium under hypoxic conditions. *Acta Pharmacol. Sin.* **2006**, *27*, 1153–1158. [CrossRef] [PubMed]

113. Wu, R.; Liu, G.; Bharadwaj, S.; Zhang, Y. Isolation and myogenic differentiation of mesenchymal stem cells for urologic tissue engineering. *Methods Mol. Biol.* **2013**, *1001*, 65–80. [PubMed]

114. Dugan, J.M.; Cartmell, S.H.; Gough, J.E. Uniaxial cyclic strain of human adipose-derived mesenchymal stem cells and C2C12 myoblasts in coculture. *J. Tissue Eng.* **2014**, *5*, 2041731414530138. [CrossRef] [PubMed]

115. Mu, M.W.; Zhao, Z.Y.; Li, C.G. Comparative study of neural differentiation of bone marrow mesenchymal stem cells by different induction methods. *Genet Mol. Res.* **2015**, *14*, 14169–14176. [CrossRef] [PubMed]

116. Jones, E.A.; Kinsey, S.E.; English, A.; Jones, R.A.; Straszynski, L.; Meredith, D.M.; Markham, A.F.; Jack, A.; Emery, P.; McGonagle, D. Isolation and characterization of bone marrow multipotential mesenchymal progenitor cells. *Arthritis Rheum.* **2002**, *46*, 3349–3360. [CrossRef] [PubMed]

117. Kaltz, N.; Ringe, J.; Holzwarth, C.; Charbord, P.; Niemeyer, M.; Jacobs, V.R.; Peschel, C.; Haupl, T.; Oostendorp, R.A. Novel markers of mesenchymal stem cells defined by genome-wide gene expression analysis of stromal cells from different sources. *Exp. Cell Res.* 2010, *316*, 2609–2617. [CrossRef] [PubMed]
118. Mendicino, M.; Bailey, A.M.; Wonnacott, K.; Puri, R.K.; Bauer, S.R. MSC-based product characterization for clinical trials: An FDA perspective. *Cell Stem. Cell* 2014, *14*, 141–145. [CrossRef] [PubMed]
119. Erdmann, G.; Suchanek, M.; Horn, P.; Graf, F.; Volz, C.; Horn, T.; Zhang, X.; Wagner, W.; Ho, A.D.; Boutros, M. Functional fingerprinting of human mesenchymal stem cells using high-throughput RNAi screening. *Genome Med.* 2015, *7*, 46. [CrossRef] [PubMed]
120. Samsonraj, R.M.; Rai, B.; Sathiyanathan, P.; Puan, K.J.; Rotzschke, O.; Hui, J.H.; Raghunath, M.; Stanton, L.W.; Nurcombe, V.; Cool, S.M. Establishing criteria for human mesenchymal stem cell potency. *Stem. Cells* 2015, *33*, 1878–1891. [CrossRef] [PubMed]
121. Sacchetti, B.; Funari, A.; Remoli, C.; Giannicola, G.; Kogler, G.; Liedtke, S.; Cossu, G.; Serafini, M.; Sampaolesi, M.; Tagliafico, E.; et al. No Identical "Mesenchymal Stem Cells" at Different Times and Sites: Human Committed Progenitors of Distinct Origin and Differentiation Potential Are Incorporated as Adventitial Cells in Microvessels. *Stem. Cell Reports* 2016, *6*, 897–913. [CrossRef] [PubMed]
122. Shahdadfar, A.; Fronsdal, K.; Haug, T.; Reinholt, F.P.; Brinchmann, J.E. In vitro expansion of human mesenchymal stem cells: Choice of serum is a determinant of cell proliferation, differentiation, gene expression, and transcriptome stability. *Stem. Cells* 2005, *23*, 1357–1366. [CrossRef] [PubMed]
123. Avanzini, M.A.; Bernardo, M.E.; Cometa, A.M.; Perotti, C.; Zaffaroni, N.; Novara, F.; Visai, L.; Moretta, A.; Del Fante, C.; Villa, R.; et al. Generation of mesenchymal stromal cells in the presence of platelet lysate: A phenotypic and functional comparison of umbilical cord blood- and bone marrow-derived progenitors. *Haematologica* 2009, *94*, 1649–1660. [CrossRef] [PubMed]
124. Torensma, R.; Prins, H.J.; Schrama, E.; Verwiel, E.T.; Martens, A.C.; Roelofs, H.; Jansen, B.J. The impact of cell source, culture methodology, culture location, and individual donors on gene expression profiles of bone marrow-derived and adipose-derived stromal cells. *Stem. Cells Dev.* 2013, *22*, 1086–1096. [CrossRef] [PubMed]
125. Steinert, A.F.; Ghivizzani, S.C.; Rethwilm, A.; Tuan, R.S.; Evans, C.H.; Noth, U. Major biological obstacles for persistent cell-based regeneration of articular cartilage. *Arthritis Res. Ther.* 2007, *9*, 213. [CrossRef] [PubMed]
126. Wakitani, S.; Nawata, M.; Tensho, K.; Okabe, T.; Machida, H.; Ohgushi, H. Repair of articular cartilage defects in the patello-femoral joint with autologous bone marrow mesenchymal cell transplantation: Three case reports involving nine defects in five knees. *J. Tissue Eng. Regen. Med.* 2007, *1*, 74–79. [CrossRef] [PubMed]
127. Huey, D.J.; Hu, J.C.; Athanasiou, K.A. Unlike bone, cartilage regeneration remains elusive. *Science* 2012, *338*, 917–921. [CrossRef] [PubMed]
128. Mackay, A.M.; Beck, S.C.; Murphy, J.M.; Barry, F.P.; Chichester, C.O.; Pittenger, M.F. Chondrogenic differentiation of cultured human mesenchymal stem cells from marrow. *Tissue Eng.* 1998, *4*, 415–428. [CrossRef] [PubMed]
129. Matsumoto, Y.; Hayashi, Y.; Schlieve, C.R.; Ikeya, M.; Kim, H.; Nguyen, T.D.; Sami, S.; Baba, S.; Barruet, E.; Nasu, A.; et al. Induced pluripotent stem cells from patients with human fibrodysplasia ossificans progressiva show increased mineralization and cartilage formation. *Orphanet J. Rare Dis.* 2013, *8*, 190. [CrossRef] [PubMed]
130. De Kroon, L.M.; Narcisi, R.; Blaney Davidson, E.N.; Cleary, M.A.; van Beuningen, H.M.; Koevoet, W.J.; van Osch, G.J.; van der Kraan, P.M. Activin Receptor-Like Kinase Receptors ALK5 and ALK1 Are Both Required for TGFbeta-Induced Chondrogenic Differentiation of Human Bone Marrow-Derived Mesenchymal Stem Cells. *PLoS ONE* 2015, *10*, e0146124. [CrossRef] [PubMed]
131. Lolli, A.; Narcisi, R.; Lambertini, E.; Penolazzi, L.; Angelozzi, M.; Kops, N.; Gasparini, S.; van Osch, G.J.; Piva, R. Silencing of Antichondrogenic MicroRNA-221 in Human Mesenchymal Stem Cells Promotes Cartilage Repair In Vivo. *Stem. Cells* 2016, *34*, 1801–1811. [CrossRef] [PubMed]
132. Lolli, A.; Narcisi, R.; Lambertini, E.; Penolazzi, L.; Angelozzi, M.; Kops, N.; Gasparini, S.; van Osch, G.J.; Piva, R. The effect of oxygen tension on human articular chondrocyte matrix synthesis: Integration of experimental and computational approaches. *Biotechnol. Bioeng.* 2014, *111*, 1876–1885.
133. Murdoch, A.D.; Hardingham, T.E.; Eyre, D.R.; Fernandes, R.J. The development of a mature collagen network in cartilage from human bone marrow stem cells in Transwell culture. *Matrix Biol.* 2016, *50*, 6–26. [CrossRef] [PubMed]

134. Van Beuningen, H.M.; Glansbeek, H.L.; van der Kraan, P.M.; van den Berg, W.B. Osteoarthritis-like changes in the murine knee joint resulting from intra-articular transforming growth factor-beta injections. *Osteoarthr. Cartil.* **2000**, *8*, 25–33. [CrossRef] [PubMed]

135. Farrell, E.; van der Jagt, O.P.; Koevoet, W.; Kops, N.; van Manen, C.J.; Hellingman, C.A.; Jahr, H.; O'Brien, F.J.; Verhaar, J.A.; Weinans, H.; et al. Chondrogenic priming of human bone marrow stromal cells: A better route to bone repair? *Tissue Eng. Part C* **2009**, *15*, 285–295. [CrossRef] [PubMed]

136. Mueller, M.B.; Fischer, M.; Zellner, J.; Berner, A.; Dienstknecht, T.; Prantl, L.; Kujat, R.; Nerlich, M.; Tuan, R.S.; Angele, P. Hypertrophy in mesenchymal stem cell chondrogenesis: Effect of TGF-beta isoforms and chondrogenic conditioning. *Cells Tissues Organs* **2010**, *192*, 158–166. [CrossRef] [PubMed]

137. Bauge, C.; Girard, N.; Lhuissier, E.; Bazille, C.; Boumediene, K. Regulation and Role of TGFbeta Signaling Pathway in Aging and Osteoarthritis Joints. *Aging Dis.* **2014**, *5*, 394–405. [PubMed]

138. Kuroda, R.; Ishida, K.; Matsumoto, T.; Akisue, T.; Fujioka, H.; Mizuno, K.; Ohgushi, H.; Wakitani, S.; Kurosaka, M. Treatment of a full-thickness articular cartilage defect in the femoral condyle of an athlete with autologous bone-marrow stromal cells. *Osteoarthr. Cartil.* **2007**, *15*, 226–231. [CrossRef] [PubMed]

139. Orozco, L.; Munar, A.; Soler, R.; Alberca, M.; Soler, F.; Huguet, M.; Sentis, J.; Sanchez, A.; Garcia-Sancho, J. Treatment of knee osteoarthritis with autologous mesenchymal stem cells: Two-year follow-up results. *Transplantation* **2014**, *97*, e66–e68. [CrossRef] [PubMed]

140. Wolfstadt, J.I.; Cole, B.J.; Ogilvie-Harris, D.J.; Viswanathan, S.; Chahal, J. Current concepts: The role of mesenchymal stem cells in the management of knee osteoarthritis. *Sports Health* **2015**, *7*, 38–44. [CrossRef] [PubMed]

141. Koh, Y.G.; Kwon, O.R.; Kim, Y.S.; Choi, Y.J.; Tak, D.H. Adipose-Derived Mesenchymal Stem Cells With Microfracture Versus Microfracture Alone: 2-Year Follow-up of a Prospective Randomized Trial. *Arthroscopy* **2016**, *32*, 97–109. [CrossRef] [PubMed]

142. Pak, J.; Lee, J.H.; Park, K.S.; Jeong, B.C.; Lee, S.H. Regeneration of Cartilage in Human Knee Osteoarthritis with Autologous Adipose Tissue-Derived Stem Cells and Autologous Extracellular Matrix. *Biores. Open Access* **2016**, *5*, 192–200. [CrossRef] [PubMed]

143. Park, Y.B.; Ha, C.W.; Lee, C.H.; Yoon, Y.C.; Park, Y.G. Cartilage Regeneration in Osteoarthritic Patients by a Composite of Allogeneic Umbilical Cord Blood-Derived Mesenchymal Stem Cells and Hyaluronate Hydrogel: Results From a Clinical Trial for Safety and Proof-of-Concept With 7 Years of Extended Follow-Up. *Stem. Cells Transl. Med.* **2016**, *6*, 613–621. [CrossRef] [PubMed]

144. Ruiz, M.; Cosenza, S.; Maumus, M.; Jorgensen, C.; Noel, D. Therapeutic application of mesenchymal stem cells in osteoarthritis. *Exp. Opin. Biol. Ther.* **2016**, *16*, 33–42. [CrossRef] [PubMed]

145. Koh, Y.G.; Choi, Y.J.; Kwon, O.R.; Kim, Y.S. Second-Look Arthroscopic Evaluation of Cartilage Lesions After Mesenchymal Stem Cell Implantation in Osteoarthritic Knees. *Am. J. Sports Med.* **2014**, *42*, 1628–1637. [CrossRef] [PubMed]

146. Davatchi, F.; Sadeghi Abdollahi, B.; Mohyeddin, M.; Nikbin, B. Mesenchymal stem cell therapy for knee osteoarthritis: 5 years follow-up of three patients. *Int. J. Rheum. Dis.* **2016**, *19*, 219–225. [CrossRef] [PubMed]

147. Xu, S.; Liu, H.; Xie, Y.; Sang, L.; Liu, J.; Chen, B. Effect of mesenchymal stromal cells for articular cartilage degeneration treatment: A meta-analysis. *Cytotherapy* **2015**, *17*, 1342–1352. [CrossRef] [PubMed]

148. Solchaga, L.A.; Penick, K.; Porter, J.D.; Goldberg, V.M.; Caplan, A.I.; Welter, J.F. FGF-2 enhances the mitotic and chondrogenic potentials of human adult bone marrow-derived mesenchymal stem cells. *J. Cell Physiol.* **2005**, *203*, 398–409. [CrossRef] [PubMed]

149. Ito, T.; Sawada, R.; Fujiwara, Y.; Tsuchiya, T. FGF-2 increases osteogenic and chondrogenic differentiation potentials of human mesenchymal stem cells by inactivation of TGF-beta signaling. *Cytotechnology* **2008**, *56*, 1–7. [CrossRef] [PubMed]

150. Solchaga, L.A.; Penick, K.; Goldberg, V.M.; Caplan, A.I.; Welter, J.F. Fibroblast growth factor-2 enhances proliferation and delays loss of chondrogenic potential in human adult bone-marrow-derived mesenchymal stem cells. *Tissue Eng. Part A* **2010**, *16*, 1009–1019. [CrossRef] [PubMed]

151. Correa, D.; Somoza, R.A.; Lin, P.; Greenberg, S.; Rom, E.; Duesler, L.; Welter, J.F.; Yayon, A.; Caplan, A.I. Sequential exposure to fibroblast growth factors (FGF) 2, 9 and 18 enhances hMSC chondrogenic differentiation. *Osteoarthr. Cartil.* **2015**, *23*, 443–453. [CrossRef] [PubMed]

152. Hellingman, C.A.; Koevoet, W.; Kops, N.; Farrell, E.; Jahr, H.; Liu, W.; Baatenburg de Jong, R.J.; Frenz, D.A.; van Osch, G.J. Fibroblast growth factor receptors in in vitro and in vivo chondrogenesis: Relating tissue engineering using adult mesenchymal stem cells to embryonic development. *Tissue Eng. Part A* **2010**, *16*, 545–556. [CrossRef] [PubMed]

153. Weiss, S.; Hennig, T.; Bock, R.; Steck, E.; Richter, W. Impact of growth factors and PTHrP on early and late chondrogenic differentiation of human mesenchymal stem cells. *J. Cell Physiol.* **2010**, *223*, 84–93. [CrossRef] [PubMed]

154. Bianchi, G.; Banfi, A.; Mastrogiacomo, M.; Notaro, R.; Luzzatto, L.; Cancedda, R.; Quarto, R. Ex vivo enrichment of mesenchymal cell progenitors by fibroblast growth factor 2. *Exp. Cell Res.* **2003**, *287*, 98–105. [CrossRef]

155. Turnbull, J.E.; Fernig, D.G.; Ke, Y.; Wilkinson, M.C.; Gallagher, J.T. Identification of the basic fibroblast growth factor binding sequence in fibroblast heparan sulfate. *J. Biol. Chem.* **1992**, *267*, 10337–10341. [PubMed]

156. Lin, X.; Buff, E.M.; Perrimon, N.; Michelson, A.M. Heparan sulfate proteoglycans are essential for FGF receptor signaling during Drosophila embryonic development. *Development* **1999**, *126*, 3715–3723. [PubMed]

157. Mohammadi, M.; Olsen, S.K.; Ibrahimi, O.A. Structural basis for fibroblast growth factor receptor activation. *Cytokine Growth Factor Rev.* **2005**, *16*, 107–137. [CrossRef] [PubMed]

158. Xu, R.; Ori, A.; Rudd, T.R.; Uniewicz, K.A.; Ahmed, Y.A.; Guimond, S.E.; Skidmore, M.A.; Siligardi, G.; Yates, E.A.; Fernig, D.G. Diversification of the structural determinants of fibroblast growth factor-heparin interactions: Implications for binding specificity. *J. Biol. Chem.* **2012**, *287*, 40061–40073. [CrossRef] [PubMed]

159. Li, Y.; Sun, C.; Yates, E.A.; Jiang, C.; Wilkinson, M.C.; Fernig, D.G. Heparin binding preference and structures in the fibroblast growth factor family parallel their evolutionary diversification. *Open Biol.* **2016**, *6*. [CrossRef] [PubMed]

160. Smith, S.M.; West, L.A.; Govindraj, P.; Zhang, X.; Ornitz, D.M.; Hassell, J.R. Heparan and chondroitin sulfate on growth plate perlecan mediate binding and delivery of FGF-2 to FGF receptors. *Matrix Biol.* **2007**, *26*, 175–184. [CrossRef] [PubMed]

161. Vincent, T.L.; McLean, C.J.; Full, L.E.; Peston, D.; Saklatvala, J. FGF-2 is bound to perlecan in the pericellular matrix of articular cartilage, where it acts as a chondrocyte mechanotransducer. *Osteoarthr. Cartil.* **2007**, *15*, 752–763. [CrossRef] [PubMed]

162. Melrose, J.; Isaacs, M.D.; Smith, S.M.; Hughes, C.E.; Little, C.B.; Caterson, B.; Hayes, A.J. Chondroitin sulphate and heparan sulphate sulphation motifs and their proteoglycans are involved in articular cartilage formation during human foetal knee joint development. *Histochem. Cell Biol.* **2012**, *138*, 461–475. [PubMed]

163. Wijesinghe, S.J.; Ling, L.; Murali, S.; Qing, Y.H.; Hinkley, S.F.; Carnachan, S.M.; Bell, T.J.; Swaminathan, K.; Hui, J.H.; van Wijnen, A.J.; et al. Affinity Selection of FGF2-Binding Heparan Sulfates for Ex Vivo Expansion of Human Mesenchymal Stem Cells. *J. Cell Physiol.* **2016**, *232*, 566–575. [PubMed]

164. Davidson, D.; Blanc, A.; Filion, D.; Wang, H.; Plut, P.; Pfeffer, G.; Buschmann, M.D.; Henderson, J.E. Fibroblast growth factor (FGF) 18 signals through FGF receptor 3 to promote chondrogenesis. *J. Biol. Chem.* **2005**, *280*, 20509–20515. [PubMed]

165. Sekiya, I.; Vuoristo, J.T.; Larson, B.L.; Prockop, D.J. In vitro cartilage formation by human adult stem cells from bone marrow stroma defines the sequence of cellular and molecular events during chondrogenesis. *Proc. Natl. Acad. Sci. USA* **2002**, *99*, 4397–4402. [PubMed]

166. McCaffrey, T.A.; Falcone, D.J.; Vicente, D.; Du, B.; Consigli, S.; Borth, W. Protection of transforming growth factor-beta 1 activity by heparin and fucoidan. *J. Cell Physiol.* **1994**, *159*, 51–59. [PubMed]

167. Lyon, M.; Rushton, G.; Gallagher, J.T. The interaction of the transforming growth factor-betas with heparin/heparan sulfate is isoform-specific. *J. Biol. Chem.* **1997**, *272*, 18000–18006. [PubMed]

168. Lee, M.J. Heparin inhibits activation of latent transforming growth factor-beta1. *Pharmacology* **2013**, *92*, 238–244. [PubMed]

169. Lee, J.; Wee, S.; Gunaratne, J.; Chua, R.J.; Smith, R.A.; Ling, L.; Fernig, D.G.; Swaminathan, K.; Nurcombe, V.; Cool, S.M. Structural determinants of heparin-transforming growth factor-beta1 interactions and their effects on signaling. *Glycobiology* **2015**, *25*, 1491–1504. [CrossRef] [PubMed]

170. Hildebrand, A.; Romaris, M.; Rasmussen, L.M.; Heinegard, D.; Twardzik, D.R.; Border, W.A.; Ruoslahti, E. Interaction of the small interstitial proteoglycans biglycan, decorin and fibromodulin with transforming growth factor beta. *Biochem. J.* **1994**, *302*, 527–534. [CrossRef] [PubMed]

171. Chang, S.C.; Hoang, B.; Thomas, J.T.; Vukicevic, S.; Luyten, F.P.; Ryba, N.J.; Kozak, C.A.; Reddi, A.H.; Moos, M., Jr. Cartilage-derived morphogenetic proteins. New members of the transforming growth factor-beta superfamily predominantly expressed in long bones during human embryonic development. *J. Biol. Chem.* **1994**, *269*, 28227–28234. [PubMed]

172. Storm, E.E.; Kingsley, D.M. GDF5 coordinates bone and joint formation during digit development. *Dev. Biol.* **1999**, *209*, 11–27. [CrossRef] [PubMed]

173. Masuya, H.; Nishida, K.; Furuichi, T.; Toki, H.; Nishimura, G.; Kawabata, H.; Yokoyama, H.; Yoshida, A.; Tominaga, S.; Nagano, J.; et al. A novel dominant-negative mutation in Gdf5 generated by ENU mutagenesis impairs joint formation and causes osteoarthritis in mice. *Hum. Mol. Genet* **2007**, *16*, 2366–2375. [CrossRef] [PubMed]

174. Kwong, F.N.; Hoyland, J.A.; Evans, C.H.; Freemont, A.J. Regional and cellular localisation of BMPs and their inhibitors' expression in human fractures. *Int. Orthop.* **2009**, *33*, 281–288. [CrossRef] [PubMed]

175. Garciadiego-Cazares, D.; Aguirre-Sanchez, H.I.; Abarca-Buis, R.F.; Kouri, J.B.; Velasquillo, C.; Ibarra, C. Regulation of alpha5 and alphaV Integrin Expression by GDF-5 and BMP-7 in Chondrocyte Differentiation and Osteoarthritis. *PLoS ONE* **2015**, *10*, e0127166. [CrossRef] [PubMed]

176. Feng, G.; Wan, Y.; Balian, G.; Laurencin, C.T.; Li, X. Adenovirus-mediated expression of growth and differentiation factor-5 promotes chondrogenesis of adipose stem cells. *Growth Factors* **2008**, *26*, 132–142. [CrossRef] [PubMed]

177. Zhang, B.; Yang, S.; Sun, Z.; Zhang, Y.; Xia, T.; Xu, W.; Ye, S. Human mesenchymal stem cells induced by growth differentiation factor 5: An improved self-assembly tissue engineering method for cartilage repair. *Tissue Eng. Part C* **2011**, *17*, 1189–1199. [CrossRef] [PubMed]

178. Yang, X.; Shang, H.; Katz, A.; Li, X. A modified aggregate culture for chondrogenesis of human adipose-derived stem cells genetically modified with growth and differentiation factor 5. *BioResour. Open Access* **2013**, *2*, 258–265. [CrossRef] [PubMed]

179. Enochson, L.; Stenberg, J.; Brittberg, M.; Lindahl, A. GDF5 reduces MMP13 expression in human chondrocytes via DKK1 mediated canonical Wnt signaling inhibition. *Osteoarthr. Cartil.* **2014**, *22*, 566–577. [CrossRef] [PubMed]

180. Coleman, C.M.; Vaughan, E.E.; Browe, D.C.; Mooney, E.; Howard, L.; Barry, F. Growth differentiation factor-5 enhances in vitro mesenchymal stromal cell chondrogenesis and hypertrophy. *Stem. Cells Dev.* **2013**, *22*, 1968–1976. [CrossRef] [PubMed]

181. Murphy, M.K.; Huey, D.J.; Hu, J.C.; Athanasiou, K.A. TGF-beta1, GDF-5, and BMP-2 stimulation induces chondrogenesis in expanded human articular chondrocytes and marrow-derived stromal cells. *Stem. Cells* **2015**, *33*, 762–773. [CrossRef] [PubMed]

182. Gandhi, N.S.; Mancera, R.L. Prediction of heparin binding sites in bone morphogenetic proteins (BMPs). *Biochim. Biophys. Acta* **2012**, *1824*, 1374–1381. [CrossRef] [PubMed]

183. Indrawattana, N.; Chen, G.; Tadokoro, M.; Shann, L.H.; Ohgushi, H.; Tateishi, T.; Tanaka, J.; Bunyaratvej, A. Growth factor combination for chondrogenic induction from human mesenchymal stem cell. *Biochem. Biophys. Res. Commun.* **2004**, *320*, 914–919. [CrossRef] [PubMed]

184. Sekiya, I.; Larson, B.L.; Vuoristo, J.T.; Reger, R.L.; Prockop, D.J. Comparison of effect of BMP-2, -4, and -6 on in vitro cartilage formation of human adult stem cells from bone marrow stroma. *Cell Tissue Res.* **2005**, *320*, 269–276. [CrossRef] [PubMed]

185. Steinert, A.F.; Proffen, B.; Kunz, M.; Hendrich, C.; Ghivizzani, S.C.; Noth, U.; Rethwilm, A.; Eulert, J.; Evans, C.H. Hypertrophy is induced during the in vitro chondrogenic differentiation of human mesenchymal stem cells by bone morphogenetic protein-2 and bone morphogenetic protein-4 gene transfer. *Arthritis Res. Ther.* **2009**, *11*, R148. [CrossRef] [PubMed]

186. Caron, M.M.; Emans, P.J.; Cremers, A.; Surtel, D.A.; Coolsen, M.M.; van Rhijn, L.W.; Welting, T.J. Hypertrophic differentiation during chondrogenic differentiation of progenitor cells is stimulated by BMP-2 but suppressed by BMP-7. *Osteoarthr. Cartil.* **2013**, *21*, 604–613. [CrossRef] [PubMed]

187. Irie, A.; Habuchi, H.; Kimata, K.; Sanai, Y. Heparan sulfate is required for bone morphogenetic protein-7 signaling. *Biochem. Biophys. Res. Commun.* **2003**, *308*, 858–865. [CrossRef]

188. Yang, H.S.; La, W.G.; Bhang, S.H.; Jeon, J.Y.; Lee, J.H.; Kim, B.S. Heparin-conjugated fibrin as an injectable system for sustained delivery of bone morphogenetic protein-2. *Tissue Eng. Part A* **2010**, *16*, 1225–1233. [CrossRef] [PubMed]

189. Bhakta, G.; Rai, B.; Lim, Z.X.; Hui, J.H.; Stein, G.S.; van Wijnen, A.J.; Nurcombe, V.; Prestwich, G.D.; Cool, S.M. Hyaluronic acid-based hydrogels functionalized with heparin that support controlled release of bioactive BMP-2. *Biomaterials* **2012**, *33*, 6113–6122. [CrossRef] [PubMed]
190. Bramono, D.S.; Murali, S.; Rai, B.; Ling, L.; Poh, W.T.; Lim, Z.X.; Stein, G.S.; Nurcombe, V.; van Wijnen, A.J.; Cool, S.M. Bone marrow-derived heparan sulfate potentiates the osteogenic activity of bone morphogenetic protein-2 (BMP-2). *Bone* **2012**, *50*, 954–964. [CrossRef] [PubMed]
191. Kraushaar, D.C.; Rai, S.; Condac, E.; Nairn, A.; Zhang, S.; Yamaguchi, Y.; Moremen, K.; Dalton, S.; Wang, L. Heparan sulfate facilitates FGF and BMP signaling to drive mesoderm differentiation of mouse embryonic stem cells. *J. Biol. Chem.* **2012**, *287*, 22691–22700. [CrossRef] [PubMed]
192. Koo, K.H.; Lee, J.M.; Ahn, J.M.; Kim, B.S.; La, W.G.; Kim, C.S.; Im, G.I. Controlled delivery of low-dose bone morphogenetic protein-2 using heparin-conjugated fibrin in the posterolateral lumbar fusion of rabbits. *Artif. Organs* **2013**, *37*, 487–494. [CrossRef] [PubMed]
193. Murali, S.; Rai, B.; Dombrowski, C.; Lee, J.L.; Lim, Z.X.; Bramono, D.S.; Ling, L.; Bell, T.; Hinkley, S.; Nathan, S.S.; et al. Affinity-selected heparan sulfate for bone repair. *Biomaterials* **2013**, *34*, 5594–5605. [CrossRef] [PubMed]
194. Hettiaratchi, M.H.; Miller, T.; Temenoff, J.S.; Guldberg, R.E.; McDevitt, T.C. Heparin microparticle effects on presentation and bioactivity of bone morphogenetic protein-2. *Biomaterials* **2014**, *35*, 7228–7238. [CrossRef] [PubMed]
195. Rai, B.; Chatterjea, A.; Lim, Z.X.; Tan, T.C.; Sawyer, A.A.; Hosaka, Y.Z.; Murali, S.; Lee, J.J.; Fenwick, S.A.; Hui, J.H.; et al. Repair of segmental ulna defects using a beta-TCP implant in combination with a heparan sulfate glycosaminoglycan variant. *Acta Biomater.* **2015**, *28*, 193–204. [CrossRef] [PubMed]
196. Church, V.; Nohno, T.; Linker, C.; Marcelle, C.; Francis-West, P. Wnt regulation of chondrocyte differentiation. *J. Cell Sci.* **2002**, *115*, 4809–4818. [CrossRef] [PubMed]
197. Bradley, E.W.; Drissi, M.H. WNT5A regulates chondrocyte differentiation through differential use of the CaN/NFAT and IKK/NF-kappaB pathways. *Mol. Endocrinol.* **2010**, *24*, 1581–1593. [CrossRef] [PubMed]
198. Narcisi, R.; Cleary, M.A.; Brama, P.A.; Hoogduijn, M.J.; Tuysuz, N.; ten Berge, D.; van Osch, G.J. Long-term expansion, enhanced chondrogenic potential, and suppression of endochondral ossification of adult human MSCs via WNT signaling modulation. *Stem. Cell. Reports* **2015**, *4*, 459–472. [CrossRef] [PubMed]
199. Studer, D.; Millan, C.; Ozturk, E.; Maniura-Weber, K.; Zenobi-Wong, M. Molecular and biophysical mechanisms regulating hypertrophic differentiation in chondrocytes and mesenchymal stem cells. *Eur. Cell Mater.* **2012**, *24*, 118–135, discussion 135. [CrossRef] [PubMed]
200. Dhoot, G.K.; Gustafsson, M.K.; Ai, X.; Sun, W.; Standiford, D.M.; Emerson, C.P., Jr. Regulation of Wnt signaling and embryo patterning by an extracellular sulfatase. *Science* **2001**, *293*, 1663–1666. [CrossRef] [PubMed]
201. Ai, X.; Do, A.T.; Lozynska, O.; Kusche-Gullberg, M.; Lindahl, U.; Emerson, C.P., Jr. QSulf1 remodels the 6-O sulfation states of cell surface heparan sulfate proteoglycans to promote Wnt signaling. *J. Cell Biol.* **2003**, *162*, 341–351. [CrossRef] [PubMed]
202. Song, H.H.; Shi, W.; Xiang, Y.Y.; Filmus, J. The loss of glypican-3 induces alterations in Wnt signaling. *J. Biol. Chem.* **2005**, *280*, 2116–2125. [CrossRef] [PubMed]
203. Liu, S.; Zhang, E.; Yang, M.; Lu, L. Overexpression of Wnt11 promotes chondrogenic differentiation of bone marrow-derived mesenchymal stem cells in synergism with TGF-beta. *Mol. Cell Biochem.* **2014**, *390*, 123–131. [CrossRef] [PubMed]
204. Enomoto-Iwamoto, M.; Kitagaki, J.; Koyama, E.; Tamamura, Y.; Wu, C.; Kanatani, N.; Koike, T.; Okada, H.; Komori, T.; Yoneda, T.; et al. The Wnt antagonist Frzb-1 regulates chondrocyte maturation and long bone development during limb skeletogenesis. *Dev. Biol.* **2002**, *251*, 142–156. [CrossRef] [PubMed]
205. Hartmann, C.; Tabin, C.J. Wnt-14 plays a pivotal role in inducing synovial joint formation in the developing appendicular skeleton. *Cell* **2001**, *104*, 341–351. [CrossRef]
206. Frisch, J.; Venkatesan, J.K.; Rey-Rico, A.; Schmitt, G.; Madry, H.; Cucchiarini, M. Influence of insulin-like growth factor I overexpression via recombinant adeno-associated vector gene transfer upon the biological activities and differentiation potential of human bone marrow-derived mesenchymal stem cells. *Stem. Cell Res. Ther.* **2014**, *5*, 103. [CrossRef] [PubMed]
207. Moller, A.V.; Jorgensen, S.P.; Chen, J.W.; Larnkjaer, A.; Ledet, T.; Flyvbjerg, A.; Frystyk, J. Glycosaminoglycans increase levels of free and bioactive IGF-I in vitro. *Eur. J. Endocrinol.* **2006**, *155*, 297–305. [CrossRef] [PubMed]

208. Kim, Y.J.; Kim, H.J.; Im, G.I. PTHrP promotes chondrogenesis and suppresses hypertrophy from both bone marrow-derived and adipose tissue-derived MSCs. *Biochem. Biophys. Res. Commun.* **2008**, *373*, 104–108. [CrossRef] [PubMed]

209. Lee, J.M.; Im, G.I. PTHrP isoforms have differing effect on chondrogenic differentiation and hypertrophy of mesenchymal stem cells. *Biochem. Biophys. Res. Commun.* **2012**, *421*, 819–824. [CrossRef] [PubMed]

210. Zak, B.M.; Crawford, B.E.; Esko, J.D. Hereditary multiple exostoses and heparan sulfate polymerization. *Biochim. Biophys. Acta* **2002**, *1573*, 346–355. [CrossRef]

211. Koziel, L.; Kunath, M.; Kelly, O.G.; Vortkamp, A. Ext1-dependent heparan sulfate regulates the range of Ihh signaling during endochondral ossification. *Dev. Cell* **2004**, *6*, 801–813. [CrossRef] [PubMed]

212. Newfeld, S.J.; Wisotzkey, R.G.; Kumar, S. Molecular evolution of a developmental pathway: Phylogenetic analyses of transforming growth factor-beta family ligands, receptors and Smad signal transducers. *Genetics* **1999**, *152*, 783–795. [PubMed]

213. Moses, H.L.; Roberts, A.B.; Derynck, R. The Discovery and Early Days of TGF-beta: A Historical Perspective. *Cold Spring Harb Perspect Biol.* **2016**, *8*. [CrossRef] [PubMed]

214. Constam, D.B.; Robertson, E.J. Regulation of bone morphogenetic protein activity by pro domains and proprotein convertases. *J. Cell Biol.* **1999**, *144*, 139–149. [CrossRef] [PubMed]

215. Griffith, D.L.; Keck, P.C.; Sampath, T.K.; Rueger, D.C.; Carlson, W.D. Three-dimensional structure of recombinant human osteogenic protein 1: Structural paradigm for the transforming growth factor beta superfamily. *Proc. Natl. Acad. Sci. USA* **1996**, *93*, 878–883. [CrossRef] [PubMed]

216. Mittl, P.R.; Priestle, J.P.; Cox, D.A.; McMaster, G.; Cerletti, N.; Grutter, M.G. The crystal structure of TGF-beta 3 and comparison to TGF-beta 2: Implications for receptor binding. *Protein Sci.* **1996**, *5*, 1261–1271. [CrossRef] [PubMed]

217. McPherron, A.C.; Lee, S.J. GDF-3 and GDF-9: Two new members of the transforming growth factor-beta superfamily containing a novel pattern of cysteines. *J. Biol. Chem.* **1993**, *268*, 3444–3449. [PubMed]

218. Corradini, E.; Babitt, J.L.; Lin, H.Y. The RGM/DRAGON family of BMP co-receptors. *Cytokine Growth Factor Rev.* **2009**, *20*, 389–398. [CrossRef] [PubMed]

219. Horiguchi, M.; Ota, M.; Rifkin, D.B. Matrix control of transforming growth factor-beta function. *J. Biochem.* **2012**, *152*, 321–329. [CrossRef] [PubMed]

220. Taipale, J.; Miyazono, K.; Heldin, C.H.; Keski-Oja, J. Latent transforming growth factor-beta 1 associates to fibroblast extracellular matrix via latent TGF-beta binding protein. *J. Cell Biol.* **1994**, *124*, 171–181. [CrossRef] [PubMed]

221. Barcellos-Hoff, M.H.; Dix, T.A. Redox-mediated activation of latent transforming growth factor-beta 1. *Mol. Endocrinol.* **1996**, *10*, 1077–1083. [PubMed]

222. Munger, J.S.; Harpel, J.G.; Gleizes, P.E.; Mazzieri, R.; Nunes, I.; Rifkin, D.B. Latent transforming growth factor-beta: Structural features and mechanisms of activation. *Kidney Int.* **1997**, *51*, 1376–1382. [CrossRef] [PubMed]

223. Yu, Q.; Stamenkovic, I. Cell surface-localized matrix metalloproteinase-9 proteolytically activates TGF-beta and promotes tumor invasion and angiogenesis. *Genes Dev.* **2000**, *14*, 163–176. [PubMed]

224. Anderson, S.B.; Goldberg, A.L.; Whitman, M. Identification of a novel pool of extracellular pro-myostatin in skeletal muscle. *J. Biol. Chem.* **2008**, *283*, 7027–7035. [CrossRef] [PubMed]

225. Harrison, C.A.; Al-Musawi, S.L.; Walton, K.L. Prodomains regulate the synthesis, extracellular localisation and activity of TGF-beta superfamily ligands. *Growth Factors* **2011**, *29*, 174–186. [CrossRef] [PubMed]

226. Akhurst, R.J.; Hata, A. Targeting the TGFbeta signalling pathway in disease. *Nat. Rev. Drug Discov.* **2012**, *11*, 790–811. [CrossRef] [PubMed]

227. Weiss, A.; Attisano, L. The TGFbeta superfamily signaling pathway. *Wiley Interdiscip. Rev. Dev. Biol.* **2013**, *2*, 47–63. [CrossRef] [PubMed]

228. Zhai, G.; Dore, J.; Rahman, P. TGF-beta signal transduction pathways and osteoarthritis. *Rheumatol. Int.* **2015**, *35*, 1283–1292. [CrossRef] [PubMed]

229. Hanyu, A.; Ishidou, Y.; Ebisawa, T.; Shimanuki, T.; Imamura, T.; Miyazono, K. The N domain of Smad7 is essential for specific inhibition of transforming growth factor-beta signaling. *J. Cell Biol.* **2001**, *155*, 1017–1027. [CrossRef] [PubMed]

230. Zhang, Y.E. Non-Smad pathways in TGF-beta signaling. *Cell Res.* **2009**, *19*, 128–139. [CrossRef] [PubMed]

231. Yamada, Y.; Miyauchi, A.; Goto, J.; Takagi, Y.; Okuizumi, H.; Kanematsu, M.; Hase, M.; Takai, H.; Harada, A.; Ikeda, K. Association of a polymorphism of the transforming growth factor-beta1 gene with genetic susceptibility to osteoporosis in postmenopausal Japanese women. *J. Bone Miner Res.* **1998**, *13*, 1569–1576. [CrossRef] [PubMed]

232. Kizawa, H.; Kou, I.; Iida, A.; Sudo, A.; Miyamoto, Y.; Fukuda, A.; Mabuchi, A.; Kotani, A.; Kawakami, A.; Yamamoto, S.; et al. An aspartic acid repeat polymorphism in asporin inhibits chondrogenesis and increases susceptibility to osteoarthritis. *Nat. Genet* **2005**, *37*, 138–144. [CrossRef] [PubMed]

233. Blaney Davidson, E.N.; Scharstuhl, A.; Vitters, E.L.; van der Kraan, P.M.; van den Berg, W.B. Reduced transforming growth factor-beta signaling in cartilage of old mice: Role in impaired repair capacity. *Arthritis Res. Ther.* **2005**, *7*, R1338–R1347. [CrossRef] [PubMed]

234. Blaney Davidson, E.N.; Vitters, E.L.; van der Kraan, P.M.; van den Berg, W.B. Expression of transforming growth factor-beta (TGFbeta) and the TGFbeta signalling molecule SMAD-2P in spontaneous and instability-induced osteoarthritis: Role in cartilage degradation, chondrogenesis and osteophyte formation. *Ann. Rheum. Dis.* **2006**, *65*, 1414–1421. [CrossRef] [PubMed]

235. Narcisi, R.; Quarto, R.; Ulivi, V.; Muraglia, A.; Molfetta, L.; Giannoni, P. TGF beta-1 administration during ex vivo expansion of human articular chondrocytes in a serum-free medium redirects the cell phenotype toward hypertrophy. *J. Cell Physiol.* **2012**, *227*, 3282–3290. [CrossRef] [PubMed]

236. Cals, F.L.; Hellingman, C.A.; Koevoet, W.; Baatenburg de Jong, R.J.; van Osch, G.J. Effects of transforming growth factor-beta subtypes on in vitro cartilage production and mineralization of human bone marrow stromal-derived mesenchymal stem cells. *J. Tissue Eng. Regen Med.* **2012**, *6*, 68–76. [CrossRef] [PubMed]

237. Campos-Xavier, B.; Saraiva, J.M.; Savarirayan, R.; Verloes, A.; Feingold, J.; Faivre, L.; Munnich, A.; Le Merrer, M.; Cormier-Daire, V. Phenotypic variability at the TGF-beta1 locus in Camurati-Engelmann disease. *Hum. Genet* **2001**, *109*, 653–658. [CrossRef] [PubMed]

238. Janssens, K.; ten Dijke, P.; Ralston, S.H.; Bergmann, C.; Van Hul, W. Transforming growth factor-beta 1 mutations in Camurati-Engelmann disease lead to increased signaling by altering either activation or secretion of the mutant protein. *J. Biol. Chem.* **2003**, *278*, 7718–7724. [CrossRef] [PubMed]

239. Van Beuningen, H.M.; van der Kraan, P.M.; Arntz, O.J.; van den Berg, W.B. Transforming growth factor-beta 1 stimulates articular chondrocyte proteoglycan synthesis and induces osteophyte formation in the murine knee joint. *Lab. Invest.* **1994**, *71*, 279–290. [PubMed]

240. Somoza, R.A.; Welter, J.F.; Correa, D.; Caplan, A.I. Chondrogenic differentiation of mesenchymal stem cells: Challenges and unfulfilled expectations. *Tissue Eng. Part B* **2014**, *20*, 596–608. [CrossRef] [PubMed]

241. Shen, B.; Wei, A.; Whittaker, S.; Williams, L.A.; Tao, H.; Ma, D.D.; Diwan, A.D. The role of BMP-7 in chondrogenic and osteogenic differentiation of human bone marrow multipotent mesenchymal stromal cells in vitro. *J. Cell Biochem.* **2010**, *109*, 406–416. [CrossRef] [PubMed]

242. Lee, P.T.; Li, W.J. Chondrogenesis of Embryonic Stem Cell-Derived Mesenchymal Stem Cells Induced by TGFbeta1 and BMP7 through Increased TGFbeta Receptor Expression and Endogenous TGFbeta1 Production. *J. Cell Biochem.* **2017**, *118*, 172–181. [CrossRef] [PubMed]

243. Handorf, A.M.; Li, W.J. Induction of mesenchymal stem cell chondrogenesis through sequential administration of growth factors within specific temporal windows. *J. Cell Physiol.* **2014**, *229*, 162–171. [CrossRef] [PubMed]

244. Denker, A.E.; Haas, A.R.; Nicoll, S.B.; Tuan, R.S. Chondrogenic differentiation of murine C3H10T1/2 multipotential mesenchymal cells: I. Stimulation by bone morphogenetic protein-2 in high-density micromass cultures. *Differentiation* **1999**, *64*, 67–76. [CrossRef] [PubMed]

245. Kobayashi, T.; Lyons, K.M.; McMahon, A.P.; Kronenberg, H.M. BMP signaling stimulates cellular differentiation at multiple steps during cartilage development. *Proc. Natl. Acad. Sci. USA* **2005**, *102*, 18023–18027. [CrossRef] [PubMed]

246. Bandyopadhyay, A.; Tsuji, K.; Cox, K.; Harfe, B.D.; Rosen, V.; Tabin, C.J. Genetic analysis of the roles of BMP2, BMP4, and BMP7 in limb patterning and skeletogenesis. *PLoS Genet.* **2006**, *2*, e216. [CrossRef] [PubMed]

247. Bian, Q.; Jia, K.; Liu, S.F.; Shu, B.; Liang, Q.Q.; Zhou, C.J.; Zhou, Q.; Wang, Y.J. Inhibitory effect of YQHYRJ recipe on osteoblast differentiation induced by BMP-2 in fibroblasts from posterior longitudinal ligament of mice. *Pharmazie* **2011**, *66*, 784–790. [PubMed]

248. Sekiya, I.; Tang, T.; Hayashi, M.; Morito, T.; Ju, Y.J.; Mochizuki, T.; Muneta, T. Periodic knee injections of BMP-7 delay cartilage degeneration induced by excessive running in rats. *J. Orthop. Res.* **2009**, *27*, 1088–1092. [CrossRef] [PubMed]

249. Hotten, G.; Neidhardt, H.; Jacobowsky, B.; Pohl, J. Cloning and expression of recombinant human growth/differentiation factor 5. *Biochem. Biophys. Res. Commun.* **1994**, *204*, 646–652. [CrossRef] [PubMed]

250. McDonald, N.Q.; Hendrickson, W.A. A structural superfamily of growth factors containing a cystine knot motif. *Cell* **1993**, *73*, 421–424. [CrossRef]

251. Luyten, F.P. Cartilage-derived morphogenetic protein-1. *Int. J. Biochem. Cell Biol.* **1997**, *29*, 1241–1244. [CrossRef]

252. Thieme, T.; Patzschke, R.; Job, F.; Liebold, J.; Seemann, P.; Lilie, H.; Balbach, J.; Schwarz, E. Biophysical and structural characterization of a folded core domain within the proregion of growth and differentiation factor-5. *FEBS J.* **2014**, *281*, 4866–4877. [CrossRef] [PubMed]

253. Storm, E.E.; Huynh, T.V.; Copeland, N.G.; Jenkins, N.A.; Kingsley, D.M.; Lee, S.J. Limb alterations in brachypodism mice due to mutations in a new member of the TGF beta-superfamily. *Nature* **1994**, *368*, 639–643. [CrossRef] [PubMed]

254. Hotten, G.C.; Matsumoto, T.; Kimura, M.; Bechtold, R.F.; Kron, R.; Ohara, T.; Tanaka, H.; Satoh, Y.; Okazaki, M.; Shirai, T.; et al. Recombinant human growth/differentiation factor 5 stimulates mesenchyme aggregation and chondrogenesis responsible for the skeletal development of limbs. *Growth Factors* **1996**, *13*, 65–74. [CrossRef] [PubMed]

255. Buxton, P.; Edwards, C.; Archer, C.W.; Francis-West, P. Growth/differentiation factor-5 (GDF-5) and skeletal development. *J. Bone Joint Surg. Am.* **2001**, *83-A* (Suppl. 1), S23–S30. [CrossRef]

256. Shwartz, Y.; Viukov, S.; Krief, S.; Zelzer, E. Joint Development Involves a Continuous Influx of Gdf5-Positive Cells. *Cell Rep.* **2016**, *15*, 2577–2587. [CrossRef] [PubMed]

257. Storm, E.E.; Kingsley, D.M. Joint patterning defects caused by single and double mutations in members of the bone morphogenetic protein (BMP) family. *Development* **1996**, *122*, 3969–3979. [PubMed]

258. Settle, S.H., Jr.; Rountree, R.B.; Sinha, A.; Thacker, A.; Higgins, K.; Kingsley, D.M. Multiple joint and skeletal patterning defects caused by single and double mutations in the mouse Gdf6 and Gdf5 genes. *Dev. Biol.* **2003**, *254*, 116–130. [CrossRef]

259. Thomas, J.T.; Kilpatrick, M.W.; Lin, K.; Erlacher, L.; Lembessis, P.; Costa, T.; Tsipouras, P.; Luyten, F.P. Disruption of human limb morphogenesis by a dominant negative mutation in CDMP1. *Nat. Genet.* **1997**, *17*, 58–64. [CrossRef] [PubMed]

260. Dawson, K.; Seeman, P.; Sebald, E.; King, L.; Edwards, M.; Williams, J., 3rd; Mundlos, S.; Krakow, D. GDF5 is a second locus for multiple-synostosis syndrome. *Am. J. Hum. Genet.* **2006**, *78*, 708–712. [CrossRef] [PubMed]

261. Miyamoto, Y.; Mabuchi, A.; Shi, D.; Kubo, T.; Takatori, Y.; Saito, S.; Fujioka, M.; Sudo, A.; Uchida, A.; Yamamoto, S.; et al. A functional polymorphism in the 5′ UTR of GDF5 is associated with susceptibility to osteoarthritis. *Nat. Genet.* **2007**, *39*, 529–533. [CrossRef] [PubMed]

262. Degenkolbe, E.; Konig, J.; Zimmer, J.; Walther, M.; Reissner, C.; Nickel, J.; Ploger, F.; Raspopovic, J.; Sharpe, J.; Dathe, K.; et al. A GDF5 point mutation strikes twice—Causing BDA1 and SYNS2. *PLoS Genet.* **2013**, *9*, e1003846. [CrossRef] [PubMed]

263. Martinez-Garcia, M.; Garcia-Canto, E.; Fenollar-Cortes, M.; Aytes, A.P.; Trujillo-Tiebas, M.J. Characterization of an acromesomelic dysplasia, Grebe type case: Novel mutation affecting the recognition motif at the processing site of GDF5. *J. Bone Miner Metab.* **2016**, *34*, 599–603. [CrossRef] [PubMed]

264. Bai, X.; Xiao, Z.; Pan, Y.; Hu, J.; Pohl, J.; Wen, J.; Li, L. Cartilage-derived morphogenetic protein-1 promotes the differentiation of mesenchymal stem cells into chondrocytes. *Biochem. Biophys. Res. Commun.* **2004**, *325*, 453–460. [CrossRef] [PubMed]

265. Katayama, R.; Wakitani, S.; Tsumaki, N.; Morita, Y.; Matsushita, I.; Gejo, R.; Kimura, T. Repair of articular cartilage defects in rabbits using CDMP1 gene-transfected autologous mesenchymal cells derived from bone marrow. *Rheumatology (Oxford)* **2004**, *43*, 980–985. [CrossRef] [PubMed]

266. Ayerst, B.I.; Smith, R.A.; Nurcombe, V.; Day, A.J.; Merry, C.L.; Cool, S.M. Growth Differentiation Factor 5-Mediated Enhancement of Chondrocyte Phenotype Is Inhibited by Heparin: Implications for the Use of Heparin in the Clinic and in Tissue Engineering Applications. *Tissue Eng. Part A* **2017**, *23*, 275–292. [CrossRef] [PubMed]

267. DeLise, A.M.; Fischer, L.; Tuan, R.S. Cellular interactions and signaling in cartilage development. *Osteoarthr. Cartil.* **2000**, *8*, 309–334. [CrossRef] [PubMed]

268. Zheng, Q.; Zhou, G.; Morello, R.; Chen, Y.; Garcia-Rojas, X.; Lee, B. Type X collagen gene regulation by Runx2 contributes directly to its hypertrophic chondrocyte-specific expression in vivo. *J. Cell Biol.* **2003**, *162*, 833–842. [CrossRef] [PubMed]

269. Tian, H.T.; Zhang, B.; Tian, Q.; Liu, Y.; Yang, S.H.; Shao, Z.W. Construction of self-assembled cartilage tissue from bone marrow mesenchymal stem cells induced by hypoxia combined with GDF-5. *J. Huazhong Univ. Sci. Technolog. Med. Sci.* **2013**, *33*, 700–706. [CrossRef] [PubMed]

270. An, B.; Heo, H.-R.; Lee, S.; Park, J.-A.; Kim, K.-S.; Yang, J.; Hong, S.-H. Supplementation of Growth Differentiation Factor-5 Increases Proliferation and Size of Chondrogenic Pellets of Human Umbilical Cord-Derived Perivascular Stem Cells. *Tissue Eng. Regen. Med.* **2015**, *12*, 181–187. [CrossRef]

271. Muraglia, A.; Cancedda, R.; Quarto, R. Clonal mesenchymal progenitors from human bone marrow differentiate in vitro according to a hierarchical model. *J. Cell Sci.* **2000**, *113*, 1161–1166. [PubMed]

272. Roelofs, A.J.; Rocke, J.P.; de Bari, C. Cell-based approaches to joint surface repair: A research perspective. *Osteoarthr. Cartil.* **2013**, *21*, 892–900. [CrossRef] [PubMed]

273. Baraniak, P.R.; McDevitt, T.C. Stem cell paracrine actions and tissue regeneration. *Regen. Med.* **2010**, *5*, 121–143. [CrossRef] [PubMed]

274. Anthony, D.F.; Shiels, P.G. Exploiting paracrine mechanisms of tissue regeneration to repair damaged organs. *Transpl. Res.* **2013**, *2*, 10. [CrossRef] [PubMed]

275. Gnecchi, M.; Melo, L.G. Bone marrow-derived mesenchymal stem cells: Isolation, expansion, characterization, viral transduction, and production of conditioned medium. *Methods Mol. Biol.* **2009**, *482*, 281–294. [PubMed]

276. Lee, R.H.; Pulin, A.A.; Seo, M.J.; Kota, D.J.; Ylostalo, J.; Larson, B.L.; Semprun-Prieto, L.; Delafontaine, P.; Prockop, D.J. Intravenous hMSCs improve myocardial infarction in mice because cells embolized in lung are activated to secrete the anti-inflammatory protein TSG-6. *Cell Stem. Cell* **2009**, *5*, 54–63. [CrossRef] [PubMed]

277. Ko, I.K.; Lee, S.J.; Atala, A.; Yoo, J.J. In situ tissue regeneration through host stem cell recruitment. *Exp. Mol. Med.* **2013**, *45*, e57. [CrossRef] [PubMed]

278. Linero, I.; Chaparro, O. Paracrine effect of mesenchymal stem cells derived from human adipose tissue in bone regeneration. *PLos ONE* **2014**, *9*, e107001. [CrossRef] [PubMed]

279. Hacker, S.; Mittermayr, R.; Nickl, S.; Haider, T.; Lebherz-Eichinger, D.; Beer, L.; Mitterbauer, A.; Leiss, H.; Zimmermann, M.; Schweiger, T.; et al. Paracrine Factors from Irradiated Peripheral Blood Mononuclear Cells Improve Skin Regeneration and Angiogenesis in a Porcine Burn Model. *Sci. Rep.* **2016**, *6*, 25168. [CrossRef] [PubMed]

280. Martino, M.M.; Briquez, P.S.; Maruyama, K.; Hubbell, J.A. Extracellular matrix-inspired growth factor delivery systems for bone regeneration. *Adv. Drug Deliv. Rev.* **2015**, *94*, 41–52. [CrossRef] [PubMed]

281. Manning, M.C.; Patel, K.; Borchardt, R.T. Stability of protein pharmaceuticals. *Pharm. Res.* **1989**, *6*, 903–918. [CrossRef] [PubMed]

282. Lauer, G.; Sollberg, S.; Cole, M.; Flamme, I.; Sturzebecher, J.; Mann, K.; Krieg, T.; Eming, S.A. Expression and proteolysis of vascular endothelial growth factor is increased in chronic wounds. *J. Investig. Dermatol.* **2000**, *115*, 12–18. [CrossRef] [PubMed]

283. Eppler, S.M.; Combs, D.L.; Henry, T.D.; Lopez, J.J.; Ellis, S.G.; Yi, J.H.; Annex, B.H.; McCluskey, E.R.; Zioncheck, T.F. A target-mediated model to describe the pharmacokinetics and hemodynamic effects of recombinant human vascular endothelial growth factor in humans. *Clin. Pharmacol. Ther.* **2002**, *72*, 20–32. [CrossRef] [PubMed]

284. Simons, M.; Annex, B.H.; Laham, R.J.; Kleiman, N.; Henry, T.; Dauerman, H.; Udelson, J.E.; Gervino, E.V.; Pike, M.; Whitehouse, M.J.; et al. Pharmacological treatment of coronary artery disease with recombinant fibroblast growth factor-2: Double-blind, randomized, controlled clinical trial. *Circulation* **2002**, *105*, 788–793. [CrossRef] [PubMed]

285. Shields, L.B.; Raque, G.H.; Glassman, S.D.; Campbell, M.; Vitaz, T.; Harpring, J.; Shields, C.B. Adverse effects associated with high-dose recombinant human bone morphogenetic protein-2 use in anterior cervical spine fusion. *Spine* **2006**, *31*, 542–547. [CrossRef] [PubMed]

286. Epstein, N.E. Complications due to the use of BMP/INFUSE in spine surgery: The evidence continues to mount. *Surg. Neurol. Int.* **2013**, *4* (Suppl. 5), S343–S352. [CrossRef] [PubMed]

287. Sreekumar, V.; Aspera-Werz, R.H.; Tendulkar, G.; Reumann, M.K.; Freude, T.; Breitkopf-Heinlein, K.; Dooley, S.; Pscherer, S.; Ochs, B.G.; Flesch, I.; et al. BMP9 a possible alternative drug for the recently withdrawn BMP7? New perspectives for (re-)implementation by personalized medicine. *Arch. Toxicol.* **2017**, *91*, 1353–1366. [CrossRef] [PubMed]

288. Devine, J.G.; Dettori, J.R.; France, J.C.; Brodt, E.; McGuire, R.A. The use of rhBMP in spine surgery: Is there a cancer risk? *Evid. Based Spine Care J.* **2012**, *3*, 35–41. [CrossRef] [PubMed]

289. Carragee, E.J.; Chu, G.; Rohatgi, R.; Hurwitz, E.L.; Weiner, B.K.; Yoon, S.T.; Comer, G.; Kopjar, B. Cancer risk after use of recombinant bone morphogenetic protein-2 for spinal arthrodesis. *J. Bone Joint Surg. Am.* **2013**, *95*, 1537–1545. [CrossRef] [PubMed]

290. Epstein, N.E. Basic science and spine literature document bone morphogenetic protein increases cancer risk. *Surg. Neurol. Int.* **2014**, *5* (Suppl. 15), S552–S560. [CrossRef] [PubMed]

291. Dettori, J.R.; Chapman, J.R.; DeVine, J.G.; McGuire, R.A.; Norvell, D.C.; Weiss, N.S. The Risk of Cancer With the Use of Recombinant Human Bone Morphogenetic Protein in Spine Fusion. *Spine* **2016**, *41*, 1317–1324. [CrossRef] [PubMed]

292. Blanquaert, F.; Saffar, J.L.; Colombier, M.L.; Carpentier, G.; Barritault, D.; Caruelle, J.P. Heparan-like molecules induce the repair of skull defects. *Bone* **1995**, *17*, 499–506. [CrossRef]

293. Uludag, H.; D'Augusta, D.; Palmer, R.; Timony, G.; Wozney, J. Characterization of rhBMP-2 pharmacokinetics implanted with biomaterial carriers in the rat ectopic model. *J. Biomed. Mater. Res.* **1999**, *46*, 193–202. [CrossRef]

294. Lafont, J.; Blanquaert, F.; Colombier, M.L.; Barritault, D.; Carueelle, J.P.; Saffar, J.L. Kinetic study of early regenerative effects of RGTA11, a heparan sulfate mimetic, in rat craniotomy defects. *Calcif. Tissue Int.* **2004**, *75*, 517–525. [CrossRef] [PubMed]

295. Wang, C.; Poon, S.; Murali, S.; Koo, C.Y.; Bell, T.J.; Hinkley, S.F.; Yeong, H.; Bhakoo, K.; Nurcombe, V.; Cool, S.M. Engineering a vascular endothelial growth factor 165-binding heparan sulfate for vascular therapy. *Biomaterials* **2014**, *35*, 6776–6786. [CrossRef] [PubMed]

296. Khan, S.; Fung, K.W.; Rodriguez, E.; Patel, R.; Gor, J.; Mulloy, B.; Perkins, S.J. The solution structure of heparan sulfate differs from that of heparin: Implications for function. *J. Biol. Chem.* **2013**, *288*, 27737–27751. [CrossRef] [PubMed]

297. Zhang, L. Glycosaminoglycan (GAG) biosynthesis and GAG-binding proteins. *Prog. Mol. Biol. Transl. Sci.* **2010**, *93*, 1–17. [PubMed]

298. Lindahl, U.; Kjellen, L. Pathophysiology of heparan sulphate: Many diseases, few drugs. *J. Intern. Med.* **2013**, *273*, 555–571. [CrossRef] [PubMed]

299. Krusius, T.; Ruoslahti, E. Primary structure of an extracellular matrix proteoglycan core protein deduced from cloned cDNA. *Proc. Natl. Acad. Sci. USA* **1986**, *83*, 7683–7687. [CrossRef] [PubMed]

300. Ng, L.; Grodzinsky, A.J.; Patwari, P.; Sandy, J.; Plaas, A.; Ortiz, C. Individual cartilage aggrecan macromolecules and their constituent glycosaminoglycans visualized via atomic force microscopy. *J. Struct. Biol.* **2003**, *143*, 242–257. [CrossRef] [PubMed]

301. Gibson, B.G.; Briggs, M.D. The aggrecanopathies; an evolving phenotypic spectrum of human genetic skeletal diseases. *Orphanet J Rare Dis.* **2016**, *11*, 86. [CrossRef] [PubMed]

302. Roughley, P.J.; Mort, J.S. The role of aggrecan in normal and osteoarthritic cartilage. *J. Exp. Orthop.* **2014**, *1*, 8. [CrossRef] [PubMed]

303. Kiani, C.; Chen, L.; Wu, Y.J.; Yee, A.J.; Yang, B.B. Structure and function of aggrecan. *Cell Res.* **2002**, *12*, 19–32. [CrossRef] [PubMed]

304. Chang, P.S.; McLane, L.T.; Fogg, R.; Scrimgeour, J.; Temenoff, J.S.; Granqvist, A.; Curtis, J.E. Cell Surface Access Is Modulated by Tethered Bottlebrush Proteoglycans. *Biophys. J.* **2016**, *110*, 2739–2750. [CrossRef] [PubMed]

305. SundarRaj, N.; Fite, D.; Ledbetter, S.; Chakravarti, S.; Hassell, J.R. Perlecan is a component of cartilage matrix and promotes chondrocyte attachment. *J. Cell Sci.* **1995**, *108*, 2663–2672. [PubMed]

306. Gu, G.; Deutch, A.Y.; Franklin, J.; Levy, S.; Wallace, D.C.; Zhang, J. Profiling genes related to mitochondrial function in mice treated with N-methyl-4-phenyl-1,2,3,6-tetrahydropyridine. *Biochem. Biophys. Res. Commun.* **2003**, *308*, 197–205. [CrossRef]

307. Echtermeyer, F.; Bertrand, J.; Dreier, R.; Meinecke, I.; Neugebauer, K.; Fuerst, M.; Lee, Y.J.; Song, Y.W.; Herzog, C.; Theilmeier, G.; et al. Syndecan-4 regulates ADAMTS-5 activation and cartilage breakdown in osteoarthritis. *Nat. Med.* **2009**, *15*, 1072–1076. [CrossRef] [PubMed]

308. Wilusz, R.E.; Defrate, L.E.; Guilak, F. A biomechanical role for perlecan in the pericellular matrix of articular cartilage. *Matrix Biol.* **2012**, *31*, 320–327. [CrossRef] [PubMed]

309. Li, L.; Ly, M.; Linhardt, R.J. Proteoglycan sequence. *Mol. Biosyst.* **2012**, *8*, 1613–1625. [CrossRef] [PubMed]

310. Caterson, B. Fell-Muir Lecture: Chondroitin sulphate glycosaminoglycans: Fun for some and confusion for others. *Int. J. Exp. Pathol.* **2012**, *93*, 1–10. [CrossRef] [PubMed]

311. Yayon, A.; Klagsbrun, M.; Esko, J.D.; Leder, P.; Ornitz, D.M. Cell surface, heparin-like molecules are required for binding of basic fibroblast growth factor to its high affinity receptor. *Cell* **1991**, *64*, 841–848. [CrossRef]

312. Yayon, A.; Klagsbrun, M.; Esko, J.D.; Leder, P.; Ornitz, D.M. Heparin is required for cell-free binding of basic fibroblast growth factor to a soluble receptor and for mitogenesis in whole cells. *Mol. Cell Biol.* **1992**, *12*, 240–247.

313. Schaefer, T.; Roux, M.; Stuhlsatz, H.W.; Herken, R.; Coulomb, B.; Krieg, T.; Smola, H. Glycosaminoglycans modulate cell-matrix interactions of human fibroblasts and endothelial cells in vitro. *J. Cell Sci.* **1996**, *109*, 479–488. [PubMed]

314. Ji, Z.S.; Pitas, R.E.; Mahley, R.W. Differential cellular accumulation/retention of apolipoprotein E mediated by cell surface heparan sulfate proteoglycans. Apolipoproteins E3 and E2 greater than e4. *J. Biol. Chem.* **1998**, *273*, 13452–13460. [CrossRef] [PubMed]

315. Linhardt, R.J.; Toida, T. Role of glycosaminoglycans in cellular communication. *Acc. Chem. Res.* **2004**, *37*, 431–438. [CrossRef] [PubMed]

316. Sadir, R.; Imberty, A.; Baleux, F.; Lortat-Jacob, H. Heparan sulfate/heparin oligosaccharides protect stromal cell-derived factor-1 (SDF-1)/CXCL12 against proteolysis induced by CD26/dipeptidyl peptidase IV. *J. Biol. Chem.* **2004**, *279*, 43854–43860. [CrossRef] [PubMed]

317. Vives, R.R.; Lortat-Jacob, H.; Chroboczek, J.; Fender, P. Heparan sulfate proteoglycan mediates the selective attachment and internalization of serotype 3 human adenovirus dodecahedron. *Virology* **2004**, *321*, 332–340. [CrossRef] [PubMed]

318. Capurro, M.I.; Xu, P.; Shi, W.; Li, F.; Jia, A.; Filmus, J. Glypican-3 inhibits Hedgehog signaling during development by competing with patched for Hedgehog binding. *Dev. Cell* **2008**, *14*, 700–711. [CrossRef] [PubMed]

319. Lewis, P.N.; Pinali, C.; Young, R.D.; Meek, K.M.; Quantock, A.J.; Knupp, C. Structural interactions between collagen and proteoglycans are elucidated by three-dimensional electron tomography of bovine cornea. *Structure* **2010**, *18*, 239–245. [CrossRef] [PubMed]

320. Ortmann, C.; Pickhinke, U.; Exner, S.; Ohlig, S.; Lawrence, R.; Jboor, H.; Dreier, R.; Grobe, K. Sonic hedgehog processing and release are regulated by glypican heparan sulfate proteoglycans. *J. Cell Sci.* **2015**, *128*, 4462. [CrossRef] [PubMed]

321. Shriver, Z.; Capila, I.; Venkataraman, G.; Sasisekharan, R. Heparin and heparan sulfate: Analyzing structure and microheterogeneity. *Handb. Exp. Pharmacol.* **2012**, *207*, 159–176.

322. Mikami, T.; Kitagawa, H. Biosynthesis and function of chondroitin sulfate. *Biochim. Biophys. Acta* **2013**, *1830*, 4719–4733. [CrossRef] [PubMed]

323. Poulain, F.E.; Yost, H.J. Heparan sulfate proteoglycans: A sugar code for vertebrate development? *Development* **2015**, *142*, 3456–3467. [CrossRef] [PubMed]

324. Langford-Smith, A.; Keenan, T.D.; Clark, S.J.; Bishop, P.N.; Day, A.J. The role of complement in age-related macular degeneration: Heparan sulphate, a ZIP code for complement factor H? *J. Innate Immun.* **2014**, *6*, 407–416. [CrossRef] [PubMed]

325. Lamanna, W.C.; Kalus, I.; Padva, M.; Baldwin, R.J.; Merry, C.L.; Dierks, T. The heparanome—The enigma of encoding and decoding heparan sulfate sulfation. *J. Biotechnol.* **2007**, *129*, 290–307. [CrossRef] [PubMed]

326. Pomin, V.H.; Mulloy, B. Current structural biology of the heparin interactome. *Curr. Opin. Struct. Biol.* **2015**, *34*, 17–25. [CrossRef] [PubMed]

327. Sasisekharan, R.; Venkataraman, G. Heparin and heparan sulfate: Biosynthesis, structure and function. *Curr. Opin. Chem. Biol.* **2000**, *4*, 626–631. [CrossRef]

328. Kreuger, J.; et al. Interactions between heparan sulfate and proteins: The concept of specificity. *J. Cell Biol.* **2006**, *174*, 323–327. [CrossRef] [PubMed]

329. Whitelock, J.; Melrose, J. Heparan sulfate proteoglycans in healthy and diseased systems. *Wiley Interdiscip. Rev. Syst. Biol. Med.* **2011**, *3*, 739–751. [CrossRef] [PubMed]

330. Nugent, M.A.; Zaia, J.; Spencer, J.L. Heparan sulfate-protein binding specificity. *Biochemistry (Moscow)* **2013**, *78*, 726–735. [CrossRef] [PubMed]

331. Johnson, C.E.; Crawford, B.E.; Stavridis, M.; Ten Dam, G.; Wat, A.L.; Rushton, G.; Ward, C.M.; Wilson, V.; van Kuppevelt, T.H.; Esko, J.D.; et al. Essential alterations of heparan sulfate during the differentiation of embryonic stem cells to Sox1-enhanced green fluorescent protein-expressing neural progenitor cells. *Stem. Cells* **2007**, *25*, 1913–1923. [CrossRef] [PubMed]

332. Baldwin, R.J.; ten Dam, G.B.; van Kuppevelt, T.H.; Lacaud, G.; Gallagher, J.T.; Kouskoff, V.; Merry, C.L. A developmentally regulated heparan sulfate epitope defines a subpopulation with increased blood potential during mesodermal differentiation. *Stem. Cells* **2008**, *26*, 3108–3118. [CrossRef] [PubMed]

333. Holley, R.J.; Pickford, C.E.; Rushton, G.; Lacaud, G.; Gallagher, J.T.; Kouskoff, V.; Merry, C.L. Influencing hematopoietic differentiation of mouse embryonic stem cells using soluble heparin and heparan sulfate saccharides. *J. Biol. Chem.* **2011**, *286*, 6241–6252. [CrossRef] [PubMed]

334. Pickford, C.E.; Holley, R.J.; Rushton, G.; Stavridis, M.P.; Ward, C.M.; Merry, C.L. Specific glycosaminoglycans modulate neural specification of mouse embryonic stem cells. *Stem. Cells* **2011**, *29*, 629–640. [CrossRef] [PubMed]

335. Meade, K.A.; White, K.J.; Pickford, C.E.; Holley, R.J.; Marson, A.; Tillotson, D.; van Kuppevelt, T.H.; Whittle, J.D.; Day, A.J.; Merry, C.L. Immobilization of heparan sulfate on electrospun meshes to support embryonic stem cell culture and differentiation. *J. Biol. Chem.* **2013**, *288*, 5530–5538. [CrossRef] [PubMed]

336. Nairn, A.V.; Aoki, K.; dela Rosa, M.; Porterfield, M.; Lim, J.M.; Kulik, M.; Pierce, J.M.; Wells, L.; Dalton, S.; Tiemeyer, M.; et al. Regulation of glycan structures in murine embryonic stem cells: Combined transcript profiling of glycan-related genes and glycan structural analysis. *J. Biol. Chem.* **2012**, *287*, 37835–37856. [CrossRef] [PubMed]

337. Suchorska, W.M.; Lach, M.S.; Richter, M.; Kaczmarczyk, J.; Trzeciak, T. Bioimaging: An Useful Tool to Monitor Differentiation of Human Embryonic Stem Cells into Chondrocytes. *Ann. Biomed. Eng.* **2016**, *44*, 1845–1859. [CrossRef] [PubMed]

338. Lin, X.; Wei, G.; Shi, Z.; Dryer, L.; Esko, J.D.; Wells, D.E.; Matzuk, M.M. Disruption of gastrulation and heparan sulfate biosynthesis in EXT1-deficient mice. *Dev. Biol.* **2000**, *224*, 299–311. [CrossRef] [PubMed]

339. Stickens, D.; Zak, B.M.; Rougier, N.; Esko, J.D.; Werb, Z. Mice deficient in Ext2 lack heparan sulfate and develop exostoses. *Development* **2005**, *132*, 5055–5068. [CrossRef] [PubMed]

340. Matsumoto, Y.; Matsumoto, K.; Irie, F.; Fukushi, J.; Stallcup, W.B.; Yamaguchi, Y. Conditional ablation of the heparan sulfate-synthesizing enzyme Ext1 leads to dysregulation of bone morphogenic protein signaling and severe skeletal defects. *J. Biol. Chem.* **2010**, *285*, 19227–19234. [CrossRef] [PubMed]

341. Vincent, T.; Hermansson, M.; Bolton, M.; Wait, R.; Saklatvala, J. Basic FGF mediates an immediate response of articular cartilage to mechanical injury. *Proc. Natl. Acad. Sci. USA* **2002**, *99*, 8259–8264. [CrossRef] [PubMed]

342. Faiyaz ul Haque, M.; King, L.M.; Krakow, D.; Cantor, R.M.; Rusiniak, M.E.; Swank, R.T.; Superti-Furga, A.; Haque, S.; Abbas, H.; Ahmad, W.; Ahmad, M.; et al. Mutations in orthologous genes in human spondyloepimetaphyseal dysplasia and the brachymorphic mouse. *Nat. Genet* **1998**, *20*, 157–162. [CrossRef] [PubMed]

343. Otsuki, S.; Taniguchi, N.; Grogan, S.P.; D'Lima, D.; Kinoshita, M.; Lotz, M. Expression of novel extracellular sulfatases Sulf-1 and Sulf-2 in normal and osteoarthritic articular cartilage. *Arthritis Res. Ther.* **2008**, *10*, R61. [CrossRef] [PubMed]

344. Otsuki, S.; Hanson, S.R.; Miyaki, S.; Grogan, S.P.; Kinoshita, M.; Asahara, H.; Wong, C.H.; Lotz, M.K. Extracellular sulfatases support cartilage homeostasis by regulating BMP and FGF signaling pathways. *Proc. Natl. Acad. Sci. USA* **2010**, *107*, 10202–10207. [CrossRef] [PubMed]

345. San Antonio, J.D.; Winston, B.M.; Tuan, R.S. Regulation of chondrogenesis by heparan sulfate and structurally related glycosaminoglycans. *Dev. Biol.* **1987**, *123*, 17–24. [CrossRef]

346. Fisher, M.C.; Li, Y.; Seghatoleslami, M.R.; Dealy, C.N.; Kosher, R.A. Heparan sulfate proteoglycans including syndecan-3 modulate BMP activity during limb cartilage differentiation. *Matrix Biol.* **2006**, *25*, 27–39. [CrossRef] [PubMed]

347. Chen, J.; Wang, Y.; Chen, C.; Lian, C.; Zhou, T.; Gao, B.; Wu, Z.; Xu, C. Exogenous Heparan Sulfate Enhances the TGF-beta3-Induced Chondrogenesis in Human Mesenchymal Stem Cells by Activating TGF-beta/Smad Signaling. *Stem. Cells Int.* **2016**, *2016*, 1520136. [CrossRef] [PubMed]

348. Jha, A.K.; Yang, W.; Kirn-Safran, C.B.; Farach-Carson, M.C.; Jia, X. Perlecan domain I-conjugated, hyaluronic acid-based hydrogel particles for enhanced chondrogenic differentiation via BMP-2 release. *Biomaterials* **2009**, *30*, 6964–6975. [CrossRef] [PubMed]

349. Sadatsuki, R.; Kaneko, H.; Kinoshita, M.; Futami, I.; Nonaka, R.; Culley, K.L.; Otero, M.; Hada, S.; Goldring, M.B.; Yamada, Y.; et al. Perlecan is required for the chondrogenic differentiation of synovial mesenchymal cells through regulation of Sox9 gene expression. *J. Orthop. Res.* **2017**, *35*, 837–846. [CrossRef] [PubMed]

350. Kim, S.H.; Turnbull, J.; Guimond, S. Extracellular matrix and cell signalling: The dynamic cooperation of integrin, proteoglycan and growth factor receptor. *J. Endocrinol.* **2011**, *209*, 139–151. [CrossRef] [PubMed]

351. Khoshgoftar, M.; Ito, K.; van Donkelaar, C.C. The influence of cell-matrix attachment and matrix development on the micromechanical environment of the chondrocyte in tissue-engineered cartilage. *Tissue Eng. Part A* **2014**, *20*, 3112–3121. [CrossRef] [PubMed]

352. Hayes, A.J.; Shu, C.C.; Lord, M.S.; Little, C.B.; Whitelock, J.M.; Melrose, J. Pericellular colocalisation and interactive properties of type VI collagen and perlecan in the intervertebral disc. *Eur. Cell Mater.* **2016**, *32*, 40–57. [CrossRef] [PubMed]

353. Schminke, B.; Frese, J.; Bode, C.; Goldring, M.B.; Miosge, N. Laminins and Nidogens in the Pericellular Matrix of Chondrocytes: Their Role in Osteoarthritis and Chondrogenic Differentiation. *Am. J. Pathol.* **2016**, *186*, 410–418. [CrossRef] [PubMed]

354. Xu, X.; Li, Z.; Leng, Y.; Neu, C.P.; Calve, S. Knockdown of the pericellular matrix molecule perlecan lowers in situ cell and matrix stiffness in developing cartilage. *Dev. Biol.* **2016**, *418*, 242–247. [CrossRef] [PubMed]

355. Hardingham, T.; Bayliss, M. Proteoglycans of articular cartilage: Changes in aging and in joint disease. *Semin. Arthritis Rheum.* **1990**, *20* (Suppl. 1), 12–33. [CrossRef]

356. Han, C.; Yan, D.; Belenkaya, T.Y.; Lin, X. Drosophila glypicans Dally and Dally-like shape the extracellular Wingless morphogen gradient in the wing disc. *Development* **2005**, *132*, 667–679. [CrossRef] [PubMed]

357. Ayerst, B.I.; Day, A.J.; Nurcombe, V.; Cool, S.M.; Merry, C.L. New strategies for cartilage regeneration exploiting selected glycosaminoglycans to enhance cell fate determination. *Biochem. Soc. Trans.* **2014**, *42*, 703–709. [CrossRef] [PubMed]

358. Coombe, D.R.; Kett, W.C. Heparan sulfate-protein interactions: Therapeutic potential through structure-function insights. *Cell Mol. Life Sci.* **2005**, *62*, 410–424. [CrossRef] [PubMed]

359. Zaia, J. Glycosaminoglycan glycomics using mass spectrometry. *Mol. Cell Proteomics* **2013**, *12*, 885–892. [CrossRef] [PubMed]

360. Fu, L.; Suflita, M.; Linhardt, R.J. Bioengineered heparins and heparan sulfates. *Adv. Drug Deliv. Rev.* **2016**, *97*, 237–249. [CrossRef] [PubMed]

361. Puvirajesinghe, T.M.; Turnbull, J.E. Glycoarray Technologies: Deciphering Interactions from Proteins to Live Cell Responses. *Microarrays (Basel)* **2016**, *5*. [CrossRef] [PubMed]

362. Smith, B.D.; Grande, D.A. The current state of scaffolds for musculoskeletal regenerative applications. *Nat. Rev. Rheumatol.* **2015**, *11*, 213–222. [CrossRef] [PubMed]

363. Kimura, T.; Yasui, N.; Ohsawa, S.; Ono, K. Chondrocytes embedded in collagen gels maintain cartilage phenotype during long-term cultures. *Clin. Orthop. Relat. Res.* **1984**, *186*, 231–239.

364. Schulz, R.M.; Zscharnack, M.; Hanisch, I.; Geiling, M.; Hepp, P.; Bader, A. Cartilage tissue engineering by collagen matrix associated bone marrow derived mesenchymal stem cells. *Biomed. Mater. Eng.* **2008**, *18* (Suppl. 1), S55–S70. [PubMed]

365. Bertolo, A.; Arcolino, F.; Capossela, S.; Taddei, A.R.; Baur, M.; Potzel, T.; Stoyanov, J. Growth Factors Cross-Linked to Collagen Microcarriers Promote Expansion and Chondrogenic Differentiation of Human Mesenchymal Stem Cells. *Tissue Eng. Part A* **2015**, *21*, 2618–2628. [CrossRef] [PubMed]

366. Vazquez-Portalatin, N.; Kilmer, C.E.; Panitch, A.; Liu, J.C. Characterization of Collagen Type I and II Blended Hydrogels for Articular Cartilage Tissue Engineering. *Biomacromolecules* **2016**, *17*, 3145–3152. [CrossRef] [PubMed]

367. Vazquez-Portalatin, N.; Kilmer, C.E.; Panitch, A.; Liu, J.C. Knee joint preservation with combined neutralising high tibial osteotomy (HTO) and Matrix-induced Autologous Chondrocyte Implantation (MACI) in younger patients with medial knee osteoarthritis: A case series with prospective clinical and MRI follow-up over 5 years. *Knee* **2012**, *19*, 431–439.

368. Ventura, A.; Memeo, A.; Borgo, E.; Terzaghi, C.; Legnani, C.; Albisetti, W. Repair of osteochondral lesions in the knee by chondrocyte implantation using the MACI(R) technique. *Knee Surg. Sports Traumatol. Arthrosc.* **2012**, *20*, 121–126. [CrossRef] [PubMed]

369. Deponti, D.; Di Giancamillo, A.; Gervaso, F.; Domenicucci, M.; Domeneghini, C.; Sannino, A.; Peretti, G.M. Collagen scaffold for cartilage tissue engineering: The benefit of fibrin glue and the proper culture time in an infant cartilage model. *Tissue Eng. Part A* **2014**, *20*, 1113–1126. [CrossRef] [PubMed]

370. Kusano, T.; Jakob, R.P.; Gautier, E.; Magnussen, R.A.; Hoogewoud, H.; Jacobi, M. Treatment of isolated chondral and osteochondral defects in the knee by autologous matrix-induced chondrogenesis (AMIC). *Knee Surg. Sports Traumatol. Arthrosc.* **2012**, *20*, 2109–2115. [CrossRef] [PubMed]

371. Gille, J.; Behrens, P.; Volpi, P.; de Girolamo, L.; Reiss, E.; Zoch, W.; Anders, S. Outcome of Autologous Matrix Induced Chondrogenesis (AMIC) in cartilage knee surgery: Data of the AMIC Registry. *Arch. Orthop. Trauma Surg.* **2013**, *133*, 87–93. [CrossRef] [PubMed]

372. Benthien, J.P.; Behrens, P. Nanofractured autologous matrix induced chondrogenesis (NAMIC(c))—Further development of collagen membrane aided chondrogenesis combined with subchondral needling: A technical note. *Knee* **2015**, *22*, 411–415. [CrossRef] [PubMed]

373. Levingstone, T.J.; Ramesh, A.; Brady, R.T.; Brama, P.A.; Kearney, C.; Gleeson, J.P.; O'Brien, F.J. Cell-free multi-layered collagen-based scaffolds demonstrate layer specific regeneration of functional osteochondral tissue in caprine joints. *Biomaterials* **2016**, *87*, 69–81. [CrossRef] [PubMed]

374. Levingstone, T.J.; Thompson, E.; Matsiko, A.; Schepens, A.; Gleeson, J.P.; O'Brien, F.J. Multi-layered collagen-based scaffolds for osteochondral defect repair in rabbits. *Acta Biomater.* **2016**, *32*, 149–160. [CrossRef] [PubMed]

375. Yuan, X.; Zhou, M.; Gough, J.; Glidle, A.; Yin, H. A novel culture system for modulating single cell geometry in 3D. *Acta Biomater.* **2015**, *24*, 228–240. [CrossRef] [PubMed]

376. Nehrer, S.; Domayer, S.; Dorotka, R.; Schatz, K.; Bindreiter, U.; Kotz, R. Three-year clinical outcome after chondrocyte transplantation using a hyaluronan matrix for cartilage repair. *Eur. J. Radiol.* **2006**, *57*, 3–8. [CrossRef] [PubMed]

377. Gobbi, A.; Kon, E.; Berruto, M.; Filardo, G.; Delcogliano, M.; Boldrini, L.; Bathan, L.; Marcacci, M. Patellofemoral full-thickness chondral defects treated with second-generation autologous chondrocyte implantation: Results at 5 years' follow-up. *Am. J. Sports Med.* **2009**, *37*, 1083–1092. [CrossRef] [PubMed]

378. Brix, M.O.; Stelzeneder, D.; Chiari, C.; Koller, U.; Nehrer, S.; Dorotka, R.; Windhager, R.; Domayer, S.E. Treatment of Full-Thickness Chondral Defects With Hyalograft C in the Knee: Long-term Results. *Am. J. Sports Med.* **2014**, *42*, 1426–1432. [CrossRef] [PubMed]

379. Methot, S.; Changoor, A.; Tran-Khanh, N.; Hoemann, C.D.; Stanish, W.D.; Restrepo, A.; Shive, M.S.; Buschmann, M.D. Osteochondral Biopsy Analysis Demonstrates That BST-CarGel Treatment Improves Structural and Cellular Characteristics of Cartilage Repair Tissue Compared With Microfracture. *Cartilage* **2016**, *7*, 16–28. [CrossRef] [PubMed]

380. Merkle, H.P. Drug delivery's quest for polymers: Where are the frontiers? *Eur. J. Pharm. Biopharm.* **2015**, *97*, 293–303. [CrossRef] [PubMed]

381. Liu, X.; Holzwarth, J.M.; Ma, P.X. Functionalized synthetic biodegradable polymer scaffolds for tissue engineering. *Macromol. Biosci.* **2012**, *12*, 911–919. [CrossRef] [PubMed]

382. Temenoff, J.S.; Mikos, A.G. Review: Tissue engineering for regeneration of articular cartilage. *Biomaterials* **2000**, *21*, 431–440. [CrossRef]

383. Gentile, P.; Chiono, V.; Carmagnola, I.; Hatton, P.V. An overview of poly(lactic-co-glycolic) acid (PLGA)-based biomaterials for bone tissue engineering. *Int. J. Mol. Sci.* **2014**, *15*, 3640–3659. [CrossRef] [PubMed]

384. Zhang, X.; Wu, Y.; Pan, Z.; Sun, H.; Wang, J.; Yu, D.; Zhu, S.; Dai, J.; Chen, Y.; Tian, N.; et al. The effects of lactate and acid on articular chondrocytes function: Implications for polymeric cartilage scaffold design. *Acta Biomater.* **2016**, *42*, 329–340. [CrossRef] [PubMed]

385. Gunatillake, P.A.; Adhikari, R. Biodegradable synthetic polymers for tissue engineering. *Eur. Cell. Mater.* **2003**, *5*, 1–16, discussion 16. [CrossRef] [PubMed]

386. Farah, S.; Anderson, D.G.; Langer, R. Physical and mechanical properties of PLA, and their functions in widespread applications—A comprehensive review. *Adv. Drug Deliv. Rev.* **2016**, *107*, 367–392. [CrossRef] [PubMed]

387. Izal, I.; Aranda, P.; Sanz-Ramos, P.; Ripalda, P.; Mora, G.; Granero-Molto, F.; Deplaine, H.; Gomez-Ribelles, J.L.; Ferrer, G.G.; Acosta, V.; et al. Culture of human bone marrow-derived mesenchymal stem cells on of poly(L-lactic acid) scaffolds: Potential application for the tissue engineering of cartilage. *Knee Surg. Sports Traumatol. Arthrosc.* **2013**, *21*, 1737–1750. [CrossRef] [PubMed]

388. Moran, J.M.; Pazzano, D.; Bonassar, L.J. Characterization of polylactic acid-polyglycolic acid composites for cartilage tissue engineering. *Tissue Eng.* **2003**, *9*, 63–70. [CrossRef] [PubMed]

389. He, X.; Feng, B.; Huang, C.; Wang, H.; Ge, Y.; Hu, R.; Yin, M.; Xu, Z.; Wang, W.; Fu, W.; et al. Electrospun gelatin/polycaprolactone nanofibrous membranes combined with a coculture of bone marrow stromal cells and chondrocytes for cartilage engineering. *Int. J. Nanomedicine* **2015**, *10*, 2089–2099. [PubMed]

390. Olubamiji, A.D.; Izadifar, Z.; Si, J.L.; Cooper, D.M.; Eames, B.F.; Chen, D.X. Modulating mechanical behaviour of 3D-printed cartilage-mimetic PCL scaffolds: Influence of molecular weight and pore geometry. *Biofabrication* **2016**, *8*, 025020. [CrossRef] [PubMed]

391. Deepthi, S.; Jayakumar, R. Prolonged release of TGF-beta from polyelectrolyte nanoparticle loaded macroporous chitin-poly(caprolactone) scaffold for chondrogenesis. *Int. J. Biol. Macromol.* **2016**, *93*, 1402–1409. [CrossRef] [PubMed]

392. Casper, M.E.; Fitzsimmons, J.S.; Stone, J.J.; Meza, A.O.; Huang, Y.; Ruesink, T.J.; O'Driscoll, S.W.; Reinholz, G.G. Tissue engineering of cartilage using poly-epsilon-caprolactone nanofiber scaffolds seeded in vivo with periosteal cells. *Osteoarthr. Cartil.* **2010**, *18*, 981–991. [CrossRef] [PubMed]

393. Pan, Z.; Ding, J. Poly(lactide-co-glycolide) porous scaffolds for tissue engineering and regenerative medicine. *Interface Focus* **2012**, *2*, 366–377. [CrossRef] [PubMed]

394. Haaparanta, A.M.; Jarvinen, E.; Cengiz, I.F.; Ella, V.; Kokkonen, H.T.; Kiviranta, I.; Kellomaki, M. Preparation and characterization of collagen/PLA, chitosan/PLA, and collagen/chitosan/PLA hybrid scaffolds for cartilage tissue engineering. *J. Mater. Sci. Mater. Med.* **2014**, *25*, 1129–1136. [CrossRef] [PubMed]

395. Chen, W.; Chen, S.; Morsi, Y.; El-Hamshary, H.; El-Newhy, M.; Fan, C.; Mo, X. Superabsorbent 3D Scaffold Based on Electrospun Nanofibers for Cartilage Tissue Engineering. *ACS Appl. Mater. Interfaces* **2016**, *8*, 24415–24425. [CrossRef] [PubMed]

396. Hou, J.; Fan, D.; Zhao, L.; Yu, B.; Su, J.; Wei, J.; Shin, J.W. Degradability, cytocompatibility, and osteogenesis of porous scaffolds of nanobredigite and PCL-PEG-PCL composite. *Int. J. Nanomedicine* **2016**, *11*, 3545–3555. [PubMed]

397. Lee, J.M.; Chae, T.; Sheikh, F.A.; Ju, H.W.; Moon, B.M.; Park, H.J.; Park, Y.R.; Park, C.H. Three dimensional poly(epsilon-caprolactone) and silk fibroin nanocomposite fibrous matrix for artificial dermis. *Mater. Sci. Eng. C Mater. Biol. Appl.* **2016**, *68*, 758–767. [CrossRef] [PubMed]

398. Sonomoto, K.; Yamaoka, K.; Kaneko, H.; Yamagata, K.; Sakata, K.; Zhang, X.; Kondo, M.; Zenke, Y.; Sabanai, K.; Nakayamada, S.; et al. Spontaneous Differentiation of Human Mesenchymal Stem Cells on Poly-Lactic-Co-Glycolic Acid Nano-Fiber Scaffold. *PLoS ONE* **2016**, *11*, e0153231. [CrossRef] [PubMed]

399. Wang, X.; Ding, B.; Li, B. Biomimetic electrospun nanofibrous structures for tissue engineering. *Mater. Today (Kidlington)* **2013**, *16*, 229–241. [CrossRef] [PubMed]

400. Bonzani, I.C.; George, J.H.; Stevens, M.M. Novel materials for bone and cartilage regeneration. *Curr. Opin. Chem. Biol.* **2006**, *10*, 568–575. [CrossRef] [PubMed]

401. Holmes, B.; Castro, N.J.; Zhang, L.G.; Zussman, E. Electrospun fibrous scaffolds for bone and cartilage tissue generation: Recent progress and future developments. *Tissue Eng. Part B* **2012**, *18*, 478–486. [CrossRef] [PubMed]

402. Wise, J.K.; Yarin, A.L.; Megaridis, C.M.; Cho, M. Chondrogenic differentiation of human mesenchymal stem cells on oriented nanofibrous scaffolds: Engineering the superficial zone of articular cartilage. *Tissue Eng. Part A* **2009**, *15*, 913–921. [CrossRef] [PubMed]

403. Kim, C.; Shores, L.; Guo, Q.; Aly, A.; Jeon, O.H.; Kim do, H.; Bernstein, N.; Bhattacharya, R.; Chae, J.J.; Yarema, K.J.; et al. Electrospun Microfiber Scaffolds with Anti-Inflammatory Tributanoylated N-Acetyl-d-Glucosamine Promote Cartilage Regeneration. *Tissue Eng. Part A* **2016**, *22*, 689–697. [CrossRef] [PubMed]

404. Tzezana, R.; Zussman, E.; Levenberg, S. A layered ultra-porous scaffold for tissue engineering, created via a hydrospinning method. *Tissue Eng. Part C* **2008**, *14*, 281–288. [CrossRef] [PubMed]

405. Rnjak-Kovacina, J.; Weiss, A.S. Increasing the pore size of electrospun scaffolds. *Tissue Eng. Part B* **2011**, *17*, 365–372. [CrossRef] [PubMed]

406. Pham, Q.P.; Sharma, U.; Mikos, A.G. Electrospun poly(epsilon-caprolactone) microfiber and multilayer nanofiber/microfiber scaffolds: Characterization of scaffolds and measurement of cellular infiltration. *Biomacromolecules* **2006**, *7*, 2796–2805. [CrossRef] [PubMed]

407. Ekaputra, A.K.; Prestwich, G.D.; Cool, S.M.; Hutmacher, D.W. Combining electrospun scaffolds with electrosprayed hydrogels leads to three-dimensional cellularization of hybrid constructs. *Biomacromolecules* **2008**, *9*, 2097–2103. [CrossRef] [PubMed]

408. Soliman, S.; Pagliari, S.; Rinaldi, A.; Forte, G.; Fiaccavento, R.; Pagliari, F.; Franzese, O.; Minieri, M.; Di Nardo, P.; Licoccia, S.; et al. Multiscale three-dimensional scaffolds for soft tissue engineering via multimodal electrospinning. *Acta Biomater.* **2010**, *6*, 1227–1237. [CrossRef] [PubMed]

409. Takanari, K.; Hong, Y.; Hashizume, R.; Huber, A.; Amoroso, N.J.; D'Amore, A.; Badylak, S.F.; Wagner, W.R. Abdominal wall reconstruction by a regionally distinct biocomposite of extracellular matrix digest and a biodegradable elastomer. *J. Tissue Eng. Regen. Med.* **2016**, *10*, 748–761. [CrossRef] [PubMed]

410. Coburn, J.; Gibson, M.; Bandalini, P.A.; Laird, C.; Mao, H.Q.; Moroni, L.; Seliktar, D.; Elisseeff, J. Biomimetics of the Extracellular Matrix: An Integrated Three-Dimensional Fiber-Hydrogel Composite for Cartilage Tissue Engineering. *Smart Struct. Syst.* **2011**, *7*, 213–222. [CrossRef] [PubMed]

411. Kim, I.L.; Mauck, R.L.; Burdick, J.A. Hydrogel design for cartilage tissue engineering: A case study with hyaluronic acid. *Biomaterials* **2011**, *32*, 8771–8782. [CrossRef] [PubMed]

412. Li, L.; He, Z.Y.; Wei, X.W.; Wei, Y.Q. Recent advances of biomaterials in biotherapy. *Regen. Biomater.* **2016**, *3*, 99–105. [CrossRef] [PubMed]

413. Ho, S.T.; Cool, S.M.; Hui, J.H.; Hutmacher, D.W. The influence of fibrin based hydrogels on the chondrogenic differentiation of human bone marrow stromal cells. *Biomaterials* **2010**, *31*, 38–47. [CrossRef] [PubMed]

414. Muller, M.; Ozturk, E.; Arlov, O.; Gatenholm, P.; Zenobi-Wong, M. Alginate Sulfate-Nanocellulose Bioinks for Cartilage Bioprinting Applications. *Ann. Biomed. Eng.* **2017**, *45*, 210–223. [CrossRef] [PubMed]

415. Hamidi, M.; Azadi, A.; Rafiei, P. Hydrogel nanoparticles in drug delivery. *Adv. Drug Deliv. Rev.* **2008**, *60*, 1638–1649. [CrossRef] [PubMed]

416. Koutsopoulos, S.; Unsworth, L.D.; Nagai, Y.; Zhang, S. Controlled release of functional proteins through designer self-assembling peptide nanofiber hydrogel scaffold. *Proc. Natl. Acad. Sci. USA* **2009**, *106*, 4623–4628. [CrossRef] [PubMed]

417. Wang, Y.; Cheetham, A.G.; Angacian, G.; Su, H.; Xie, L.; Cui, H. Peptide-drug conjugates as effective prodrug strategies for targeted delivery. *Adv. Drug. Deliv. Rev.* **2016**. [CrossRef] [PubMed]

418. Wang, Y.; Cheetham, A.G.; Angacian, G.; Su, H.; Xie, L.; Cui, H. Self-assembled peptide-based hydrogels as scaffolds for anchorage-dependent cells. *Biomaterials* **2009**, *30*, 2523–2530.

419. Zhou, M.; Ulijn, R.V.; Gough, J.E. Extracellular matrix formation in self-assembled minimalistic bioactive hydrogels based on aromatic peptide amphiphiles. *J. Tissue Eng.* **2014**, *5*. [CrossRef] [PubMed]

420. Saiani, A.; Frielinghaus, H. Self-assembly and gelation properties of a-helix versus b-sheet forming peptides. *Soft Matter* **2009**, *5*, 193–202. [CrossRef]

421. Zhou, M.; Smith, A.M.; Das, A.K.; Hodson, N.W.; Collins, R.F.; Ulijn, R.V.; Gough, J.E. Self-assembled octapeptide scaffolds for in vitro chondrocyte culture. *Acta Biomater.* **2013**, *9*, 4609–4617.

422. King, P.J.; Giovanna Lizio, M.; Booth, A.; Collins, R.F.; Gough, J.E.; Miller, A.F.; Webb, S.J. A modular self-assembly approach to functionalised beta-sheet peptide hydrogel biomaterials. *Soft Matter* **2016**, *12*, 1915–1923. [CrossRef] [PubMed]

423. Coxon, T.P.; Fallows, T.W.; Gough, J.E.; Webb, S.J. A versatile approach towards multivalent saccharide displays on magnetic nanoparticles and phospholipid vesicles. *Org. Biomol. Chem.* **2015**, *13*, 10751–10761. [CrossRef] [PubMed]

424. Freudenberg, U.; Liang, Y.; Kiick, K.L.; Werner, C. Glycosaminoglycan-Based Biohybrid Hydrogels: A Sweet and Smart Choice for Multifunctional Biomaterials. *Adv. Mater.* **2016**, *28*, 8861–8891. [CrossRef] [PubMed]

425. Kim, M.; Erickson, I.E.; Choudhury, M.; Pleshko, N.; Mauck, R.L. Transient exposure to TGF-beta3 improves the functional chondrogenesis of MSC-laden hyaluronic acid hydrogels. *J. Mech. Behav. Biomed. Mater.* **2012**, *11*, 92–101. [CrossRef] [PubMed]

426. Getgood, A.; Henson, F.; Skelton, C.; Herrera, E.; Brooks, R.; Fortier, L.A.; Rushton, N. The Augmentation of a Collagen/Glycosaminoglycan Biphasic Osteochondral Scaffold with Platelet-Rich Plasma and Concentrated Bone Marrow Aspirate for Osteochondral Defect Repair in Sheep: A Pilot Study. *Cartilage* **2012**, *3*, 351–363. [CrossRef] [PubMed]
427. Kim, Y.J.; Kang, I.K.; Huh, M.W.; Yoon, S.C. Surface characterization and in vitro blood compatibility of poly(ethylene terephthalate) immobilized with insulin and/or heparin using plasma glow discharge. *Biomaterials* **2000**, *21*, 121–130. [CrossRef]
428. Ji, Y.; Ghosh, K.; Shu, X.Z.; Li, B.; Sokolov, J.C.; Prestwich, G.D.; Clark, R.A.; Rafailovich, M.H. Electrospun three-dimensional hyaluronic acid nanofibrous scaffolds. *Biomaterials* **2006**, *27*, 3782–3792. [CrossRef] [PubMed]
429. Wang, K.; Chen, X.; Pan, Y.; Cui, Y.; Zhou, X.; Kong, D.; Zhao, Q. Enhanced vascularization in hybrid PCL/gelatin fibrous scaffolds with sustained release of VEGF. *Biomed. Res. Int.* **2015**, *2015*, 865076. [CrossRef] [PubMed]
430. Hua, Q.; Knudson, C.B.; Knudson, W. Internalization of hyaluronan by chondrocytes occurs via receptor-mediated endocytosis. *J. Cell Sci.* **1993**, *106*, 365–375. [PubMed]
431. Sorensen, V.; Nilsen, T.; Wiedlocha, A. Functional diversity of FGF-2 isoforms by intracellular sorting. *Bioessays* **2006**, *28*, 504–514. [CrossRef] [PubMed]
432. Payne, C.K.; Jones, S.A.; Chen, C.; Zhuang, X. Internalization and trafficking of cell surface proteoglycans and proteoglycan-binding ligands. *Traffic* **2007**, *8*, 389–401. [CrossRef] [PubMed]
433. Mahoney, D.J.; Whittle, J.D.; Milner, C.M.; Clark, S.J.; Mulloy, B.; Buttle, D.J.; Jones, G.C.; Day, A.J.; Short, R.D. A method for the non-covalent immobilization of heparin to surfaces. *Anal. Biochem.* **2004**, *330*, 123–129. [CrossRef] [PubMed]
434. Keselowsky, B.G.; Collard, D.M.; Garcia, A.J. Surface chemistry modulates fibronectin conformation and directs integrin binding and specificity to control cell adhesion. *J. Biomed. Mater. Res. A* **2003**, *66*, 247–259. [CrossRef] [PubMed]
435. Robinson, D.E.; Buttle, D.J.; Short, R.D.; McArthur, S.L.; Steele, D.A.; Whittle, J.D. Glycosaminoglycan (GAG) binding surfaces for characterizing GAG-protein interactions. *Biomaterials* **2012**, *33*, 1007–1016. [CrossRef] [PubMed]
436. Rinsch, C.L.; Chen, X.; Panchalingam, V.; Eberhart, R.C.; Wang, J.H.; Timmons, R.B. Pulsed radio frequency plasma polymerization of allyl alcohol: Controlled deposition of surface hydroxyl groups. *Langmuir* **1996**, *12*, 2995–3002. [CrossRef]
437. Marson, A.; Robinson, D.E.; Brookes, P.N.; Mulloy, B.; Wiles, M.; Clark, S.J.; Fielder, H.L.; Collinson, L.J.; Cain, S.A.; Kielty, C.M.; et al. Development of a microtiter plate-based glycosaminoglycan array for the investigation of glycosaminoglycan-protein interactions. *Glycobiology* **2009**, *19*, 1537–1546. [CrossRef] [PubMed]
438. Robinson, D.E.; Marson, A.; Short, R.D.; Buttle, D.J.; Day, A.J.; Parry, K.L.; Wiles, M.; Highfield, P.; Mistry, A.; Whittle, J.D. Surface gradient of functional heparin. *Adv. Mater.* **2008**, *20*, 1166–1169. [CrossRef]
439. Yang, Z.; Tu, Q.; Wang, J.; Huang, N. The role of heparin binding surfaces in the direction of endothelial and smooth muscle cell fate and re-endothelialization. *Biomaterials* **2012**, *33*, 6615–6625. [CrossRef] [PubMed]
440. Kim, M.; Hong, B.; Lee, J.; Kim, S.E.; Kang, S.S.; Kim, Y.H.; Tae, G. Composite system of PLCL scaffold and heparin-based hydrogel for regeneration of partial-thickness cartilage defects. *Biomacromolecules* **2012**, *13*, 2287–2298. [CrossRef] [PubMed]
441. Wang, J.; An, Q.; Li, D.; Wu, T.; Chen, W.; Sun, B.; El-Hamshary, H.; Al-Deyab, S.S.; Zhu, W.; Mo, X. Heparin and Vascular Endothelial Growth Factor Loaded Poly(L-lactide-co-caprolactone) Nanofiber Covered Stent-Graft for Aneurysm Treatment. *J. Biomed. Nanotechnol.* **2015**, *11*, 1947–1960. [CrossRef] [PubMed]
442. Sackler, J.P.; Liu, L. Heparin-induced osteoporosis. *Br. J. Radiol.* **1973**, *46*, 548–550. [CrossRef] [PubMed]
443. Bounameaux, H.; Schneider, P.A.; Mossaz, A.; Suter, P.; Vasey, H. Severe vasospastic reactions (ergotism) during prophylactic administration of heparin-dihydroergotamine. *Vasa* **1987**, *16*, 370–372. [PubMed]
444. Mazziotti, G.; Canalis, E.; Giustina, A. Drug-induced osteoporosis: Mechanisms and clinical implications. *Am. J. Med.* **2010**, *123*, 877–884. [CrossRef] [PubMed]
445. Bambrah, R.K.; Pham, D.C.; Zaiden, R.; Vu, H.; Tai, S. Heparin-induced thrombocytopenia. *Clin. Adv. Hematol. Oncol.* **2011**, *9*, 594–599. [PubMed]

446. Ling, L.; Camilleri, E.T.; Helledie, T.; Samsonraj, R.M.; Titmarsh, D.M.; Chua, R.J.; Dreesen, O.; Dombrowski, C.; Rider, D.A.; Galindo, M.; et al. Effect of heparin on the biological properties and molecular signature of human mesenchymal stem cells. *Gene* **2016**, *576*, 292–303. [CrossRef] [PubMed]

447. Ling, L.; Camilleri, E.T.; Helledie, T.; Samsonraj, R.M.; Titmarsh, D.M.; Chua, R.J.; Dreesen, O.; Dombrowski, C.; Rider, D.A.; Galindo, M.; et al. Oversulfated chondroitin sulfate is a contaminant in heparin associated with adverse clinical events. *Nat. Biotechnol.* **2008**, *26*, 669–675.

448. Mulloy, B.; Wu, N.; Gyapon-Quast, F.; Lin, L.; Zhang, F.; Pickering, M.C.; Linhardt, R.J.; Feizi, T.; Chai, W. Abnormally High Content of Free Glucosamine Residues Identified in a Preparation of Commercially Available Porcine Intestinal Heparan Sulfate. *Anal. Chem.* **2016**, *88*, 6648–6652. [CrossRef] [PubMed]

449. Liu, J.; Linhardt, R.J. Chemoenzymatic synthesis of heparan sulfate and heparin. *Nat. Prod. Rep.* **2014**, *31*, 1676–1685. [CrossRef] [PubMed]

450. Liu, R.; Xu, Y.; Chen, M.; Weiwer, M.; Zhou, X.; Bridges, A.S.; DeAngelis, P.L.; Zhang, Q.; Linhardt, R.J.; Liu, J. Chemoenzymatic design of heparan sulfate oligosaccharides. *J. Biol. Chem.* **2010**, *285*, 34240–34249. [CrossRef] [PubMed]

451. Peterson, S.; Frick, A.; Liu, J. Design of biologically active heparan sulfate and heparin using an enzyme-based approach. *Nat. Prod. Rep.* **2009**, *26*, 610–627. [CrossRef] [PubMed]

452. Chen, Y.; Li, Y.; Yu, H.; Sugiarto, G.; Thon, V.; Hwang, J.; Ding, L.; Hie, L.; Chen, X. Tailored design and synthesis of heparan sulfate oligosaccharide analogues using sequential one-pot multienzyme systems. *Angew. Chem. Int. Ed. Engl.* **2013**, *52*, 11852–11856. [CrossRef] [PubMed]

453. Xu, Y.; Cai, C.; Chandarajoti, K.; Hsieh, P.H.; Li, L.; Pham, T.Q.; Sparkenbaugh, E.M.; Sheng, J.; Key, N.S.; Pawlinski, R.; et al. Homogeneous low-molecular-weight heparins with reversible anticoagulant activity. *Nat. Chem. Biol.* **2014**, *10*, 248–250. [CrossRef] [PubMed]

454. Ori, A.; Wilkinson, M.C.; Fernig, D.G. A systems biology approach for the investigation of the heparin/heparan sulfate interactome. *J. Biol. Chem.* **2011**, *286*, 19892–19904. [CrossRef] [PubMed]

455. Kim, M.; Kim, S.E.; Kang, S.S.; Kim, Y.H.; Tae, G. The use of de-differentiated chondrocytes delivered by a heparin-based hydrogel to regenerate cartilage in partial-thickness defects. *Biomaterials* **2011**, *32*, 7883–7896. [CrossRef] [PubMed]

456. Kuo, Y.C.; Tsai, Y.T. Heparin-conjugated scaffolds with pore structure of inverted colloidal crystals for cartilage regeneration. *Coll. Surf. B Biointerfaces* **2011**, *82*, 616–623. [CrossRef] [PubMed]

457. Fernandez-Muinos, T.; Recha-Sancho, L.; Lopez-Chicon, P.; Castells-Sala, C.; Mata, A.; Semino, C.E. Bimolecular based heparin and self-assembling hydrogel for tissue engineering applications. *Acta Biomater.* **2015**, *16*, 35–48. [CrossRef] [PubMed]

458. Liu, Y.; Deng, L.Z.; Sun, H.P.; Xu, J.Y.; Li, Y.M.; Xie, X.; Zhang, L.M.; Deng, F.L. Sustained dual release of placental growth factor-2 and bone morphogenic protein-2 from heparin-based nanocomplexes for direct osteogenesis. *Int. J. Nanomedicine* **2016**, *11*, 1147–1158. [CrossRef] [PubMed]

459. Recha-Sancho, L.; Semino, C.E. Heparin based self-assembling peptide scaffold reestablish chondrogenic phenotype of expanded de-differentiated human chondrocytes. *J. Biomed. Mater. Res. A* **2016**, *104*, 1694–1706. [CrossRef] [PubMed]

460. Zwingenberger, S.; Langanke, R.; Vater, C.; Lee, G.; Niederlohmann, E.; Sensenschmidt, M.; Jacobi, A.; Bernhardt, R.; Muders, M.; Rammelt, S.; et al. The effect of SDF-1alpha on low dose BMP-2 mediated bone regeneration by release from heparinized mineralized collagen type I matrix scaffolds in a murine critical size bone defect model. *J. Biomed. Mater. Res. A* **2016**, *104*, 2126–2134. [CrossRef] [PubMed]

461. Salek-Ardakani, S.; Arrand, J.R.; Shaw, D.; Mackett, M. Heparin and heparan sulfate bind interleukin-10 and modulate its activity. *Blood* **2000**, *96*, 1879–1888. [PubMed]

462. Kanzaki, S.; Takahashi, T.; Kanno, T.; Ariyoshi, W.; Shinmyouzu, K.; Tujisawa, T.; Nishihara, T. Heparin inhibits BMP-2 osteogenic bioactivity by binding to both BMP-2 and BMP receptor. *J. Cell Physiol.* **2008**, *216*, 844–850. [CrossRef] [PubMed]

463. Hirsh, J.; Anand, S.S.; Halperin, J.L.; Fuster, V. AHA Scientific Statement: Guide to anticoagulant therapy: Heparin: A statement for healthcare professionals from the American Heart Association. *Arterioscler. Thromb. Vasc. Biol.* **2001**, *21*, E9. [CrossRef] [PubMed]

464. Kan, A.; Ikeda, T.; Fukai, A.; Nakagawa, T.; Nakamura, K.; Chung, U.I.; Kawaguchi, H.; Tabin, C.J. SOX11 contributes to the regulation of GDF5 in joint maintenance. *BMC Dev. Biol.* **2013**, *13*, 4. [CrossRef] [PubMed]

465. Fujise, M.; Takeo, S.; Kamimura, K.; Matsuo, T.; Aigaki, T.; Izumi, S.; Nakato, H. Dally regulates Dpp morphogen gradient formation in the Drosophila wing. *Development* **2003**, *130*, 1515–1522. [CrossRef] [PubMed]

466. Bornemann, D.J.; Duncan, J.E.; Staatz, W.; Selleck, S.; Warrior, R. Abrogation of heparan sulfate synthesis in Drosophila disrupts the Wingless, Hedgehog and Decapentaplegic signaling pathways. *Development* **2004**, *131*, 1927–1938. [CrossRef] [PubMed]

467. Ornitz, D.M. FGFs, heparan sulfate and FGFRs: Complex interactions essential for development. *Bioessays* **2000**, *22*, 108–112. [CrossRef]

468. Pellegrini, L. Role of heparan sulfate in fibroblast growth factor signalling: A structural view. *Curr. Opin. Struct. Biol.* **2001**, *11*, 629–634. [CrossRef]

469. Kuo, W.J.; Digman, M.A.; Lander, A.D. Heparan sulfate acts as a bone morphogenetic protein coreceptor by facilitating ligand-induced receptor hetero-oligomerization. *Mol. Biol. Cell.* **2010**, *21*, 4028–4041. [CrossRef] [PubMed]

470. Irimura, T.; Nakajima, M.; Nicolson, G.L. Chemically modified heparins as inhibitors of heparan sulfate specific endo-beta-glucuronidase (heparanase) of metastatic melanoma cells. *Biochemistry* **1986**, *25*, 5322–5328. [CrossRef] [PubMed]

471. Bar-Ner, M.; Eldor, A.; Wasserman, L.; Matzner, Y.; Cohen, I.R.; Fuks, Z.; Vlodavsky, I. Inhibition of heparanase-mediated degradation of extracellular matrix heparan sulfate by non-anticoagulant heparin species. *Blood* **1987**, *70*, 551–557. [PubMed]

472. Parish, C.R.; Coombe, D.R.; Jakobsen, K.B.; Bennett, F.A.; Underwood, P.A. Evidence that sulphated polysaccharides inhibit tumour metastasis by blocking tumour-cell-derived heparanases. *Int. J. Cancer* **1987**, *40*, 511–518. [CrossRef] [PubMed]

473. Huegel, J.; Enomoto-Iwamoto, M.; Sgariglia, F.; Koyama, E.; Pacifici, M. Heparanase stimulates chondrogenesis and is up-regulated in human ectopic cartilage: A mechanism possibly involved in hereditary multiple exostoses. *Am. J. Pathol.* **2015**, *185*, 1676–1685. [CrossRef] [PubMed]

474. Cardin, A.D.; Weintraub, H.J. Molecular modeling of protein-glycosaminoglycan interactions. *Arteriosclerosis* **1989**, *9*, 21–32. [CrossRef] [PubMed]

475. Ori, A.; Free, P.; Courty, J.; Wilkinson, M.C.; Fernig, D.G. Identification of heparin-binding sites in proteins by selective labeling. *Mol. Cell Proteom.* **2009**, *8*, 2256–2265. [CrossRef] [PubMed]

476. Chang, S.C.; Mulloy, B.; Magee, A.I.; Couchman, J.R. Two distinct sites in sonic Hedgehog combine for heparan sulfate interactions and cell signaling functions. *J. Biol. Chem.* **2011**, *286*, 44391–44402. [CrossRef] [PubMed]

477. Uniewicz, K.A.; Ori, A.; Ahmed, Y.A.; Yates, E.A.; Fernig, D.G. Characterisation of the interaction of neuropilin-1 with heparin and a heparan sulfate mimetic library of heparin-derived sugars. *PeerJ* **2014**, *2*, e461. [CrossRef] [PubMed]

478. Tatsinkam, A.J.; Mulloy, B.; Rider, C.C. Mapping the heparin-binding site of the BMP antagonist gremlin by site-directed mutagenesis based on predictive modelling. *Biochem. J.* **2015**, *470*, 53–64. [CrossRef] [PubMed]

479. Esko, J.D.; Kimata, K.; Lindahl, U. Proteoglycans and Sulfated Glycosaminoglycans. In *Essentials of Glycobiology*; Varki, A., Ed.; Cold Spring Harbor: New York, NY, USA, 2009.

480. Powell, A.K.; Yates, E.A.; Fernig, D.G.; Turnbull, J.E. Interactions of heparin/heparan sulfate with proteins: Appraisal of structural factors and experimental approaches. *Glycobiology* **2004**, *14*, 17R–30R. [CrossRef] [PubMed]

481. Mosier, P.D.; Krishnasamy, C.; Kellogg, G.E.; Desai, U.R. On the specificity of heparin/heparan sulfate binding to proteins. Anion-binding sites on antithrombin and thrombin are fundamentally different. *PLoS ONE* **2012**, *7*, e48632. [CrossRef] [PubMed]

482. Gallagher, J. Fell-Muir Lecture: Heparan sulphate and the art of cell regulation: A polymer chain conducts the protein orchestra. *Int. J. Exp. Pathol.* **2015**, *96*, 203–231. [CrossRef] [PubMed]

483. Olson, S.T.; Halvorson, H.R.; Bjork, I. Quantitative characterization of the thrombin-heparin interaction. Discrimination between specific and nonspecific binding models. *J. Biol. Chem.* **1991**, *266*, 6342–6352. [PubMed]

484. Xu, D.; Esko, J.D. Demystifying heparan sulfate-protein interactions. *Annu. Rev. Biochem.* **2014**, *83*, 129–157. [CrossRef] [PubMed]

485. Petitou, M.; van Boeckel, C.A. A synthetic antithrombin III binding pentasaccharide is now a drug! What comes next? *Angew. Chem. Int. Ed. Engl.* **2004**, *43*, 3118–3133. [CrossRef] [PubMed]

486. Atha, D.H.; Lormeau, J.C.; Petitou, M.; Rosenberg, R.D.; Choay, J. Contribution of monosaccharide residues in heparin binding to antithrombin III. *Biochemistry* **1985**, *24*, 6723–6729. [CrossRef] [PubMed]

487. Xu, Y.; Wang, Z.; Liu, R.; Bridges, A.S.; Huang, X.; Liu, J. Directing the biological activities of heparan sulfate oligosaccharides using a chemoenzymatic approach. *Glycobiology* **2012**, *22*, 96–106. [CrossRef] [PubMed]

488. Lortat-Jacob, H.; Turnbull, J.E.; Grimaud, J.A. Molecular organization of the interferon gamma-binding domain in heparan sulphate. *Biochem. J.* **1995**, *310*, 497–505. [CrossRef] [PubMed]

489. Merry, C.L.; Bullock, S.L.; Swan, D.C.; Backen, A.C.; Lyon, M.; Beddington, R.S.; Wilson, V.A.; Gallagher, J.T. The molecular phenotype of heparan sulfate in the Hs2st-/- mutant mouse. *J. Biol. Chem.* **2001**, *276*, 35429–35434. [CrossRef] [PubMed]

490. Skidmore, M.A.; Guimond, S.E.; Rudd, T.R.; Fernig, D.G.; Turnbull, J.E.; Yates, E.A. The activities of heparan sulfate and its analogue heparin are dictated by biosynthesis, sequence, and conformation. *Connect. Tissue Res.* **2008**, *49*, 140–144. [CrossRef] [PubMed]

491. Catlow, K.R.; Deakin, J.A.; Wei, Z.; Delehedde, M.; Fernig, D.G.; Gherardi, E.; Gallagher, J.T.; Pavao, M.S.; Lyon, M. Interactions of hepatocyte growth factor/scatter factor with various glycosaminoglycans reveal an important interplay between the presence of iduronate and sulfate density. *J. Biol. Chem.* **2008**, *283*, 5235–5248. [CrossRef] [PubMed]

492. Raman, R.; Sasisekharan, V.; Sasisekharan, R. Structural insights into biological roles of protein-glycosaminoglycan interactions. *Chem. Biol.* **2005**, *12*, 267–277. [CrossRef] [PubMed]

493. Capila, I.; Linhardt, R.J. Heparin-protein interactions. *Angew. Chem. Int. Ed. Engl.* **2002**, *41*, 391–412. [CrossRef]

494. Thompson, L.D.; Pantoliano, M.W.; Springer, B.A. Energetic characterization of the basic fibroblast growth factor-heparin interaction: Identification of the heparin binding domain. *Biochemistry* **1994**, *33*, 3831–3840. [CrossRef] [PubMed]

495. Asensio, J.L.; Arda, A.; Canada, F.J.; Jimenez-Barbero, J. Carbohydrate-aromatic interactions. *Acc. Chem. Res.* **2013**, *46*, 946–954. [CrossRef] [PubMed]

496. Sarkar, A.; Desai, U.R. A Simple Method for Discovering Druggable, Specific Glycosaminoglycan-Protein Systems. Elucidation of Key Principles from Heparin/Heparan Sulfate-Binding Proteins. *PLoS ONE* **2015**, *10*, e0141127. [CrossRef] [PubMed]

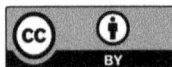

pharmaceuticals

MDPI

Article
Precipitation and Neutralization of Heparin from Different Sources by Protamine Sulfate

John Hogwood [1,*], Barbara Mulloy [2] and Elaine Gray [1,2]

[1] National Institute for Biological Standards and Control (NIBSC), Blanche Lane, South Mimms, Herts EN6 3QG, UK; elaine.gray@nibsc.org
[2] Institute for Pharmaceutical Sciences, King's College London, 10 Stamford Street, London SE1 9HN, UK; barbara.mulloy@kcl.ac.uk
* Correspondence: john.hogwood@nibsc.org; Tel.: +44-1707-641-480

Academic Editor: Jean Jacques Vanden Eynde
Received: 8 June 2017; Accepted: 29 June 2017; Published: 2 July 2017

Abstract: Current therapeutic unfractionated heparin available in Europe and US is of porcine mucosal origin. There is now interest, specifically in the US, to use bovine mucosa as an additional source for the production of heparin. The anticoagulant action of heparin can be neutralized by protamine sulfate, and in this study the ability of protamine to bind and neutralize the anticoagulant activities of heparin from porcine mucosa, bovine mucosa and bovine lung were assessed. Protamine sulfate was able to bind and precipitate similar amounts of heparins from different sources on a mass basis. However, differential amounts of anticoagulant activities were neutralized by protamine sulfate, with neutralization of porcine mucosa more effective than for bovine lung and bovine mucosa. For all heparins, potentiation of thrombin inhibition by antithrombin and heparin cofactor II was preferentially neutralized over antithrombin-mediated inhibition of factor Xa or plasma clotting time. Whole blood thromboelastography showed that neutralization by protamine sulfate was more effective than the antithrombin dependent thrombin inhibition assays indicated. While there was no absolute correlation between average or peak molecular weight of heparin samples and neutralization of anticoagulant activity, correlation was observed between proportions of material with high affinity to antithrombin, specific activities and neutralization of activity.

Keywords: heparin; protamine sulfate; neutralization

1. Introduction

Contamination of porcine heparin with oversulfated chondroitin sulfate in 2007/2008 [1] led to rapid revisions to pharmacopoeial monographs. The principal changes made to the United States Pharmacopeia (USP) and European Pharmacopeia (EP) monographs for heparin included specifying the source as porcine intestinal mucosa, adoption of a purified reagent assay based on antithrombin inhibition of thrombin for potency determination and a specific activity of not less than 180 IU/mg [2]. Furthermore, the contamination issue highlighted the primary reliance on a single source for clinical heparin, porcine mucosa, in Europe and the US. There is now interest in diversifying the supply of heparin, with bovine mucosa suggested as an alternative source [3].

Heparin is a complex heterogeneous and polydisperse anionic polysaccharide, consisting of alternating glucosamine and uronic acid monosaccharide residues [4]. Its primary use is as an anticoagulant and antithrombotic agent for surgery and extracorporeal circuits [5]. Heparin is the anticoagulant of choice for these indications as it can be readily reversed by protamine sulfate [6], an arginine rich basic protein [7]. The use of protamine sulfate is not without some risk [8], and there has been interest in alternative compounds which can neutralize heparin activity [9–12]. However, such investigations have been limited in scope, primarily involving in vitro experimentation. In an animal model [10], a synthetic compound with lower immunogenicity was found to be able to neutralize heparin comparably to protamine. Despite the interest in alternatives to protamine sulfate, until clinical evaluations are carried out it will remain the heparin neutralization agent of choice.

Porcine intestinal mucosa (PM) heparins have been used extensively for over 50 years, with gradual improvements in quality and specific activity [13]. Bovine heparins, whilst clinically used in South America, have not been subjected to extensive study until recently [14,15]. Primary observations are that bovine and porcine heparins have structural differences [14] such as lower weight average molecular weight for bovine lung (BL) heparin, and a lower proportion of 6-O-sulfo groups in bovine intestinal mucosa (BM) heparin. Bovine heparins also have lower specific activities [16], with values consistently below the new minimum monograph potency requirement. The lower specific activity would mean that greater amounts by mass of bovine heparin would be required to achieve the same dose in units of activity.

There is limited information on the ability of protamine sulfate to neutralize the activity of heparin from different sources. Recent interest in the interaction between protamine sulfate and heparin has centered on the possible immunogenic nature of large macromolecular protamine–heparin complexes [17]. Some previous work has shown that high molecular weight heparins have a higher affinity for protamine [18,19], with these studies carried out with porcine unfractionated or low molecular weight heparins. Independent of molecular weight, protamine sulfate has also been shown to neutralize more effectively antithrombin dependent inhibition of thrombin than the antithrombin inhibition of factor Xa [19]. The clinical dosage of protamine sulfate as recommended by the manufacturers is related to the pharmacopoeial methods for bioidentity of protamine sulfate which specify that 1 mg of protamine should precipitate not less than 100 international units (IU) of heparin reference standards. However, it is not clear how the precipitation of heparin relates to neutralization of anticoagulant activity of heparin.

The main objective of this study was to investigate the relationship between precipitation and neutralization of porcine and bovine heparins with protamine sulfate. Accurate anticoagulant activities were determined for a range of PM, BM and BL heparins and used to ascertain whether the units of heparin as measured by heparin/protamine sulfate precipitation related to neutralization of activity. The results from the current study indicate that there are differences in the precipitation and neutralization of biological activity of the heparins by protamine sulfate, and that neutralization of anticoagulant activities by the same amount of protamine sulfate is different for heparin from different sources.

2. Results

2.1. Anticoagulant Activity of Heparin Samples

The anticoagulant activities were estimated against the 6th International Standard for Unfractionated Heparin (07/328, NIBSC, South Mimms, UK), a PM heparin. All activity assays: antithrombin-dependent anti-Xa (AT:aXa), antithrombin-dependent anti-IIa (AT:aIIa), human plasma anticoagulant activated thromboplastin time (APTT) and heparin cofactor II dependent anti-IIa (HCII:aIIa) were valid by parallelism and linearity criteria using the statistical package, Combistats 5.0 (EDQM, Strasbourg, France). The activities of fifty-two PM heparins (Figure 1) were similar (AT:aXa 190, AT:aIIa 186, APTT 185, HCII:aIIa 193 IU/mg) irrespective of the method used (ANOVA, $p = 0.23$). For twenty-six batches of BM heparin samples, there was significant difference between the different assay methods (ANOVA $p < 0.0001$). However, there was no significant difference between results for AT:aXa (127 IU/mg) and APTT (133 IU/mg) activities when considered independently of the other assay methods ($p > 0.01$). AT:aIIa potencies (107 IU/mg) were lower and the HCII:aIIa activities (165 IU/mg) were higher than AT:aXa and APTT estimates. For ten batches of bovine lung heparin, the AT:aXa, AT:aIIa and APTT (130, 127, 121 IU/mg respectively) activities were similar (ANOVA,

$p > 0.01$), but HCII:aIIa (220 IU/mg) activity was significantly higher than all other activities (ANOVA, $p < 0.0001$).

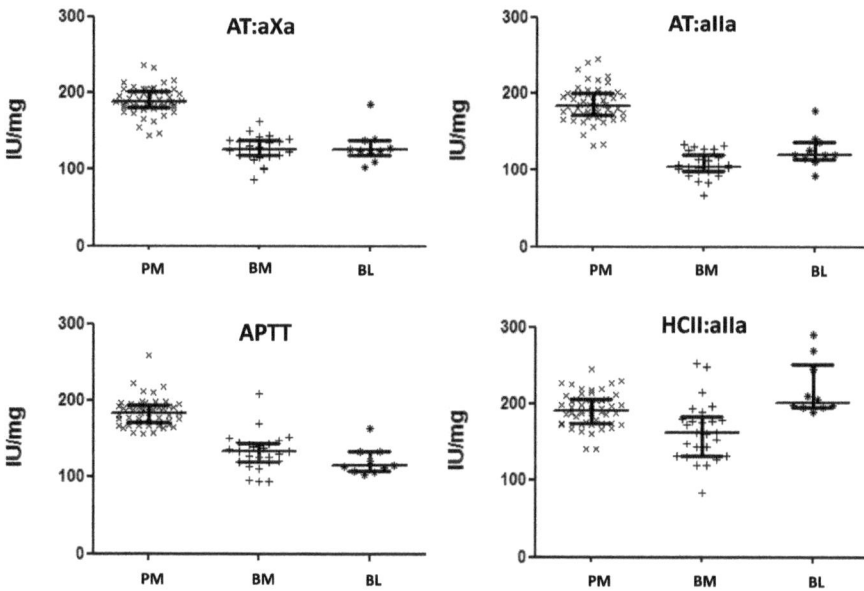

Figure 1. Scatter Plots of specific activities, and interquartile range for porcine intestinal mucosa (PM), bovine intestinal mucosa (BM) and bovine lung (BL) heparin samples. Activities have been calculated relative to the 6th International standard for Unfractionated Heparin (porcine heparin) using parallel line bioassay model for all assays. All samples compared validly to the standard, passing the ANOVA criteria for parallelism and linearity. AT:aXa—antithrombin dependent anti-Xa; AT:aIIa—antithrombin dependent anti-IIa, APTT—plasma APTT assay; HCII:aIIa—heparin cofactor II dependent anti-IIa.

With the exception of HCII:aIIa for bovine lung heparin, PM heparin had higher anticoagulant activities (Figure 1) than BM and BL heparins. BM and BL heparins had similar activities by AT:aXa (127 to 131 IU/mg), but different activities by AT:aIIa (107 to 127 IU/mg) and by APTT (133 to 121 IU/mg). The higher average HCII:aIIa activity of BL heparin (220 IU/mg) compared to PM heparin (193 IU/mg) and BM heparin (165 IU/mg) was influenced by three out of 10 BL heparin samples having exceptionally high activities, thus raising the overall average HCII:aIIa value. When the median HCII:aIIa activity is compared, BL heparin (203 IU/mg) is only slightly higher than PM heparin (191 IU/mg).

2.2. Protamine Sulfate Precipitation Assay

The European Pharmacopeia (EP) monograph states that 1 mg of protamine sulfate precipitates not less than 100 IU of Biological Reference Preparation (BRP) heparin standard. A selection of 16 PM, 16 BM and 4 BL heparin samples were used in the precipitation assay (Figure 2). For this set of experiments, the quantity of heparin (based on AT:aIIa unitage) needed to precipitate 1 mg protamine sulfate was measured. Broadly, greater amounts of PM heparins by activity (average of 126 AT:aIIa IU, ranging 103–142 AT:aIIa IU) were required to precipitate protamine sulfate than BM heparin (an average of 79 IU AT:aIIa, ranging from 48–96 AT:aIIa IU) and BL heparins (an average of 84, ranging from 79–95 AT:aIIa IU).

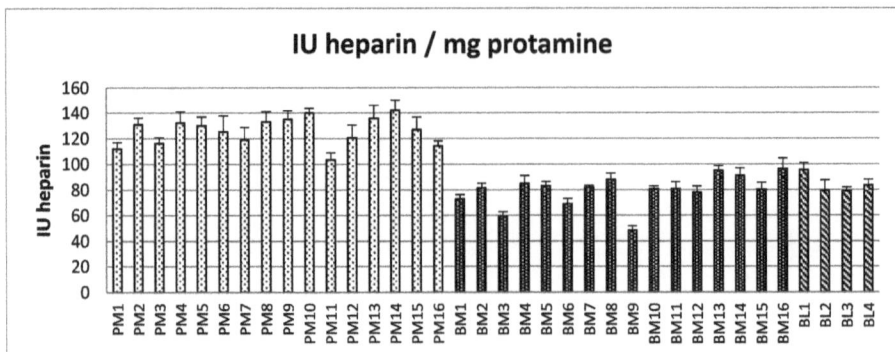

Figure 2. Amount of heparin in International Units (anti-IIa) that is required to precipitate 1 mg of protamine sulfate, estimated according to the European Pharmacopeia assay for protamine sulfate. (error bars = standard deviation, *n* = 9).

Based on the AT:aIIa specific activity estimated, the corresponding amounts of heparin in terms of mass were recalculated from the amount in IU. The heparin by mass which precipitated 1 mg of protamine sulfate is shown in Figure 3. By contrast, the average mass concentration required to precipitate the same amount of protamine sulfate was the same for all the heparins, PM 0.76 mg, BM 0.76 mg and BM 0.74 mg. Table 1 shows that on an IU basis PM and BM are clearly different ($p < 0.001$), but on an mg basis the same amount of heparin was needed to precipitate 1 mg of protamine sulfate.

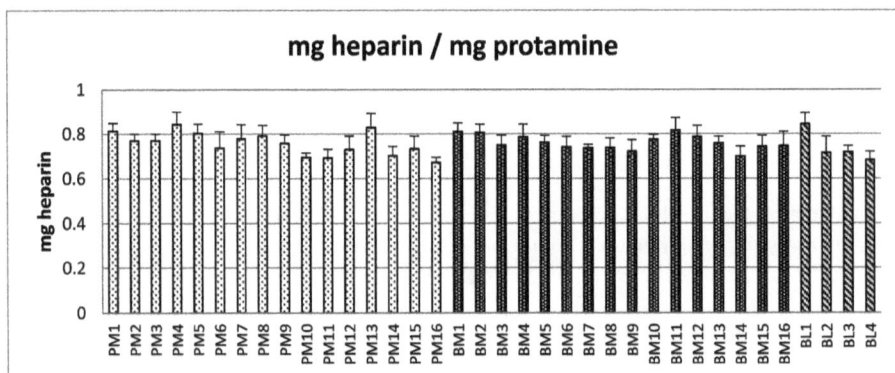

Figure 3. Amount of heparin in mg (calculated from anti-IIa specific activity) that is required to precipitate out 1 mg of protamine sulfate, estimated according to the European Pharmacopeia assay for protamine sulfate. (error bars = standard deviation, *n* = 9).

Table 1. Protamine Sulfate precipitation results for heparin samples by IU/mg and mg/mg. Results show the mean and range for each heparin type for IU (anti-IIa) to mg protamine and recalculated for mg (anti-IIa) to mg protamine.

	PM (*n* = 16)	BM (*n* = 16)	BL (*n* = 4)	*p*-Values
IU/mg PS Mean (range)	126 (103–142)	79.4 (48.4–96.2)	84.3 (79.0–95.3)	PM–BM < 0.001; PM–BL < 0.001; BM–BL = 0.233
mg/mg PS Mean (range)	0.76 (0.67–0.84)	0.76 (0.70–0.82)	0.74 (0.68–0.84)	PM–BM = 0.403; PM–BL = 0.289; BM–BL = 0.188

2.3. Neutralization of Heparin Activity

Four samples each of PM, BM and BL heparin, spanning the range of specific activities by AT:aIIa assays, were investigated further (Table 2) for neutralization of activities. With a fixed amount of heparin mixed with a fixed concentration of protamine sulfate, the remaining amount of heparin by precipitation and by anticoagulant activity was estimated (Figure 4).

Table 2. Selected heparins (four each of PM, BM and BL heparins) IU (AT:aIIa) required to precipitate 1 mg protamine sulfate. Samples here are not PM 1–4 or BM 1–4 as indicated in Figures 2 and 3.

	Sample Code and IU Heparin/mg Protamine			
PM	P1 142	P2 135	P3 121	P4 127
BM	B1 81	B2 91	B3 69	B4 59
BL	L1 81	L2 79	L3 79	L4 95

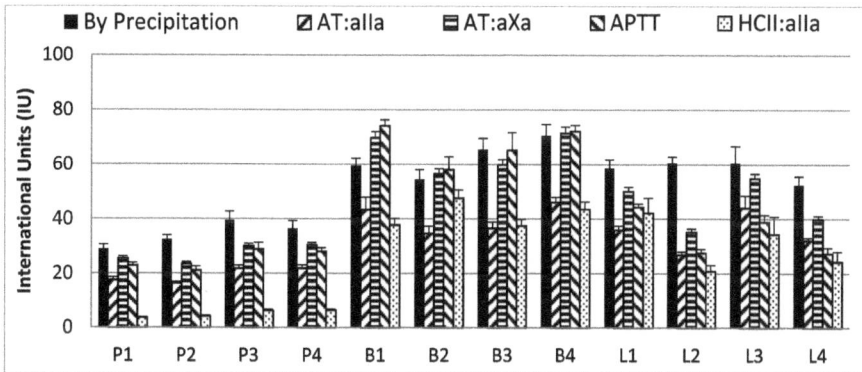

Figure 4. Remaining activity from precipitation and neutralization assays for each heparin sample. Potency shown above has been calculated from mixture of 100 IU/mL heparin with 0.5 mg/mL protamine sulfate, precipitation assay value has been calculated from the protamine sulfate assay, AT:aIIa, AT:aXa, APTT and HCII:aIIa are residual potency estimations. AT:aIIa—antithrombin dependent anti-IIa, AT:aXa—antithrombin dependent anti-Xa, APTT—plasma APTT clotting assay, HCII:aIIa—Heparin Cofactor II dependent anti-IIa. Error bars are SD for precipitation assay, and upper 95% confidence limit for other assays.

In general, for all the samples, protamine sulfate was able to neutralize more biological activity than the precipitation assays indicated. For PM heparin, the anticoagulant activity through HCII was more readily neutralized than antithrombin dependent activity or plasma based activity (Figure 4). For example, for sample P1, the remaining activities by AT:aIIa, AT:aXa, APTT and HCII:aIIa were 17.5, 25.6, 28.5 and 3.5 IU respectively. The ranking order for neutralization was HCII:aIIa > AT:aIIa > AT:aXa = APTT across the four samples. For BM heparin, HCII and AT:aIIa were neutralized to a similar extent, and AT:aXa and APTT neutralization were also similar to each other. For example, for sample B1 the remaining activities by AT:aIIa, AT:aXa, APTT and HCII:aIIa were 43.4, 69.7, 74.1 and 37.7 IU respectively. The ranking order for neutralization was HCII:aIIa = AT:aIIa > AT:aXa = APTT. The BL heparin ranking order for neutralization was HCII:aIIa > AT: aIIa > APTT > AT:aXa. When comparing the differences between neutralization and precipitation, only the BM samples had values which were similar. This is illustrated by the remaining level of anticoagulant activity in BM samples by AT:aXa (69.7, 56.5, 59.8, 71.4 IU) and APTT (74.1, 57.9, 65.2, 72.0 IU) were similar to the precipitation values (59.5, 54.5, 65.5, 70.5 IU).

The average amount of heparin which protamine sulfate can precipitate or neutralize is shown in Table 3. Protamine sulfate neutralized more activity in BM, 123 AT:aIIa IU/mg, than indicated by precipitation, 75 IU/mg, a 64% difference. The difference between neutralization and precipitation for BL heparin was 56%, 131 and 84 IU/mg respectively. Neutralization of PM heparin by protamine sulfate was also higher than precipitation indicated, 161 IU/mg from 131 IU/mg. For all heparins, neutralization of anticoagulant activity measured by AT:aIIa was higher than indicated by precipitation. Calculation using the specific activities of the heparins for a mass/mass interaction between the heparins and protamine sulfate showed that by neutralization the amount of heparin required was no longer similar as shown by the precipitation assay.

Table 3. Average amount of heparin which 1 mg of protamine sulfate can precipitate or neutralize. (±SDs).

Ave (*n* = 4)	By EP Precipitation Assay		By Neutralization of Biological Activity	
	IU anti-IIa/mg protamine	mg heparin/mg protamine	IU anti-IIa/mg protamine	mg heparin/mg protamine
PM	131 (±9)	0.73 (±0.02)	161 (±6)	0.90 (±0.06)
BM	75 (±14)	0.75 (±0.04)	123 (±9)	1.26 (±0.19)
BL	84 (±8)	0.74 (±0.07)	131 (±15)	1.16 (±0.15)

2.4. Thromboelastography

The thromboelastography activated clotting time (ACT) and whole blood APTT clotting time is shown in Figure 5. For both ACT and APTT, the clotting times were different for each donor (*n* = 6) with and without heparin (data not shown). The reported clotting times for each heparin sample are the averaged clotting times from all donors and have each been blank corrected (heparin clotting times minus heparin-free clotting time).

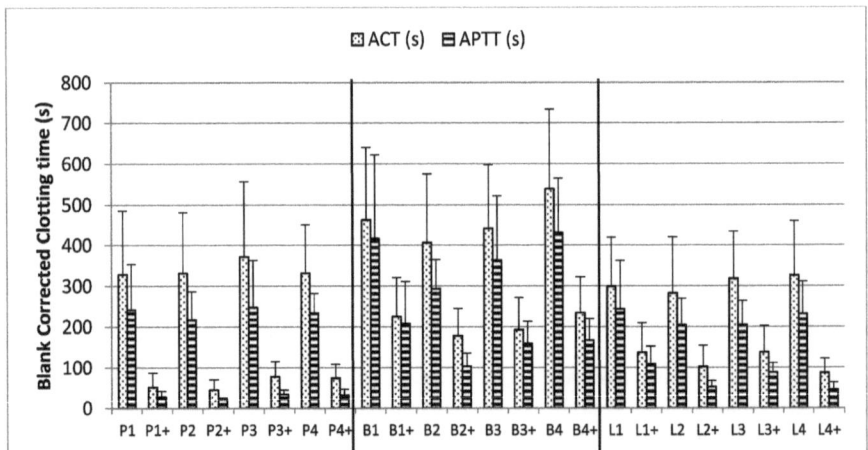

Figure 5. Activated clotting from thromboelastography and clotting times from APTT assay of heparin samples at 1 IU/mL without (P1, B1, B2 etc.) or with 0.05 mg/mL protamine sulfate added (P1+, B1+, B2+ etc.) in whole blood. Data shown are the blank corrected clotting times averaged from six individual blood donors, a 0 s time would indicate that all heparin present has been neutralized. (*n* = 6, error bars = SDs).

The same amount by AT:aIIa activity of each heparin was used to prepare the samples using each donor's blood. The ACT measured was significantly different between the samples, PM to BM $p = 0.002$, PM to BL $p = 0.046$, and BM to BL $p = 0.001$. In the APTT assays, there was a difference between the PM and BM ($p = 0.004$), the BM and BL ($p = 0.001$) but not between PM and BL ($p = 0.157$).

The addition of protamine sulfate reduced the anticoagulant activity in all heparin samples. The reduction in clotting times was more pronounced for PM than BM or BL (average ACTs decreased from 341 to 62s, 462 to 207s and 306 to 116s respectively). The order of neutralization was PM, BL and BM, the same as that seen in the anticoagulant assays (Figure 4).

2.5. Molecular Weight

Molecular weights for the heparin samples are shown in Table 4. Except for one BM sample, B2, porcine heparins had higher molecular weights than the bovine heparin samples. The peak molecular weight, number average and weight average molecular weights for the bovine lung samples were lower than BM heparin. The polydispersity for all the heparins was comparable for each heparin type, ranging from 1.20 to 1.29.

Table 4. Molecular Weight of heparin samples, determined against the USP Unfractionated Heparin Molecular Weight Standard, results are average from two determinations. Mp = peak molecular weight, Mn = number average molecular weight, Mw weight average molecular weight, PD = polydispersity.

		Mp	Mn	Mw	PD	% < 8 kDa
Porcine Mucosa	P1	15,800	13,820	17,870	1.29	8.7
	P2	16,110	13,900	17,290	1.24	7.7
	P3	16,320	14,140	17,390	1.23	6.5
	P4	15,080	13,080	15,720	1.2	8.4
Bovine Mucosa	B1	13,230	11,660	14,750	1.27	15.5
	B2	16,140	14,980	17,950	1.2	4.4
	B3	14,130	12,920	15,920	1.23	9.4
	B4	13,940	12,670	15,430	1.22	9.8
Bovine Lung	L1	9700	11,280	14,450	1.28	18.1
	L2	8770	10,570	13,380	1.27	22.7
	L3	8810	9740	12,160	1.25	28
	L4	9720	11,310	14,360	1.27	17.5

2.6. Antithrombin Titration Assay

The amount of antithrombin high affinity binding material in each heparin sample is shown in Figure 6. The PM samples had a similar quantity of high affinity material to each other, with the average level 52%. The BM heparins had an average 30% high affinity material with little difference between the samples. The level of high affinity material in BL heparin was more variable, ranging from 25 to 40% and an average of 33%. The amount of antithrombin binding high affinity material was higher in PM heparin than both BM and BL (about 70% and 60% more respectively).

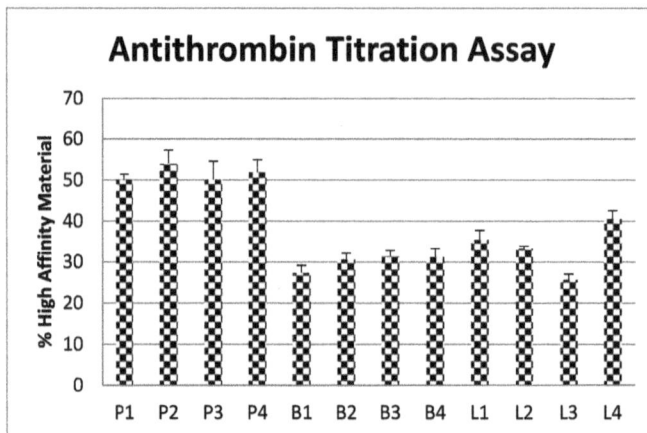

Figure 6. Antithrombin fluorescent titration assay with % high affinity antithrombin binding material within each heparin preparations. High affinity material calculated using the number average molecular weight Mn for each heparin and the concentration of heparin required to titrate antithrombin to generate a maximum change in fluorescent signal. (n = 4, error bars = SDs).

3. Discussion

In this study, we show that the specific activities of PM, BM and BL heparins are different. The potency labelling assay, antithrombin dependent inhibition of thrombin (AT:aIIa), gave much lower values for both BM heparin and BL heparin samples when compared to PM heparin which confirms previous observations [14,20]. Of note, all the samples tested gave statistically valid results for all the activity assays against the 6th International Standard for Unfractionated Heparin. This indicates that the International Standard, a PM heparin, is a suitable potency standard not only for PM heparin but also for BM and BL heparins.

The pharmacopoeial specifications for PM heparin are for potency, a specific activity not less than 180 IU/mg or USP U/mg, and for identity a ratio of AT:aIIa/AT:aXa values within 0.9 to 1.1. All PM heparins passed the identity criterion and most passed the specific activity requirement of >180 IU/mg. PM heparins also gave anticoagulant activities by APTT and HCII:aIIa assays that were similar to the antithrombin dependent assays. Both BM and BL heparins have lower specific activity than the >180 IU/mg required for PM heparin. Furthermore, BM heparin had an AT:aIIa/AT:aXa ratio that was outside the 0.9–1.1 criteria, with a calculated average of 1.2. It has been suggested that it will be unlikely for manufacturers to achieve the 180 IU/mg criteria for bovine heparin samples [20] and the data here support this. It should be noted that the lower specific activities of the bovine heparins indicate that more heparin in terms of mass would be required to achieve a similar anticoagulant effect to PM heparin.

The reversal of PM heparin post-operatively by protamine sulfate has been well established [21]. Protamine sulfate quality is assessed by a straightforward titration assay with heparin, with the minimal requirement that 1 mg precipitates not less than 100 IU of the pharmacopoeial reference preparations which are porcine heparins. However, it is unclear whether 1 mg protamine sulfate will precipitate as much as 100 IU of BM or BL heparin. The current study has shown that 1 mg protamine sulfate precipitated less than 100 IU of bovine heparins.

Irrespective of the specific activities of the samples, the amount of heparin in mass needed to precipitate a given quantity of protamine sulfate is the same for all heparins. In terms of activity units however, the ability of heparin to precipitate protamine sulfate was linked to the specific activities of the various heparins. A lower specific activity results in an increased concentration in units of heparin being required to precipitate a given amount of protamine sulfate.

The precipitation assay for protamine sulfate assesses the quality of protamine sulfate (a bio-identity test) and does not provide an indication of its ability to neutralize heparin activity. The use of a fixed activity of heparin for all preparations along with a fixed amount of protamine sulfate allowed for the estimation of the amount of activity neutralized. For all samples, the ability of protamine sulfate to neutralize activity was higher than would be predicted from the amount of heparin that can be precipitated. As expected, the use of fixed activity with a fixed amount of protamine showed that PM heparins, with have higher specific activities, were more effectively neutralized than BM and BL heparins.

Broadly, the thrombin based assays were more readily neutralized which may be due to the extended heparin chain length being more critical for these methods [22]. However, despite PM heparins having higher molecular weight than the BM and BL heparins, there is no significant correlation between the neutralization of activity and the molecular weight profiles of the heparin tested. The anti-Xa and plasma APTT anticoagulant activities were neutralized to a similar degree. The interaction between negatively charged heparin and positively charged protamine sulfate will favour the longer oligosaccharides in heparin [19] and as shown here influence antithrombin dependent thrombin inhibition activity which requires a minimum heparin molecular weight of about 5400 [16].

Clinically protamine sulfate will be administered by perfusion in order to neutralize heparin, and neutralization can be assessed using thromboelastography. This point-of-care technique is used with patient whole blood, where success of heparin neutralization is assessed by observing the time at which responses return to baseline. In this study, a controlled approach with the same amount of heparin, 1 IU anti-IIa, spiked into whole blood was used. We showed that the clotting times for each heparin type were different. In addition, at the same potency (AT:aIIa units), BM heparin gave longer activated clotting times than both PM and BL. The addition of protamine sulfate gave a reduction in clotting times for all samples, with the greatest reduction in PM, then BL and finally BM. This matched the profile of responses for the anticoagulant assays.

Fluorescence titration with antithrombin showed that PM heparin has a higher proportion of high affinity binding material than both BL and BM heparins. This correlates with the higher specific activity seen for PM heparin, and also explains the greater effectiveness of protamine sulfate at neutralizing the activity of PM heparin. Whilst having similar proportions of high affinity binding material and antithrombin dependent inhibition, BM and BL heparins show some differences in neutralization profiles. Neutralization of BL heparin is slightly greater than for BM heparin, which coincides with the slightly higher anti-IIa specific activity for bovine lung heparin.

For therapeutic purposes, an increase in mass of BM or BL heparin would be required to achieve the same therapeutic dose in International or USP Units of PM heparin. Based on the results of this study, it would be important to assess whether the current regimen of neutralization by protamine sulfate would need to be revised.

4. Materials and Methods

4.1. Materials

PM, BM and BL heparin samples were from the NIBSC archive of heparin samples, donated by several manufacturers. All heparin samples were subjected to a freeze dry step for 24 h prior to testing. Protamine sulfate was from Wockhardt UK Ltd, Wrexham, UK.

4.2. Anticoagulant Assays

Anticoagulant activity was estimated against the 6th International Standard for Unfractionated Heparin (07/328, NIBSC, South Mimms, UK). Antithrombin dependent anti-Xa (AT:aXa) and anti-IIa (AT:aIIa) activities were carried out in accordance to the USP Monograph (USP 34 NF 29). Briefly, heparin samples are mixed with purified antithrombin (NIBSC, South Mimms, UK) prior to the addition of thrombin (FIIa) (NIBSC, South Mimms, UK) or factor Xa (Diagnostic Reagents, Thame, UK). After incubation a specific chromogenic substrate (S2238 and S2765 respectively, Werfen Ltd, Warrington, UK) was added, and the colour developed is inversely proportional to the amount of heparin. APTT assay was carried out in accordance with the European Monograph (01/2008:20705) but with human pooled plasma used instead of sheep plasma. Briefly, heparin samples are mixed with plasma to which an APTT regent (APTT-SP, Werfen Ltd, Warrington, UK) is added. After incubation, calcium chloride was added and the clotting time measured, which is directly proportional to the amount of heparin present. Heparin cofactor II dependent activity (HCII:aIIa) was measured by substitution of antithrombin with heparin cofactor II (Enzyme Research, Swansea, UK) in the USP anti-IIa method, and prolongation of the incubation steps from one to seven minutes [23].

All activities were estimated and assessed for statistical validity using the parallel line model in the statistics package Combistats 5.0 (EDQM, Strasbourg, France).

4.3. Protamine Sulfate Precipitation Assay

The titration method, as described in the European Monograph for protamine sulfate (01/2017:0569), was adapted for use with the heparin samples. This method as described is a titration assay for protamine sulfate, where the requirement is that 1 mg of protamine sulfate precipitates not less than 100 IU of heparin sodium BRP. The method was adapted to allow for the calculation of heparin IU which precipitates 1 mg of protamine sulfate. Briefly, increasing volumes of heparin were added to a fixed concentration of protamine sulfate until a sharp increase in optical density was observed (wavelength is not critical). The sharp increase was then used to calculate the amount of heparin which has precipitated protamine sulfate.

4.4. Heparin/Protamine Sulfate Complex

Several heparin samples, 4 each of PM, BM and BL, were diluted to 200 anti-IIa IU/mL and either mixed with an equal volume of 1 mg/mL protamine sulfate or deionised water. Anticoagulant activity, as above, was then measured for all prepared samples.

4.5. Whole Blood Assays

Citrated whole blood was obtained through the National Blood and Transfusion Service (NBTS, New Brunswick, NJ, USA) and used to dilute samples of heparin (100 IU/mL) and heparin/protamine sulfate (100 IU/mL, 0.5 mg/mL) as described in Section 4.4. The clotting time of each sample, diluted 100 fold in whole blood, was measured by Activated Partial Thromboplastin Time (APTT) in a KC4 coagulometer. The activated clotting time was measured using thromboelastography (TEG, Haemonetics, Coventry, UK) with tissue factor (14/302, NIBSC, South Mimms, UK) and calcium chloride as the activating reagent.

4.6. Molecular Weights

Molecular weights for all samples were determined using size-exclusion chromatography with the USP Heparin Sodium Molecular Weight Calibrant RS (US Pharmacopeial Convention, MD, USA) as the broad standard calibrant as previously described [24].

4.7. Antithrombin Fluorescent Titration

The binding of heparin to antithrombin was assessed using a fluorescence titration assay [25]. This method, which relies on a change in intrinsic fluorescence of antithrombin when bound to heparin, was adapted for use in a microtitre plate. All materials were diluted in 50 mM TRIS, 150 mM NaCl, 10 mM EDTA, 0.05% Tween-20 pH 7.4 buffer (all reagents from, Sigma, UK). A fixed concentration of antithrombin (NIBSC, South Mimms, UK) was placed into each well in a microplate, and increasing concentrations of heparin, 0 to 100 µg/mL, or fondaparinux (USP Fondaparinux Sodium for Assay, USP, Rockville, MD, USA), 0 to 6 µg/mL were added across wells. The increase in fluorescence (λ_{EX} 280 nm, λ_{EM} 340 nm) was measured and using the equation: $\Delta F_{[H]} = (F_{[H]}-F0)/(Fm-F0)$, where $F_{[H]}$ is measured fluorescence at a concentration of heparin [H], F0 is basal fluorescence and Fm is maximum fluorescence, a chart was plotted of $\Delta F_{[H]}$ vs heparin concentration. From this chart, the amount of high affinity material in heparin which binds to antithrombin was calculated as the heparin concentration value at $\Delta F_{[H]} = Fm$ on an extrapolated straight line fitted to the first five heparin concentration points. The percentage high affinity material was then calculated using the concentration of antithrombin, where the molar concentration was estimated based on the assumption of 1:1 binding between antithrombin and fondaparinux, and molar concentration of heparin, calculated using number average molecular weight.

Acknowledgments: Heparin manufacturers who donated heparin samples to the NIBSC heparin panel: Aspen Oss BV; Biolberica SA; Kin Master Produtos Quimicos Ltda; Opocrin SpA; Pfizer; Sanofi Aventis; Welding GmbH & Co; Wockhardt Ltd. Peter Rigsby, Head of BioStatistics at NIBSC for helpful advice on analysis of data.

Author Contributions: John Hogwood and Elaine Gray conceived and designed the experiments; John Hogwood performed the experiments and analyzed the data; Barbara Mulloy provided guidance on antithrombin titration assays and analysis of data; John Hogwood, Elaine Gray and Barbara Mulloy wrote the manuscript.

Conflicts of Interest: The authors declare no conflict of interest.

References

1. Kishimoto, T.K.; Viswanathan, K.; Ganguly, T.; Elankumaran, S.; Smith, S.; Pelzer, K.; Lansing, J.C.; Sriranganathan, N.; Zhao, G.; Galcheva-Gargova, Z.; et al. Contaminated heparin associated with adverse clinical events and activation of the contact system. *N. Engl. J. Med.* **2008**, *358*, 2457–2467. [CrossRef] [PubMed]
2. Szajek, A.Y.; Chess, E.; Johansen, K.; Gratzl, G.; Gray, E.; Keire, D.; Linhardt, R.J.; Liu, J.; Morris, T.; Mulloy, B.; et al. The us regulatory and pharmacopeia response to the global heparin contamination crisis. *Nat. Biotechnol.* **2016**, *34*, 625–630. [CrossRef] [PubMed]
3. Keire, D.A.; Mulloy, B.; Chase, C.; Al-Hakim, A.; Cairatti, D.; Gray, E.; Hogwood, J.; Morris, T.; Mourao, P.; Soares, M.; et al. Diversifying the global heparin supply chain reintroduction of bovine heparin in the united states? *Pharm. Technol.* **2015**, *39*, 2–8.
4. Lindahl, U.; Backstrom, G.; Thunberg, L. The antithrombin-binding sequence in heparin. Identification of an essential 6-O-sulfate group. *J. Biol. Chem.* **1983**, *258*, 9826–9830. [PubMed]
5. Gresele, P.; Busti, C.; Paganelli, G. Heparin in the prophylaxis and treatment of venous thromboembolism and other thrombotic diseases. *Handb. Exp. Pharmacol.* **2012**, *207*, 179–209.
6. Pai, M.; Crowther, M.A. Neutralization of heparin activity. *Handb. Exp. Pharmacol.* **2012**, *207*, 265–277.
7. Chang, L.C.; Lee, H.F.; Yang, Z.; Yang, V.C. Low molecular weight protamine (LMWP) as nontoxic heparin/low molecular weight heparin antidote (i): Preparation and characterization. *AAPS PharmSci.* **2001**, *3*, E17. [CrossRef] [PubMed]
8. Nybo, M.; Madsen, J.S. Serious anaphylactic reactions due to protamine sulfate: A systematic literature review. *Basic Clin. Pharmacol. Toxicol.* **2008**, *103*, 192–196. [CrossRef] [PubMed]
9. Mecca, T.; Consoli, G.M.; Geraci, C.; La Spina, R.; Cunsolo, F. Polycationic calix[8]arenes able to recognize and neutralize heparin. *Org. Biomol. Chem.* **2006**, *4*, 3763–3768. [CrossRef] [PubMed]
10. Kalaska, B.; Kaminski, K.; Sokolowska, E.; Czaplicki, D.; Kujdowicz, M.; Stalinska, K.; Bereta, J.; Szczubialka, K.; Pawlak, D.; Nowakowska, M.; et al. Nonclinical evaluation of novel cationically modified polysaccharide antidotes for unfractionated heparin. *PLoS ONE* **2015**, *10*, e0119486. [CrossRef] [PubMed]
11. Shenoi, R.A.; Kalathottukaren, M.T.; Travers, R.J.; Lai, B.F.; Creagh, A.L.; Lange, D.; Yu, K.; Weinhart, M.; Chew, B.H.; Du, C.; et al. Affinity-based design of a synthetic universal reversal agent for heparin anticoagulants. *Sci. Transl. Med.* **2014**, *6*, 260ra150. [CrossRef] [PubMed]
12. Valimaki, S.; Khakalo, A.; Ora, A.; Johansson, L.S.; Rojas, O.J.; Kostiainen, M.A. Effect of peg-pdmaema block copolymer architecture on polyelectrolyte complex formation with heparin. *Biomacromolecules* **2016**, *17*, 2891–2900. [CrossRef] [PubMed]

13. Mulloy, B.; Gray, E.; Barrowcliffe, T.W. Characterization of unfractionated heparin: Comparison of materials from the last 50 years. *Thromb. Haemost.* **2000**, *84*, 1052–1056. [PubMed]

14. St Ange, K.; Onishi, A.; Fu, L.; Sun, X.; Lin, L.; Mori, D.; Zhang, F.; Dordick, J.S.; Fareed, J.; Hoppensteadt, D.; et al. Analysis of heparins derived from bovine tissues and comparison to porcine intestinal heparins. *Clin. Appl. Thromb. Hemost.* **2016**, *22*, 520–527. [CrossRef] [PubMed]

15. Bertini, S.; Fareed, J.; Madaschi, L.; Risi, G.; Torri, G.; Naggi, A. Characterization of pf4-heparin complexes by photon correlation spectroscopy and zeta potential. *Clin. Appl. Thromb. Hemost.* **2017**. [CrossRef] [PubMed]

16. Tovar, A.M.; Capille, N.V.; Santos, G.R.; Vairo, B.C.; Oliveira, S.N.; Fonseca, R.J.; Mourao, P.A. Heparin from bovine intestinal mucosa: Glycans with multiple sulfation patterns and anticoagulant effects. *Thromb. Haemost.* **2012**, *107*, 903–915. [CrossRef] [PubMed]

17. Sommers, C.D.; Ye, H.; Liu, J.; Linhardt, R.J.; Keire, D.A. Heparin and homogeneous model heparin oligosaccharides form distinct complexes with protamine: Light scattering and zeta potential analysis. *J. Pharm. Biomed. Anal.* **2017**, *140*, 113–121. [CrossRef] [PubMed]

18. Ramamurthy, N.; Baliga, N.; Wakefield, T.W.; Andrews, P.C.; Yang, V.C.; Meyerhoff, M.E. Determination of low-molecular-weight heparins and their binding to protamine and a protamine analog using polyion-sensitive membrane electrodes. *Anal. Biochem.* **1999**, *266*, 116–124. [CrossRef] [PubMed]

19. Schroeder, M.; Hogwood, J.; Gray, E.; Mulloy, B.; Hackett, A.M.; Johansen, K.B. Protamine neutralisation of low molecular weight heparins and their oligosaccharide components. *Anal. Bioanal. Chem.* **2011**, *399*, 763–771. [CrossRef] [PubMed]

20. Tovar, A.M.; Santos, G.R.; Capille, N.V.; Piquet, A.A.; Glauser, B.F.; Pereira, M.S.; Vilanova, E.; Mourao, P.A. Structural and haemostatic features of pharmaceutical heparins from different animal sources: Challenges to define thresholds separating distinct drugs. *Sci. Rep.* **2016**, *6*, 35619. [CrossRef] [PubMed]

21. Dhakal, P.; Rayamajhi, S.; Verma, V.; Gundabolu, K.; Bhatt, V.R. Reversal of anticoagulation and management of bleeding in patients on anticoagulants. *Clin. Appl. Thromb. Hemost.* **2016**. [CrossRef] [PubMed]

22. Gray, E.; Hogwood, J.; Mulloy, B. The anticoagulant and antithrombotic mechanisms of heparin. *Handb. Exp. Pharmacol.* **2012**, *207*, 43–61.

23. Panagos, C.G.; Thomson, D.S.; Moss, C.; Hughes, A.D.; Kelly, M.S.; Liu, Y.; Chai, W.; Venkatasamy, R.; Spina, D.; Page, C.P.; et al. Fucosylated chondroitin sulfates from the body wall of the sea cucumber holothuria forskali: Conformation, selectin binding, and biological activity. *J. Biol. Chem.* **2014**, *289*, 28284–28298. [CrossRef] [PubMed]

24. Mulloy, B.; Hogwood, J. Chromatographic molecular weight measurements for heparin, its fragments and fractions, and other glycosaminoglycans. *Methods Mol. Biol.* **2015**, *1229*, 105–118. [PubMed]

25. Boothello, R.S.; Al-Horani, R.A.; Desai, U.R. Glycosaminoglycan-protein interaction studies using fluorescence spectroscopy. *Methods Mol. Biol.* **2015**, *1229*, 335–353. [PubMed]

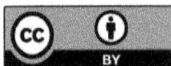

pharmaceuticals

MDPI

Review
Heparin Mimetics: Their Therapeutic Potential

Shifaza Mohamed [1,2] and Deirdre R. Coombe [1,*]

[1] School of Biomedical Sciences, Curtin Health Innovation Research Institute, Faculty of Health Sciences, Curtin University, Perth 6102, Western Australia; Shifaza.Mohamed@curtin.edu.au
[2] School of Applied Chemistry, Faculty of Science and Engineering, Curtin University, Perth 6102, Western Australia
* Correspondence: D.Coombe@curtin.edu.au; Tel.: +61-8-9266-9708

Received: 5 July 2017; Accepted: 22 September 2017; Published: 2 October 2017

Abstract: Heparin mimetics are synthetic and semi-synthetic compounds that are highly sulfated, structurally distinct analogues of glycosaminoglycans. These mimetics are often rationally designed to increase potency and binding selectivity towards specific proteins involved in disease manifestations. Some of the major therapeutic arenas towards which heparin mimetics are targeted include: coagulation and thrombosis, cancers, and inflammatory diseases. Although Fondaparinux, a rationally designed heparin mimetic, is now approved for prophylaxis and treatment of venous thromboembolism, the search for novel anticoagulant heparin mimetics with increased affinity and fewer side effects remains a subject of research. However, increasingly, research is focusing on the non-anticoagulant activities of these molecules. Heparin mimetics have potential as anti-cancer agents due to their ability to: (1) inhibit heparanase, an endoglycosidase which facilitates the spread of tumor cells; and (2) inhibit angiogenesis by binding to growth factors. The heparin mimetic, PI-88 is in clinical trials for post-surgical hepatocellular carcinoma and advanced melanoma. The anti-inflammatory properties of heparin mimetics have primarily been attributed to their ability to interact with: complement system proteins, selectins and chemokines; each of which function differently to facilitate inflammation. The efficacy of low/non-anticoagulant heparin mimetics in animal models of different inflammatory diseases has been demonstrated. These findings, plus clinical data that indicates heparin has anti-inflammatory activity, will raise the momentum for developing heparin mimetics as a new class of therapeutic agent for inflammatory diseases.

Keywords: heparin mimetics; heparin; heparan sulfate; glycosaminoglycan; anticoagulant; cancer; anti-inflammatory

1. Introduction

Sulfated glycosaminoglycans (GAGs) are glycans present on mammalian cell surfaces and in the extracellular matrix (ECM). They are synthesized covalently attached to their specific core proteins and the resulting proteoglycans may be transmembrane, linked to the membrane by a glycosylphosphatidylinositol anchor, or they may be secreted and comprise an integral part of the ECM. The GAG chains are responsible for much of the activities of proteoglycans as they can bind selectively to a variety of proteins and pathogens making them very relevant to many disease processes, such as inflammation [1], angiogenesis [2], neurodegeneration [3], cardiovascular disorders [4], cancers [5] and infectious diseases [6]. Heparin is perhaps the best known member of the GAG family. It is a highly negatively-charged, linear polysaccharide found in the secretory granules of connective tissue mast cells where it is the GAG chains of the proteoglycan, serglycin [7]. Heparin/heparan sulfate (HS) are composed of 1-4 linked repeating disaccharide units comprising a uronic acid (D-glucuronic acid (GlcA) or L-iduronic acid (IdoA)) and D-glucosamine (GlcN) (Figure 1). Heparin and HS chains are remarkably heterogeneous as during biosynthesis they are modified by epimerization of GlcA to

IdoA, and by sulfation at different positions on mainly GlcN and IdoA residues. HS contains a greater proportion of GlcA, whereas heparin contains more IdoA. Heparin, with its high content of sulfo and carboxyl groups, is a polyelectrolyte, having the highest negative charge density of any known biological macromolecule [8].

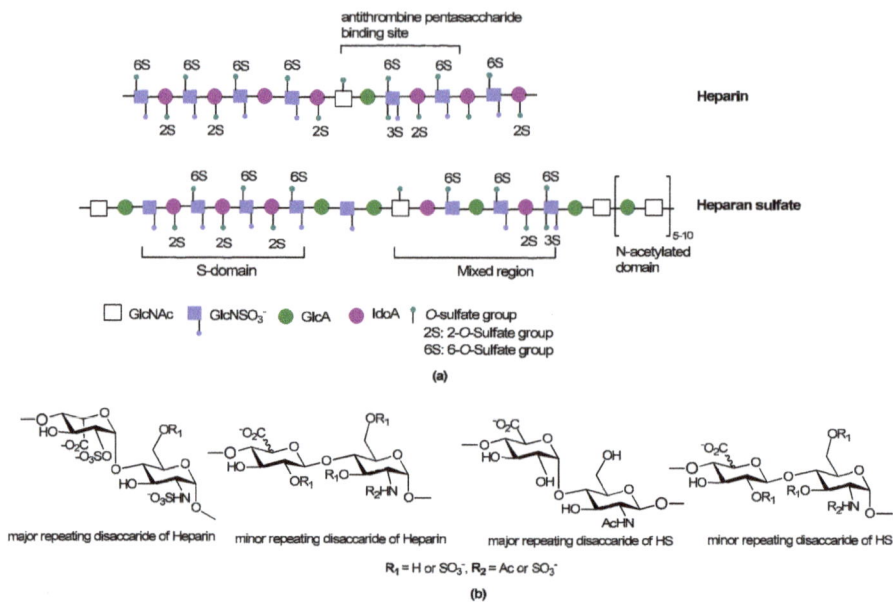

Figure 1. (a) Cartoon illustration of heparin and heparan sulfate structure; (b) Major and minor disaccharide repeating units in heparin and heparan sulfate.

Heparin is often said to have been discovered in 1916 by Jay McLean, a medical student of Johns Hopkin Medical School, to whom has also been attributed the discovery of heparin's anticoagulant effects in in vitro experiments [9]. However, the first descriptions of heparin as an anticoagulant were a little earlier and are summarized in a 1912 publication by Maurice Doyon [10]. In the 1930s clinical trials were conducted for heparin as an anticoagulant. Since then heparin has been used as a major clinical anticoagulant for many decades. However, its precise chemical structure, the range of its biological activities, and its Structure Activity Relationships (SAR) are not fully understood. Although biological functional studies of heparin were initially focused on its anticoagulant properties, in recent years the extent of its involvement in a range of other fundamental biological processes essential for normal mammalian development and physiology has been recognized. As such, heparin binds a multitude of proteins in addition to antithrombin III, giving rise to its well-appreciated polypharmacy [10].

For over 50 years, heparin gained widespread popularity and was extensively used in clinical practice. However, low-molecular-weight-heparin (LMWH) preparations have largely replaced heparin for clinical use over the past decade. This can be attributed to their superior pharmacokinetic profiles and their potential use in a wider range of clinical applications. However, LMWHs are not entirely free from the clinical disadvantages of its parent drug [11]. Heparin preparations have the potential to cause heparin-induced thrombocytopaenia type 2 which is an immunological response that involves generation of antibodies against a heparin-platelet factor 4 complex. Furthermore, non-specific binding to clotting factors by long chain heparin is believed to contribute to hemorrhagic side effects of the drug. Another disadvantage of heparin therapy is that its size and charge make parenteral administration a necessity.

In its natural state, heparin is a heterogeneous mixture of polysaccharide chains of different lengths and with different sulfation patterns; some of these chains are up to 100 saccharides in length [12]. Over the years there has been considerable debate as to whether distinct heparin sulfation motifs are required for the binding of different proteins. The current consensus is that the degree of structural specificity of motifs within heparin for protein binding is dependent upon the particular protein. Some of these interactions are highly specific and require the rare 3-*O*-sulfate group, whereas most proteins use *N*- and 2-*O*-sulfates, which in heparin are extremely common [13]; the most abundant disaccharide unit being a 2-*O*-sulfated iduronate linked to an *N*- and 6-*O*-sulfated glucosamine [14]. Importantly, the fact that heparin structures can bind a particular protein does not imply that the structure can necessarily modulate that protein's function. Modulation of a protein's function can depend on (1) where the heparin structure binds the protein; or (2) whether binding is of sufficient affinity to trigger a conformational change in the protein, as is the case when antithrombin III binds the pentasaccharide sequence from heparin containing the rare 3-*O*-sulfated glucosamine. In relation to the first point we have shown that a number of structurally different heparin tetrasaccharides can bind the chemokine, CCL5, but only those tetrasaccharides with a particular sulfation pattern preferentially bound CCL5 at a site that interfered with its ability to bind its cell surface receptor [15]. Consequently, success with developing heparin inspired therapeutic agents relies not only on identifying heparin-like structures, or heparin mimetics, that bind the protein of interest, but also in determining the effects of these structures on the biological functions of the protein target.

Heparin mimetics are synthetic or semi-synthetic compounds that are highly sulfated (usually), anionic, structurally distinct analogues of GAGs. Compounds (not other types of GAGs) that perform similar functions as heparin such as binding to the heparin-binding site on a protein may also be characterized as a heparin mimetic. Despite the increased understanding of the complex structure of heparin, the synthesis of clinically useful heparin mimetics is a relatively recent achievement.

The rational for development of heparin mimetics are numerous and varied, but a key consideration is that the mimetics are expected to overcome many of the problems associated with the parent molecule. The prospect of developing mimetics that display a higher relative potency and greater selectivity of action than its parent molecule is a major driving factor in this field of research. The need to curtail (but not necessarily eliminate) heparin's polypharmacy and its anticoagulant activity is another prime consideration for mimetic design. Furthermore, heparin mimetics are designed to tackle the heterogeneity of heparin, the rational being homogeneous structures could lead to enhanced potency and greater specificity. The ultimate goal in designing heparin mimetics is the removal of unwanted biological activities and to maximize their therapeutic benefits for the disease being targeted.

Major advances in the field of carbohydrate synthesis such as building block preparation (one-pot multi-step procedures), coupling reactions, and the development of convergent strategies for coupling key building blocks, has led to an increase in the synthesis of complex oligosaccharides which can act as heparin mimetics [16–20]. Such synthetic methods allow the preparation of tailor-made saccharides, with customized sizes and functional groups. These tailor-made saccharides can be used for SAR studies on a specific biological target. A number of discovery programs, including our own, have used this approach for hit optimization of heparin/heparan sulfate mimetics for various therapeutic uses such as anticoagulation, angiogenesis modulation, anti-cancer metastasis, and anti-inflammation.

This review will highlight the advances in the development of heparin mimetics for various clinical purposes, with a focus on the potential of using these compounds as drugs.

2. Structure and Diversity of Heparin Mimetics

There is great diversity in the structure and biological activities of the heparin mimetics that have been reported in the literature. Most of the mimetics created to date are carbohydrate based mimetics, although non-carbohydrate mimetics have also been reported and there is a growing number of mimetics that are a combination of carbohydrates and aglycones. The anionic charge of heparin mimetics has generally been introduced by sulfation and rarely by phosphorylation or carboxylation.

The main classes of heparin mimetics that have been reported in the literature are: (a) modified polysaccharides; (b) synthetically sulfated oligosaccharides; (c) oligosaccharide-aglycone conjugates; and (d) non-carbohydrate-based sulfated mimetics. For a detailed description of these classes the reader is directed to the review by Coombe and Kett [21].

When developing mimetics that are directed towards particular therapeutic needs certain structural features are a necessity for modulating biological function. Some such structural features include:

- Size/molecular weight: The first step in any synthetic strategy for a heparin mimetic directed towards a specific target is to determine the size of the structure that is most likely to have the required biological activity. This decision requires knowledge of the shape and size of the heparin binding site on the protein target. Not all heparin binding sites resemble the small pockets on proteins surfaces that are traditionally targeted by drugs; for example, they may be a face on a protein surface. If the latter is true, the size of the heparin-like structure that is required for binding, and for modulating the protein's function, will be larger than a disaccharide or a tetrasaccharide. It can also be that larger structures are required to provide the correct orientation of the entity that actively engages with the protein. Hence, smaller analogues may not always produce the anticipated increase in selectivity and potency.

- Heterogeneity: Heterogeneous mixtures are more likely to display a broad range of biological activities than structurally similar homogeneous products, but the technical challenges associated with their reproducible synthesis and the characterization of heterogeneous mixtures are far greater. This means proof of reproducible synthesis is required once a heterogeneous mimetic enters clinical development. Accordingly, current trends are towards the synthesis of structurally homogeneous heparin mimetics.

- Pattern and extent of sulfation: It is well known that the extent of sulfation influences the strength with which heparin or HS fragments bind proteins. This was concluded from studies where HS fragments were eluted off protein affinity columns with varying salt concentrations; the highly sulfated structures eluting at higher salt concentrations [22]. These studies also showed that when HS fragments bound some proteins, like Fibroblast growth factor-1 (FGF-1), a higher degree of sulfation did not necessarily translate into the fragments displaying higher affinity binding. Thus, not only the number of sulfates but also the positions of the sulfates were important [22]. We have also shown that the pattern and extent of sulfation has a marked effect on the location on a protein where heparin fragments prefer to bind and that not all fragments that bind affect the protein's activity in the same way [15]. Given these findings with heparin fragments, it is probable that heparin mimetics will similarly vary in their activities in accordance with the patterns of sulfation. Techniques to control the degree of sulfation include; the choice of starting material, selective sulfation and limiting reaction conditions. Similarly, careful selection of different carbohydrate starting materials can result in different patterns of sulfation in a mimetic.

- Linkage patterns: The influence of anomers, or of linkage patterns on the biological activity of a polysaccharide can also be explored by careful selection of the starting material. Both of these aspects of GAG structure contribute profoundly to their solution structures, and in all probability also to the structures GAG fragments adopt when bound to proteins. The torsion angle values are altered by glycosidic linkages and the anomeric configuration of the linkage, and even small differences in these angles can contribute to differences of the structure in solution. This is illustrated by the more bent solution structure of HS compared to that of heparin [23], although here sulfation and monosaccharide differences also contribute.

- Flexibility of the backbone: Polysaccharide chains are relatively inflexible due to the limited rotations allowed about a glycosidic linkage. Thus, more flexible heparin mimetics are synthesized by chemical modifications such as glycol splitting. Furthermore, synthetic non-carbohydrate chemical linkers of varying degrees of flexibility can be employed to link short carbohydrate chains, resulting in more flexible heparin mimetics. This approach was used to produce HS-mimics that bound interferon-γ. Two highly sulfated octasaccharide HS fragments linked by a spacer of 10 polyethylene glycol repeats were found to efficiently bind interferon-γ [24]. It was argued that when linked, the sulfated regions acted in a concerted manner and formed a functional unit, whereas when unlinked the octasaccharides did not bind efficiently.

Heparin mimetics are a group of compounds that have been created to combat the promiscuity and polypharmacy of heparin. Possible strategies that can be used to address this problem include; increasing the potency of a particular mimetic such that the dosage can be decreased to a point where harmful side effects are insignificant. Alternatively, increasing binding selectivity could eliminate undesired protein interactions of a mimetic.

3. Heparin Mimetics as Anticoagulants

Heparin in its unfractionated form has been used as an anticoagulant drug for over 80 years. SAR studies have shown that a unique pentasaccharide sequence, termed the "antithrombin III-binding domain", is primarily responsible for the anticoagulant activity of heparin. The antithrombin III-binding domain contains a very specific pattern of negatively charged groups (*O*-sulfonates and carboxylates) surrounded in standard heparin by a repetitive sequence composed of 2-*O*-sulfated IdoA linked to a 6-*O* sulfated glucosamine (Figure 2a). Although heparin is highly effective and inexpensive, it has several undesirable qualities as a therapeutic. Firstly, it is a heterogeneous mixture of compounds extracted from porcine or bovine mucosa, and it carries a potential risk of contamination as is illustrated by the incident which occurred in 2007–2008 [25,26]. Secondly, heparin chains vary in size, anticoagulant activity, and in their ability to bind various plasma proteins; as a consequence heparin displays a variable dose-response relationship amongst patients and requires active monitoring to fine-tune the dosage [27]. Third, approximately 3% of patients undergoing prolonged heparin therapy experience severe autoimmune responses [28]. These limitations have led to the development of a variety of low molecular weight heparin like anticoagulants with more homogenous composition and predictable pharmacokinetic properties.

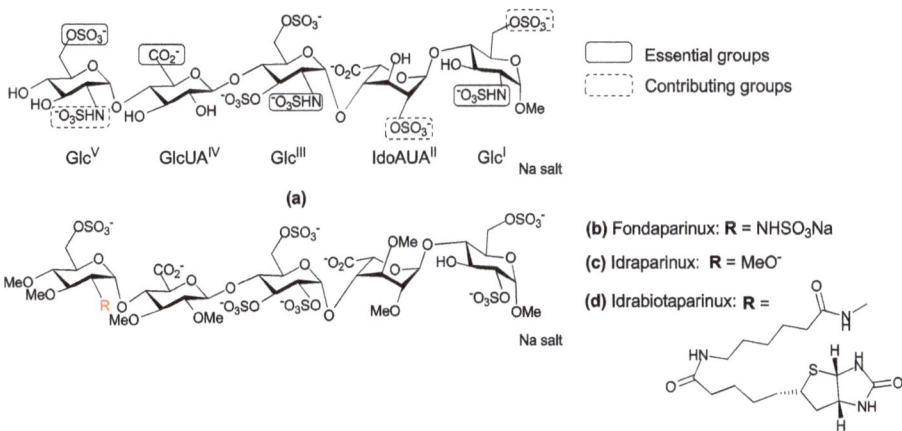

Figure 2. Chemical structure of heparin pentasccharide derivatives. (**a**) The antithrombin III binding pentasccharide motif of heparin; (**b**–**d**) Structure of synthetic analogues of the antithrombin III binding site of heparin.

Anticoagulants based on heparin are the drugs of choice in the therapy and prophylaxis of thromboembolic diseases. The anticoagulant market for heparin mimetics has been very active over the past few decades due to the development of new compounds. Several reviews have been published describing the SAR and mechanism of action of these heparin mimetic anticoagulants [29–31].

In 2001, GlaxoSmithKline (GSK; Brentford, UK) registered Fondaparinux as a new antithrombin III drug under the name Arixtra [32]. It is the methyl glycoside analogue of the natural antithrombin III binding pentasaccharide in which the acetamido is replaced by a sulfoamino group on the GlcV unit (Figure 2b). The specificity and the binding strength of Fondaparinux to antithrombin III, can be attributed to the presence of the methyl groups which prevent non-specific binding to plasma proteins. Fondaparinux has a linear pharmacokinetic profile and a longer half-life, compared to LHWHs. In addition, it does not induce immune thrombocytopenia. Fondaparinux is now approved for the prophylaxis and treatment of venous thromboembolism (VTE) in virtually all Western countries, and is increasingly being used as a substitute for LMWHs. In the search for antithrombotic carbohydrates with reduced synthetic complexity and tailor-made pharmacological properties, attention was directed to a novel class of 'non-glycosaminoglycan' analogues. Initially the synthesis of Fondaparinux was performed in about 50 chemical steps [33], and other synthetic methods have been explored to obtain a straightforward synthetic sequence with fewer steps that could also be used to obtain analogues. Indraparinux (Figure 2c) is a synthetic pentasaccharide analogue of Fondaparinux, in which the hydroxyl groups are methylated and the *N*-sulfate groups are replaced by *O*-sulfates [34]. It can be prepared from glucose in approximately 25 synthetic steps in a highly convergent manner. The strategy used for the synthesis of Idraparinux consists of assembling the Glc^V on a suitably protected $GlcUA^{IV}$-Glc^{III}-$IdoUA^{II}$-Glc^I tetrasaccharide [35]. Idraparinux was not only synthesized using fewer synthetic steps but it also gave rise to a new class of antithrombotic agent that specifically inhibited Factor Xa and lacked activity against thrombin. It was developed for the treatment and secondary prevention of VTE, as well as for the prevention of thromboembolic events associated with atrial fibrillation. Some of the clinical advantages of Idrapainux include: (1) A linear pharmacokinetic profile and a longer half-life than Fondaparinux; (2) It has consistent effects as it is not metabolized and is completely bioavailable; (3) It does not bind to plasma proteins and in particular does not bind platelet factor 4 (PF4), which makes the development of immune thrombocytopenia extremely unlikely [36]. However, Idrapainux has no neutralizing agent thus its antithrombotic activity cannot be reversed, unlike heparin. This can lead to severe complications in some cases.

Idrabiotaparinux (Figure 2d) is a novel, long-acting, synthetic anticoagulant, which has a similar chemical structure to Idrapainux but with an added biotin segment. The biotin segment of Idrabiotaparinux enables the neutralization of the drug using avidin as a neutralizing agent. Avidin is a tetrameric protein derived from the egg white of many species. Injection of avidin can trigger the immediate elimination of biotinylated Idrabiotapariux from the blood stream of humans and animals, resulting in neutralization of the antithrombic activity [37,38]. However, a systematic review reported a lack of sufficient evidence to clarify whether Idraparinux and Idrabiotaparinux are as effective and safe as the standard warfarin treatment for VTE [39]. As a result, Sanofi-Aventis (Paris, France, now known as Sanofi) halted the development of Idrabiotaparinux for arterial fibrillation at the phase III clinical trial stage.

A number of years ago now Petitou et al. synthesized a family of heparin mimetic oligosaccharides that were able to inhibit thrombin as well as bind antithrombin III, the aim being to obtain more potent, well-tolerated antithrombic drugs [40]. Unfortunately, like thrombin inhibition, undesirable interactions with plasma proteins are directly correlated with the charge and the size of the oligosaccharide. So the compounds were designed to discriminate between thrombin and other proteins, particularly PF4. A multistep converging synthesis was used to obtain sulfated oligosaccharides that met these requirements. Petitou et al. reasoned that thrombin inhibition should be obtained when the saccharide was long enough to accommodate antithrombin III and thrombin at the same time. Accordingly, they synthesized a "non-GAG" series in which *N*-sulfate groups were replaced by *O*-sulfate groups, and hydroxyls were alkylated. These structural modifications fully preserved the specific binding to antithrombin III yet they drastically simplified the synthesis. This work led to the synthesis of a 17-mer oligosaccharide (Figure 3a) which was 5- to 10-fold more potent than standard heparin and LMWHs in models of both venous and arterial thrombosis. The design of this oligosaccharide was based on the following considerations: (1) a pentasaccharide sequence is required to bind and activate antithrombin III towards Factor Xa (FXa) and thrombin inhibition; (2) the separate thrombin binding-domain must be two to three disaccharides long; (3) a chain length of 17 saccharide units is required for notable thrombin inhibition meaning the two binding domains could be separated by a spacer; and (4) as the six or eight units of the central saccharide spacer were not critically involved in interacting with either antithrombin III or with thrombin, the charge on these units could be suppressed without affecting the anticoagulant activity. The 17-mer saccharide that resulted displayed a very simple elimination profile compared to heparin and LMWHs, owing to the limited number of proteins with which it interacted. The publication describing this 17-mer saccharide attracted a lot of excitement, and at the time it was thought such longer oligosaccharides had the potential to address some of side effects of other anticoagulant drugs that were on the market [40,41].

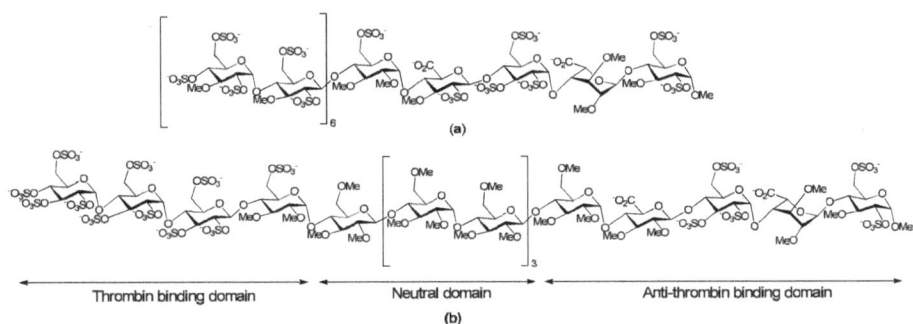

Figure 3. Chemical structure of (**a**) 17-mer saccharide; (**b**) SR123781.

SR123781 is a short acting synthetic hexadecasaccharide, developed from the work of Petitou et al. [40]. It is an indirect antithrombin III dependent inhibitor of FXa (Figure 3b). SR123781 is an analogue of heparin and was obtained from glucose through a convergent synthesis; it comprises an antithrombin binding pentasaccharide, a thrombin binding sulfated tetrasaccharide, and a neutral methylated hexasaccharide linker sequence, with *N*-sulfated groups replaced by *O*-sulfates, and alkylated hydroxyl groups in the antithrombin III binding domain. SR123781 was found to be more potent than heparin and Fondaparinux in a number of different animal models for arterial venous thrombosis with a high affinity for human antithrombin [42]. Furthermore, SR123781 displayed prolonged anti-FXa and antithrombin activity after intravenous and subcutaneous administration to rats, rabbits and baboons. It also inhibited thrombus formation in experimental in vivo models and had a favorable antithrombotic:bleeding ratio compared to heparin [43]. Even though SR123781 progressed to phase IIb clinical trials, its development was discontinued following the success of the heparin mimetic AV5026.

AV5026 (Semuloparin, Sanofi-Aventis) is a complex mixture of oligomeric ultra-low-molecular-weight heparin fragments (molecular weight 2000–3000 Da) with a polydispersity index of approximately 1.0. It is synthesized by partial and controlled chemoselective depolymerization of porcine unfractionated heparin. It has a novel antithrombotic profile resulting from high anti-FXa activity and residual anti-Factor IIa (FIIa or thrombin) activity in comparison to heparin and LMWH [44]. This unique physiochemical profile of AV5026 is the result of a highly selective depolymerization of heparin by a phosphazene base. AV5026 demonstrated a dose-dependent antithrombic effect with similar activity compared to the marketed LMWH, enoxaparin, in well-established thrombosis models in rats, rabbits and dogs [45]. Clinical evaluation of AV5026 in patients undergoing orthopedic surgery (TREK-study) demonstrated a significant dose response for the prevention of venous thromboembolism [46]. Although, clinical data suggested that AV5026 could represent a new alternative for the prevention of thrombosis with an improved benefit-risk profile compared with classic heparinoids and LMWHs, its development was stopped in 2012.

Several decades of intensive research has led to the discovery of several synthetic heparin mimetics with anticoagulant activity. Structure based approaches gave insights into the mechanism of heparin-induced activation of antithrombin III and identification of the pentasaccharide sequence in heparin that bind antithrombin III with high affinity. This then led to the discovery of LMWH or fragments of heparin with higher potency and a longer half-life with fewer side effects. However, the search for novel heparin mimetics with increased affinity have proven to be a formidable challenge and constructing simplified analogues of the unique heparin binding pentasccharide is a complicated endeavor. Recently the notion of synthesizing glycopolymers with hydrocarbon backbones that carry pendant well defined heparin disaccharides was explored. The aim was to achieve efficient synthesis of defined heparin-like compounds that retained the anticoagulation activity of intact heparin. Hsieh-Wilson and her colleagues synthesized a compound that surpassed the anticoagulant activity of heparin (Figure 4) [47], showing greater anti-Factor Xa and 100-fold greater anti-FIIa activity. This compound comprised tetrasulfated disaccharides consisting of 2-*O*-sulfated L-iduronic acid and glucosamine with 3-*O* and 6-*O*-sulfation as well as *N*-sulfation. The sulfation reactions were performed prior to polymerization and the polymerization was controlled to produce a glycopolymer of 45 repeats. This compound also strongly bound PF4, a result in accordance with other reports indicating that long negatively charged species that are not glycosaminoglycans may bind this chemokine [48,49]. When the polymerization was restricted to 30 repeats anti-FXa and anti-FIIa activities were markedly lower than that of both heparin and the longer polymer. Moreover, loss of the 3-*O*-sulfate from the glucosamine abrogated the anti-FXa activity [47], pointing to the importance of this sulfation pattern for antithrombin III binding. It is particularly interesting that a collection of disaccharides carrying this motif arranged in a pendant fashion on a polymeric scaffold are sufficient to bind antithrombin III and trigger anti-FXa activity, as previous studies with heparin have indicated that a pentasaccharide structure containing a 3-*O*-sulfated glucosamine was required [40]. Nevertheless, it remains to be seen as to the clinical usefulness of this anticoagulant heparin mimicking glycopolymer.

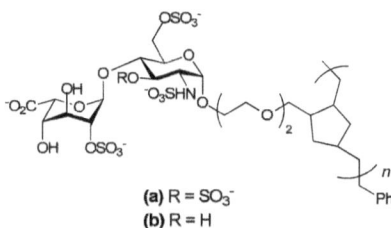

Figure 4. Chemical structure of tailored glycopolymers as anticoagulant heparin mimetics.

4. Heparin Mimetics in Cancer

HS are present on the surface of all eukaryotic cells, including tumor cells and the stromal cells surrounding a tumor, which are important for tumor survival. The HS on tumor cell surfaces have been shown to be vital for many aspects of tumor phenotype and tumor development, including cell transformation, tumor growth, cell invasion and metastasis. Both clinical and animal model studies indicate that heparin mediates anti-tumor activity [50–53]. Furthermore, a number of retrospective and prospective clinical studies have shown that heparin therapy may prolong the survival of cancer patients across a variety of solid tumor types [54,55]. However, exploitation of heparin's anti-tumor activities are limited by its anticoagulant activity. Therefore, research has been directed at developing heparin mimetics with limited anticoagulant activity but with the retention of heparin's anti-tumor activity.

Heparanase is an endoglycosidase which cleaves the HS side chains of heparan sulfate proteoglycans (HSPG) in the ECM surrounding tumor cells. The degradation of ECM facilitates the spread of tumor cells by enabling them to enter into, and escape from, blood vessels and lymphatics. In addition, heparanase is known to exhibit pro-angiogenic properties, i.e., stimulate the growth of new blood vessels from pre-existing blood vessels that surround tumors [56]. Thus, drugs targeting heparanase have been under investigation by both academic and industry based laboratories. As a result, numerous sulfated sugar molecules including heparin mimetics have been identified as selective inhibitors of heparanase [57]. In addition to heparanase, fibroblast growth factors (FGFs) and vascular endothelial growth factor (VEGF) are essential mediators of angiogenesis and thus are also attractive targets for drug discovery [58]. These growth factors are sequestered to the extracellular matrix by binding to HS in the matrix associated HSPGs, and they are released by heparanase. FGFs and VEGF initiate the cell signaling cascades that lead to angiogenesis by forming ternary complexes with HS and their particular cognate cell surface receptors. Thus, inhibiting angiogenesis by targeting the HS and heparin binding sites on these growth factors with heparin mimetics is considered to be a viable therapeutic strategy for cancer [59–61].

PI-88 (Progen Pharmaceuticals Ltd. (Brisbane, Australia) is one such inhibitor. It is the product of exhaustive sulfation of the oligosaccharide phosphate fraction of the extracellular phosphomannan (derived from the yeast *Pichia (Hansenula) holstii* NRRL Y-2448) [62,63]. It is a heterogeneous material being primarily composed of sulfated phosphomannopentaose and phosphomannotetraose oligosaccharides carrying variously 10–13 sulfates [14,64]. A detailed analysis of the non-sulfated starting material from which PI-88 was prepared has recently been published [65]. PI-88 exerts its antimetastatic effects by inhibiting heparanase and so the cleavage of HS in the ECM and the release of angiogenic growth factors. PI-88 also binds competitively to growth factors, such as FGF-1 and FGF-2 and VEGF to exert an anti-angiogenetic effect [66]. PI-88 has been tested in phase II clinical trials for liver cancer and has shown efficacy as an adjuvant for postsurgical hepatocellular carcinoma (HCC) [67,68]. It is currently in phase III HCC clinical studies, but has not yet been approved for routine clinical use. Phase I and Phase III clinical trials of PI-88 in patients with advanced melanoma also demonstrated noteworthy activity [69]. PI-88 is generally well tolerated, but is does have the common toxicity issues of thrombocytopenia and thrombosis, injection site hemorrhage and other bleeding events. Several analogues of PI-88 have been synthesized with the aim of altering the pharmacokinetic properties in a favorable manner to result in less frequent dosing whilst maintaining biological activity. As such, the analogues were based on a single pentasaccharide backbone for ease of synthesis and evaluation of biological activity. The compounds in the initial series of analogues were mostly glycosides of the major pentasaccharide found in **a** (Figure 5) [70,71]. Compounds such as **b c**, and **d** (Figure 5) exhibited biological activity similar to that of **a**, but with improved pharmacokinetics in a rat model. Furthermore, both compounds **a** and **b** were shown to be potent inhibitors of in vivo angiogenesis in two separate murine models. Additionally, the introduction of lipophilic modifications resulted in significant attenuation of anticoagulant activity, a common side effect of heparin/HS mimetics including PI-88. This data supports the continued development of heparin/HS mimetics of this type as antiangiogenic, anti-cancer agents.

Progen Pharmaceuticals Ltd. then designed a series of compounds named PG500, which are second-generation versions of PI-88. The PG500 series of compounds are anomerically pure, fully sulfated and are single entity oligosaccharides attached to a lipophilic moiety, e.g., aglycone, at the reducing end of the molecule [72]. Some of the compounds from this series are more potent inhibitors of angiogenesis and metastasis than PI-88 and have shown strong anti-tumor activity in some aggressive tumor models [73]. These compounds are believed to interfere with angiogenesis via inhibition of VEGF and FGFs, and with metastasis via inhibition of heparanase. The lead molecule of this series is PG545, which was selected based on its efficacy, pharmacokinetics, toxicology and ease of manufacture [74].

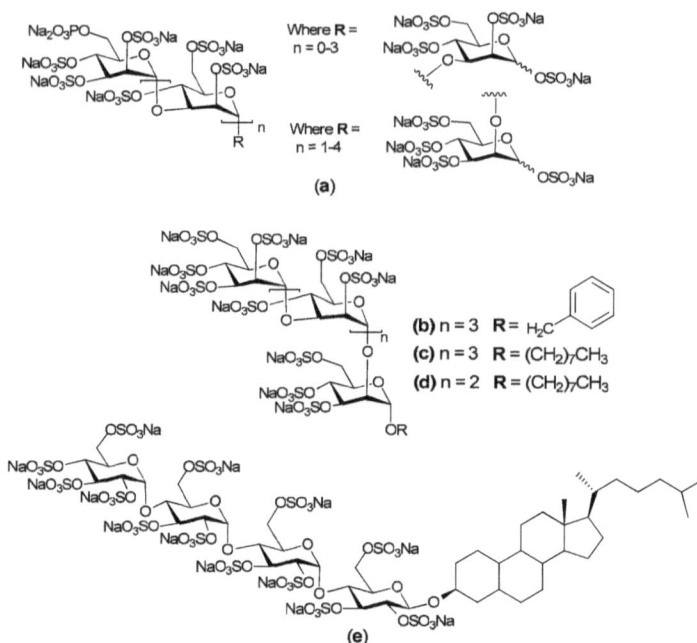

Figure 5. (**a**) Generalized chemical structure of PI-88; (**b**–**d**) Analogues of PI-88; (**e**) Chemical structure of PG545.

PG454 is a synthetic, fully sulfated tetrasaccharide functionalized with a cholestanyl aglycone (Figure 5e) [75]. It is currently in phase I clinical trials and has shown potent inhibition of heparanase with low anti-coagulant properties. Interestingly, the cholestanyl group increased the affinity of PG545 for heparanase over that of a non-functionalized derivative. It appears this hydrophobic group allows PG545 to bind to a hydrophobic pocket near to the active site of the enzyme in addition to binding to the basic amino acids that are involved in HS binding [76]. PG545 has been shown to exhibit a long plasma half-life and shows activity in multiple murine models of the cancers of breast, prostate, liver, lung and colon, as well as head and neck cancers and melanoma [75]. Recent publications have shown that PG545 has activities in addition to those attributed to its effects on heparanase and the growth factors VEGF and FGF-2. For example, the anti-lymphoma effect of PG545 in vivo seems to require NK (natural killer) cell activation and this activation involves PG545 acting via TLR9 (toll-like receptor-9) to trigger dendritic cells to release IL-12, which is necessary for PG545 activation of NK cells [77]. In addition, PG545 was shown to act on the Wnt pathway in a pancreatic ductal adenocarcinoma model. PG545 bound directly to Wnt3a and Wnt7a, thereby blocking their interactions with their receptors. This inhibition of Wnt signaling within tumor cells led to reduced levels of β-catenin, which caused a reduction in the expression of VEGF, matrix metalloproteinase (MMP)-7 and Cyclin D1, as well as triggering apoptosis of the tumor cells [78]. The multiple activities of PG545 mirror the ability of heparin to also act on multiple pathways and points to the likely polypharmacy of most heparin mimetics.

Heparin/HS binding proteins interact with particular preferred structural motifs within heparin and HS, and the extent to which a particular motif is a requirement for binding varies from one heparin binding protein to another. Some heparin binding proteins are very specific in their requirements (e.g., antithrombin III), whereas others are less specific (e.g., compare FGF-1 and FGF-2 [79]); thus heparin/HS mimetics are often designed with a view of selectively blocking protein-GAG interactions.

To explore this, Parish and co-workers synthesized a homogenous structurally well define HS mimetic family of sulfated linked cyclitols. They then compared the ability of 15 different sulfated linked cyclitols to bind to 10 functionally diverse proteins [80]. This relatively simple panel of mimetics provided considerable information regarding the patterns and orientations of anionic groups that are recognized by different proteins. Specifically, it demonstrated that spatial separation of anionic groups within the HS mimetics plays a critical role in determining the specificity of interactions. For example, compounds **a** and **b** (Figure 6), which only differ by the length of their alkyl chain spacer exhibited different inhibitory activity towards growth factors. Compound **a** was found to be strong inhibitor of FGF-1, with modest inhibition of FGF-2. Whereas compound **b** was a strong inhibitor of FGF-2 and VEGF with modest inhibition of FGF-1. Ferro and co-workers extended this work by synthesizing a library of mimetics with simple ionic binding motifs on a monosaccharide scaffold based on D-mannopyranose that could "anchor" the ligand to the HS-binding site on the targeted protein [81]. This library of mimetics was synthesized by harnessing the powerful Ugi four component reaction for decorating the scaffold with linkers containing a diverse range of functional groups. The affinities of these monosaccharide mimetics for angiogenic HS-binding growth factors were close to those generally observed for polysulfated di-or tetrasccharides. From this study a clear trend for proteins to prefer particular structures was evident, for example the presence of an aromatic group was favored by FGF-1 and VEGF. This supported the previous observation that lipophilic modifications can improve affinity for VEGF and FGF-1 but not FGF-2 [82].

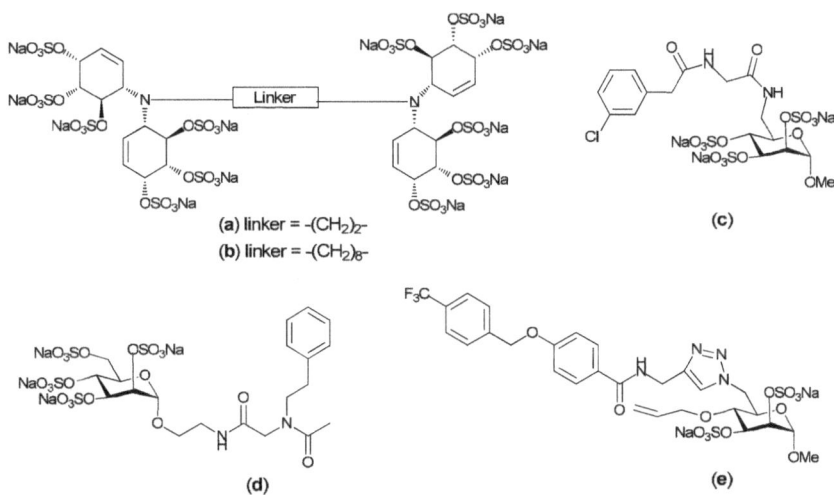

Figure 6. Small molecule heparin/heparan sulfate (HS) mimetics as potential inhibitors of fibroblast growth factors (FGF)-and/or vascular endothelial growth factor (VEGF) mediated angiogenesis for the development of novel cancer therapeutics; Structure of potent (**a,b**) linked cyclitol; (**c,d**) compounds from Ugi library; (**e**) compounds synthesized via click chemistry.

Ferro and co-workers also synthesized an 18-membered library of small molecule HS mimetics via click chemistry. These mimetics were targeted against the angiogenic growth factors FGF-1, FGF-2 and VEGF [83]. The library of mimetics was designed with the specific aims of firstly, identifying the critical sulfate groups for binding on the monosaccharide ring, with the view to decreasing the overall sulfation without loss of activity, and secondly, to enable the exploration of possible non-ionic binding surfaces around the primary binding site on the proteins; the primary binding site being comprised of clusters of basic, positively charged amino acids. 6-azido-6-deoxy-α-D-mannopyranoside was selected as the building block for the synthesis of this library of heparin mimetics. The library was made more diverse by incorporating various alkyne derivatives into functional motifs and by employing a Swern oxidation-Witting olefination sequence to synthesize functional motifs (e.g., aromatic groups) with varied geometrical representation to produce different isomers. Collectively this diversity allowed exploration of the size and position of hydrophobic or hydrogen bonding regions near to the basic amino acids which comprised the primary binding site. The binding studies indicated that affinity and structural specificity of the mimetic was increased by the incorporation of non-anionic motifs. A lead compound was identified from the library with micromolar binding affinity towards FGF-1 and VEGF and good selectivity over FGF-2 [83]. This work illustrates the power of combining an anionic sugar structure with an aromatic spacer, of an appropriate length and rigidity, to position a polar group at a site on the protein removed from the binding hot-spot that recognizes the sulfate groups, for enhancing the specificity of the heparin mimetic. Interestingly, this strategy provided a rapid method to probe the chemical space around a binding hot-spot, which could then be used to differentiate a family of similar proteins by their mimetic binding capability.

Recently, "small glycol" drugs which are heparin mimetics have been identified as exhibiting anti-cancer properties. These molecules are small, synthetic oligosaccharides with potent affinity and selective inhibition of several growth factors and proteins involved in tumor growth and propagation. As such, a library of more than 100 synthetic oligosaccharides of different sizes containing various substitutions has been evaluated for their specificity and efficacy in inhibiting cell proliferation and migration and in vitro endothelial tubule formation. EP80061 is the lead compound in this series which has shown potent anti-metastatic effects in a disseminated tumor model in C571B1/6 mice [84]. The structure of this series is yet to be disclosed.

Sigma-Tau Pharmaceuticals (Gaithersburg, MD, USA) developed a heparin mimetic, SST0001 (Roneparstat, Figure 7a) which is currently in phase I clinical studies for advanced multiple myeloma. SST001 is an *N*-acetylated, glycol-split high molecular weight heparin that also exhibits low anticoagulant activity and selective inhibition of heparanase [85]. It is obtained from standard porcine mucosal heparin after total *N*-desulfation, *N*-acetylation, controlled periodate oxidation, and finally borohydride reduction (the sequence of the last two steps is called glycol-splitting). In preclinical studies, SST0001 showed a significant anti-myeloma effect in in vivo models of multiple myeloma [86]. The combination of SST0001 with irinotecan, a cytotoxic agent, exhibited potent activity against sarcoma xenografts with all animals showing marked tumour regression and a number of animals had no apparent disease at the completion of the experiment, whereas either drug alone only delayed tumour growth [87]. The latter study demonstrated that in vivo SST0001 administration caused reduced phosphorylation of a number of receptor tyrosine kinases (EGFR, ERBB4, INSR and IGF1R), providing evidence that this heparin mimetic may influence intracellular signaling as well as block heparanase.

Momenta pharmaceuticals presented anti-metastatic preclinical data for a heparin mimetic, M402 (Necuparanib, Figure 7b). M402 is a low molecular weight heparin, resulting from depolymerization of heparin and further oxidation and borohydride reduction. In vitro and in vivo studies of M402 showed reduced anticoagulant activity and inhibition of tumor metastasis through the modulation of factors, such as P-selectin, VEGF, and FGFs [88]. M402 has shown statistically significant survival benefits in animal models when used as a monotherapy or in a combination with other chemotherapeutics. Furthermore, mice treated with M402 showed reduced epithelial-to-mesenchymal transition, a key step in the progression of tumor cells towards a more invasive phenotype. Currently, M402 is in phase II clinical trial for pancreatic cancer.

(a) n+p+m = 25-30 R = 30%H, 70% SO$_3^-$; R$_2$ = 91% H, 9% SO$_3^-$

(b) n+p+m 10 R = 30%H, 70% SO$_3^-$; R$_1$ = 80% SO$_3^-$, 20% Ac; R$_2$ = 91% H, 9% SO$_3^-$

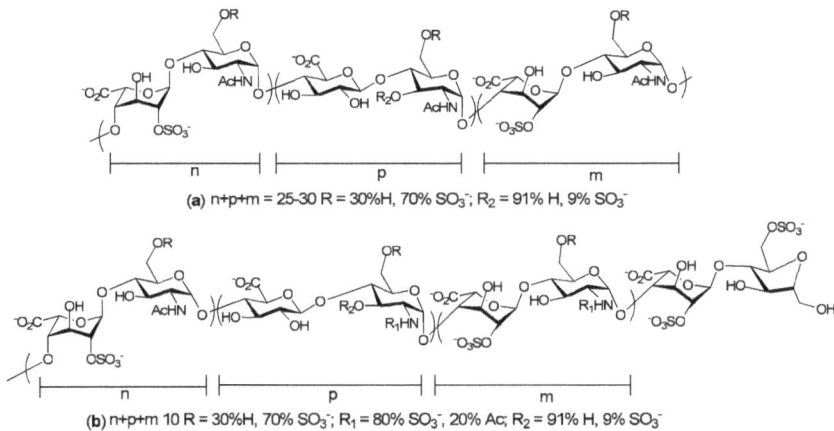

Figure 7. Schematic representation of **(a)** SST0001 (roneoparstat) **(b)** M402 (necuparanib). The actual structures may retain the microheterogeneity of the original heparin and low-molecular-weight-heparin (LMWH) [89].

Endotis Pharma (Romainville, France) reported the synthesis of an octasaccharide-based heparin mimetic capable of antagonising angiogenic proteins that are known to be involved in cancer progression and angiogenesis associated with tumor growth [90,91]. The mimetic is expected to interfere with two major processes in tumor progression: (1) angiogenesis, in part mediated by growth factors, or endothelial progenitor cell recruitment; and (2) metastasis mediated by heparanase activity. The octasaccharide was assembled from three different disaccharide units which were synthesized from three different monosaccharides in sufficient quantities and with appropriate protecting groups. A fluoropyridinilated derivative of the sulfated octasaccharide heparin mimetic was then prepared by linking a triazole conjugated with FPyME to the reducing terminus (Figure 8). The use of [^{18}F]FPyMe allowed the incorporation of radiolabeled fluorine-18 which allows in vivo evaluation of the compound and is extremely useful for performing the ADMET assays required for drug development. Pharmacodistribution studies revealed that following injection into rats this heparin mimetic accumulated in the kidneys and to a lesser extent the liver and at later time points the bladder, indicating likely urinary excretion. Radioactivity in other organs was low but clearance from the blood vascular system was slow (t$_{1/2}$ was greater than 90 min). The in vivo properties of this mimetic are appropriate for an anti-cancer drug.

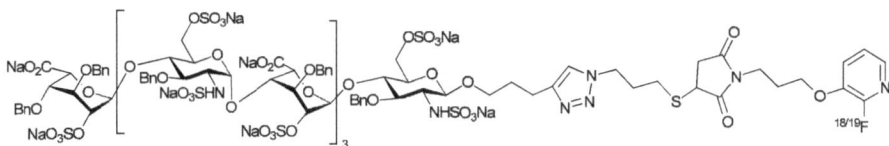

Figure 8. Chemical structure of the conjugated and radiolabeled octasaccharide-based HS mimetic.

Heparin mimetics designed for specific targets are expected to act preferentially on specific proteins such as growth factors of the FGF family and VEGF, and heparanase, which are overexpressed in cancer, but as was seen with PG545 other activities may well be detected for some of these compounds. The design of precisely tailored heparin mimetics is likely to require both anionic and non-anionic structures, the latter structures binding to the protein target outside of the basic region that is recognized by heparin and other GAGs.

5. Heparin Mimetics as Anti-Inflammatories

It has long being recognized that heparin has range of biological effects in addition to its well characterized anticoagulant properties, and possibly one of its best known non-anticoagulant activities are its anti-inflammatory effects [92–94]. The anti-inflammatory properties of heparin and heparin mimetics have primarily, but not exclusively, been linked to their ability to interact with three different types of proteins: complement system proteins, selectins and chemokines; each of which function in different ways to facilitate inflammation [95–97]. The potential of heparin as an anti-inflammatory drug is supported by a number of small, and several modestly sized clinical trials. Heparin has been shown to benefit patients with arthritis [98], inflammatory bowel disease [99,100], allergic rhinitis [101] and bronchial asthma [102,103]. However, the use of heparin as an anti-inflammatory agent has been hindered by its anticoagulant proprieties. Since the anti-inflammatory potential of heparin is independent of its anticoagulant properties, the development of novel non-anticoagulant heparin mimetics but with the anti-inflammatory properties of heparin is an attractive possibility. Thus, considerable effort has been directed towards the development of heparin mimetics with the potential to act as anti-inflammatory agents.

It is well known that selectins play a key role in the early stages of an inflammatory response [104], and so antagonists of selectins have the potential for being valuable therapeutic agents for various inflammatory diseases. The Sialyl Lewis^x (sLe^x) motif provides a lead structure for the search of E-selectin antagonists since it is a component of all the physiological receptors of the selectins. This motif, NeuAcα2-3Galβ1-4(Fucα1-3)GlcNAc, on its own is not a selectin receptor, rather additional structures are also required for binding. For example, P-selectin binds sLe^x on a threonine residue and an adjacent sulfated tyrosine on its ligand, P-selectin glycoprotein ligand-1; L-selectin binds O-linked SLe^x with a sulfate on the 6-hydroxyl of the SLe^x GlcNAc, and E-selectin binds glycosphingolipids carrying the terminal glycan structure: NeuAcα2-3Galβ1-4GlcNAcβ1-3 [Galβ1-4Fucα1-3)GlcNAcβ1-3]$_2$-R [105]. GMI-1070 (Rivipansel, developed by GlycoMimetics Inc., Rockville, MD, USA. Figure 9b) is a novel small molecule sLe^x mimetic pan-selectin antagonist [106]. GMI-1070 was developed by rational design, focusing on the conformation of sLe^x when it is bound to E-selectin, as determined by nuclear magnetic resonance. In GMI-1070 the oligosaccharide fragments of sLe^x were replaced with a conformationally restricted linker which reproduced the three-dimensional (3D) features of sLe^x. GMI-1070 contains a cyclohexane core structure with a carbohydrate branching motif linked to a benzyl amino sulfonic acid residue [107]. The extended sulfated domain was designed to allow binding of P- and L-selectins as well as E-selectin. Although it binds all three selectins its ability to block the binding of the natural selectin ligands, sLe^a and sLe^x to immobilized selectins was far greater with E-selectin than with L-selectin or P-selectin, being approximately 10-fold more sensitive with an IC$_{50}$ of 4.3 μM. Selectins facilitate leukocyte rolling on endothelial cells of the vasculature, which is the first step in leukocyte migration from the blood and into the tissues in an inflammatory response. The administration of GMI-1070 into mice with sickle cell disease caused an increase in leukocyte rolling, which is a characteristic of E-selectin inhibition. Moreover, GMI-1070 reduced the number of leukocytes adhering to the venular endothelium and also inhibited red blood cell-leukocyte interactions and vascular occlusion. It is currently undergoing clinical trials for treatment of vaso-occlusive crisis in people with sickle cell disease. It has been demonstrated to have a good safety profile, a serum half-life of 7–8 h and greater than 90% of the drug is excreted intact [106,108]. Phase II studies revealed the drug reduced the time to resolution of vaso-occlusive events (not considerably significant) and improvements were also observed in other aspects, like time to hospital discharge [109]. Phase III trials have commenced for this drug.

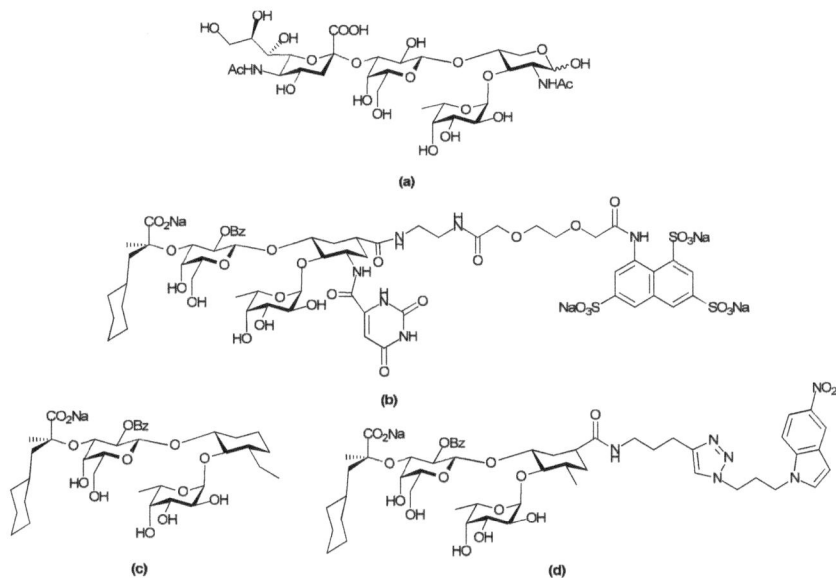

Figure 9. Chemical structure of (**a**) Sialyl Lewis^x (sLe^x); (**b**) GM-1070, sLe^x mimic in clinical trials for treatment of vaso-occlusive crisis in sickle cell disease patients; (**c**) sLe^x mimic that maximizes conformational pre-organization of the binding determinants; (**d**) sLe^x mimic designed using fragment based discovery techniques with improved binding kinetics.

Recently, Ernst and co-workers dissected the role of the cyclohexane core structure of the natural SLe^x ligand and correlated (by nuclear magnetic resonance spectroscopy (NMR) and molecular dynamic calculations) the affinities with which it binds E-selectin with the flexibility and the degree of pre-organization of the pharmacophores in the bioactive conformation [110]. In SLe^x, the hydroxyl groups of the fucose moiety, the 4- and the 6-hydroxyl of the galactose moiety and carboxylic acid group of the sialic acid residue act as pharmacophores. Whereas the *N*-acetylglucosamine (GlcNAc) moiety serves as 3D spacer to position L-fucose underneath the β-face of D-galactose. This 3D orientation and pre-organization of the pharmacophores are extremely important for high affinity binding [111]. Ernst and co-workers used a molecular design strategy which involves introducing conformational restriction which then limits the degrees of freedom a molecule can lose upon binding, to synthesize a library of high-affinity E-selectin antagonists. These antagonists were synthesized with a cyclohexane linker which acts as GlcNAc mimic of the native SLe^x ligand. Using Surface Plasmon Resonance (SPR) and Saturation Transfer Difference NMR experiments, they showed that addition of hydrophobic substituents on the cyclohexane linker improved the affinity by forcing the adjacent fucose moiety into the bioactive conformation. In this manner, the affinity of the native SLe^x (Figure 9a) was improved more than 660-fold (Figure 9c: dissociation constant, $K_D = 1.5$ μM, $IC_{50} = 4.0$ μM), predominantly by pre-organizing the SLe^x-core with a novel GlcNAc mimetic and leaving the pharmacophores as present in native SLe^x [110].

Ernst and co-workers further optimized E-selectin antagonists using fragment based discovery techniques to select ligands able to bind in a second site near the sLe^x mimic binding site [112]. Fragments were screened for E-selectin binding using spin-lock filtered NMR experiments. The hits were then retested in the presence of the first site ligand which was labeled with a spin-label probe. This then enabled the identification of fragments which were binding in the vicinity of the spin-label via paramagnetic relaxation enhancement spectroscopy. These fragments were then connected to the sLe^x mimic through flexible linkers of variable length and tested by SPR for interaction with E-selectin.

The most potent antagonists so obtained had K_D values between 30 and 89 nM and a half-life of the ligand protein complex in the range 4–5 min (e.g., Figure 9d: K_D = 30 nM, $t_{1/2}$ = 4.1 min). This was a substantial improvement with respect to affinity and half-life as carbohydrate-lectin interactions are generally characterized by micro- to millimolar affinities and half-lives in the seconds [113].

Others have also developed heparin mimetics that target the selectins [114]. Some of these were produced by varying the degree of sulfation of natural linear glucans with varying degrees of polymerization and different linkages between their monosaccharide units. This work revealed that charge density (degree of sulfation), rather than molecular weight is the more important factor in determining whether the various sulfated glucans inhibit P-selectin activity. The monomer glycosidic linkage also seemed to play a role, as mimetics of comparable length and degree of sulfation but with a backbone of β-1,3-linked glucose units, were inferior to mimetics with a backbone consisting of α-1,4/1,6-glucans. The increased activity was attributed to the greater flexibility of the latter mimetics. A kinetic study, on the binding interactions of some of these compounds with P-selectin, was quite informative [115]. This work revealed that mimetic occupancy time on P-selectin was critical for inhibitory activity, and mimetics with a disassociation rate markedly slower than the natural ligand should be good inhibitors. One of these compounds was PS3 (Figure 10), a low polydispersity β-1,3-glucan sulfate in which the primary hydroxyl group at position 6 was fully sulfated, the secondary hydroxyl groups at positions 2 and 4 were equally sulfated to about 60%, giving an overall degree of sulfation of 2.2 sulfates per glucose unit, and the degree of polymerization was about 25. This compound significantly inhibited peripheral blood mononuclear cell interactions with endothelial cells under flow conditions, an effect attributed to its inhibition of both L-selectin and P-selectin, but not E-selectin [116]. It was also shown to act as an anti-inflammatory agent in a murine model of contact hypersensitivity, but it's in vivo potency was not investigated at concentrations other than 25 mg kg^{-1}, which is quite a high dose.

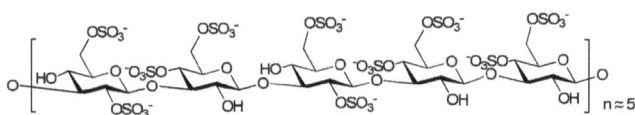

Figure 10. Structure of PS3; the sodium salt of a β-1,3-glucan sulfate with a degree of sulfation of 2.2 and a polydispersity of 25 corresponding to a mean molecular weight of 10,000.

The notion that greater potency against the selectins may be achieved by multivalent, dendritic compounds of polyglycerol anions has also been investigated. A variety of different compounds were made using dendritic polyglycerols of different molecular weights as the starting material. The dendritic polyglycerols were synthesized by one-step anionic ring-opening multibranching polymerization of glycidol on a polyol initiator. These compounds were functionalized with different polyanions with a high degree of functionalization (>80%) using click chemistry (Figure 11A). Those with a core size of 6000 Da and functionalized with sulfates most effectively inhibited L-selectin with low nanomolar range IC_{50} values [117]. Importantly, the in vivo pharmacokinetics of the best of these compounds has also been examined via radiolabeling. The radiolabeling of the dendritic polyglycerol candidate was accomplished by an oxidation-reduction process with sodium periodate and [^{3}H]-borohydride followed by sulfation using SO_3.pyridine complex. This method represents a mild straight forward labelling technique for the introduction of titrium into 1,2-diol containing molecules without the use of radioactive monomers. An optimized radiochemical yield of >80% was achieved for this reaction, proving its efficacy. ^{64}Cu-labeled compounds were synthesized by conjugating Cu(II) chelators to the partially aminated dendrimer (Figure 11B). A radiolabelling yield of >99% was achieved within 5 min with a high radiochemical purity, eliminating the need for further purification [118]. These radiolabelling methods are likely to be applicable to other heparin mimetics as they move into the pre-clinical phase. In this case, the biodistribution studies in healthy mice and rats revealed that the polysulfated dendrimers accumulated in the liver and spleen and although small amounts were excreted via the kidneys there was still evidence of organ accumulation after 3 weeks, which was not a favorable distribution pattern for a drug.

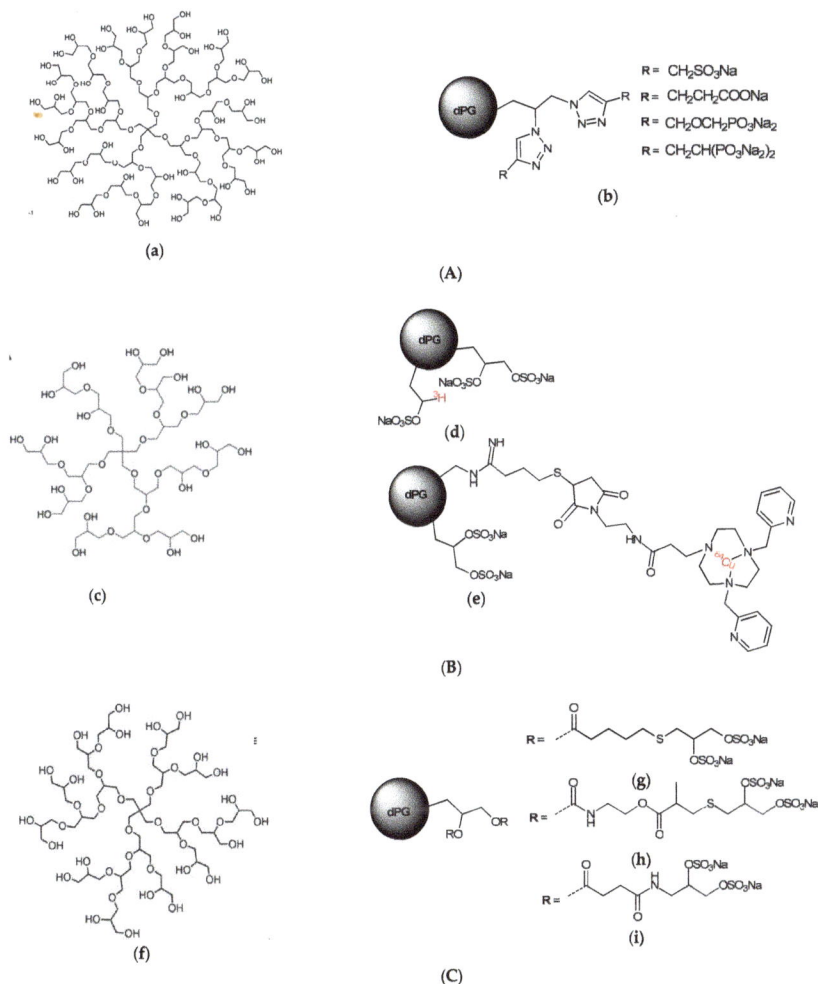

Figure 11. Structure of dendritic polyglycerol heparin mimetics: The structure of dendritic polyglycerols (dPG) scaffold illustrates an idealized fragment of the polymer. (**A**) Structure of (**a**) dendritic polyglycerol starting material and (**b**) dendritic polyglycerol heparin mimetics synthesized via click coupling by Weinhart et al. [117]; (**B**) Structure of (**c**) dendritic polyglycerol starting material and (**d,e**) radiolabeled dendritic polyglycerol heparin mimetics synthesized by Pant et al. [118]; (**C**) Structure of (**f**) dendritic polyglycerol starting material and (**g–i**) shell cleavable dendritic polyglycerol heparin mimetics synthesized by Reimann et al. [95].

To overcome this problem shell cleavable polysulfated dendrimers were synthesized and investigated for competitive L-selectin binding, blood coagulation, complement activation and degradation in vitro. This synthesis and the biological activities are described in the report by Reimann et al. [95]. This work revealed that two of these compounds dPG-thioglyceryl pentanoatyl sulfate (Figure 11C(h)) and pPG-thioglyceryl methylpropanoatyl sulfate (Figure 11C(g)) containing long flexible hydrophobic linkers which included respectively, either an ester functionality, or a carbamate and an ester functionality, had potent complement pathway inhibition activity, minimal anticoagulant activity and high picomolar IC_{50} values in the L-selectin binding assay. These two compounds also degraded quite readily and so were considered as interesting compounds for long term treatment of chronic inflammation or as a new class of anti-complement therapeutic for preventing tissue damage within inflammatory disease [95].

Heparin and HS are known to interact with numerous proteins in all three pathways of the complement cascade. Most of these interactions have a regulatory role and most result in the inhibition of the complement cascade [97]. Structure-activity relationships of more than 40 structurally distinct sulfated glycans with the serpin C1 inhibitor (C1-INH) and the serine protease, C1s, have been examined [119]. C1-INH inactivates the initiating enzymes of the complement classical pathway, C1r and C1s, as well as the initiating serine proteases of the mannose-binding lectin pathway, Mannose binding lectin Associated Serine Protease (MASP)-1 and MASP-2. C1-INH is also the most important inhibitor of the plasma proteases kallikrein, Factor XIa and Factor XIIa of the intrinsic coagulation pathway. It was found that the sulfated glycans potentiated C1-INH activity and shortened the time for C1s inhibition by about 50% and this potentiating effect was dependent on degree of sulfation and molecular weight, but glycan structure was also important. The linear β-1,3-glucan structure was favored over the branched α-1,6-glucan structure of dextrans, and the former structure was also favored over heparin. The dependence on degree of sulfation and size was linked so that a small compound like the pentasaccharide Fondaparinux, which is highly sulfated, was slightly potentiating, whereas if the degree of sulfation was low, a much larger sulfated glycan was required for any C1-INH potentiation. It is believed that the polyanion links the basic surfaces of C1s and C1-INH like the filling in a protein sandwich [120], which is different from the "bridging" mechanism of antithrombin III and thrombin whereby these two proteins bind adjacent regions on a single heparin chain. It could be argued that as the entire "top" face of C1-INH is positively charged, longer polyanions of low sulfation are required for charge neutralization of this face on C1-INH and trimer formation. Schoenfeld et al., used this rational, plus the argument that C1-INH amplifiers should have both: low anticoagulant activity, and the improved pharmacokinetics of a rather low molecular size, to promote the β-1,3-glucan sulfates as promising candidates for further investigation [119].

Additionally, a number of GAG analogues that bind to chemokines are under development as novel anti-inflammatory drugs. In one study compounds were developed based on two different approaches. Firstly, a structure based approach was used after initial screening of potential small molecule binders using protein NMR on a target chemokine, in this case CCL5 (or RANTES) [96]. Two small molecules shown to bind to separate sites on CCL5 by NMR and X-ray crystallography were linked to form a chimera, the hope being that the chimera would have better anti-inflammatory activity than the separate molecules. In the second approach by the same group, commercially available short oligosaccharides were persulfated. In vitro, the molecules prevented chemokine-GAG binding and chemokine receptor activation without disrupting coagulation. However, in vivo variable results were seen in a murine peritoneal recruitment assay, with the chimeric molecule enhancing cell recruitment in this assay [96]. In this study, the crystallography was performed at low pH. However, our work with CCL5 revealed that the sites where heparin tetrasaccharides bind this chemokine vary depending on the pH [15]. Thus, the crystallography data would have indicated where the heparin mimetics bound CCL5 at low pH (pH 3.5), rather than where they bind at the pH encountered in vivo, and as this was unlikely to have been the same site the structural data may have provided misleading information. Nevertheless, some of the persulfated oligosaccharides were shown to inhibit inflammation in a delayed-type hypersensitivity model and in an antigen-induced arthritis model [96], the reasons for the different activities in the different models is unknown.

Other workers have examined heparin mimicking glycopolymers for their ability to bind CCL5. The rational was that a HS disaccharide epitope presented as a multivalent, pendant array on a polynorbornene backbone might antagonize CCL5 if the binding affinity was enhanced by increased avidity [121]. Controlling the sulfation pattern before polymerization allowed the production of four different glycopolymers each with a different pattern of sulfation on the disaccharide. These sulfation patterns were: 2-*O*-sulfated IdoA 1,4-linked to *N*- and 6-*O*-sulfated GlcN; 2-*O*-sulfated IdoA 1,4-linked to *N*-acetylated, 6-*O*-sulfated GlcN; IdoA 1,4-linked to *N*-acetylated GlcN, and IdoA 1,4-linked to *N*- and 6-*O*-sulfated GlcN. The resulting mimetics were variations on the structures shown in Figure 4. Of these mimetics the glycopolymer carrying the trisulfated disaccharide most effectively competed with heparin for binding CCL5, and not surprisingly, the non-sulfated glycopolymer was without activity. Chemotactic activity mediated by CCL5 binding its receptor CCR3 was also inhibited by both heparin and trisulfated disaccharide glycopolymer, but chemotaxis of cells bearing the alternative CCL5 receptor, CCR5, was not inhibited. Unfortunately the efficacy of this glycopolymer in an in vivo inflammation model was not reported, nor is it clear how the glycopolymer would bind CCL5 oligomers.

CCL5 is not the only chemokine that has been studied for its interaction with heparin mimetics. A recent study using synthetic heparin/HS-like dodecasaccharides has revealed that that addition of a single 6-*O*-sulfate to the glucosamine at the non-reducing terminus of the mimetic alters which chemokine binds [122]. The use of the 3 homogeneous, synthetic dodecasaccharides of known structures indicated that the presence or absence of this site-specific 6-*O*-sulfation determined whether the signaling of either of the chemokines CXCL8 (or IL-8) or CXCL12 was inhibited. The dodecasaccharides were of the following structures: (1) non-reducing terminal *N*- and 4-*O*-sulfated GlcN 1,4 linked 2-*O*-sulfated IdoA 1,4 linked [*N*-sulfated GlcN 1,4-linked 2-*O*-sulfated IdoA]₅ (Figure 12a); (2) non-reducing terminal *N*-sulfated,4,6-*O*-sulfated GlcN 1,4-linked 2-*O*-sulfated IdoA 1,4-linked [*N*-sulfated GlcN 1,4-linked 2-*O*-sulfated IdoA]₅ (Figure 12b); and (3) fully 6-*O*-sulfated dodecasaccharide (Figure 12c). Interestingly the fully 6-*O*-sulfated dodecasaccharide did not preferentially inhibit either CXCL8, or CXCL12, but its biological activity resembled that of a native dp12 arising from digesting commercial heparin. The mimetics also demonstrated these behaviors in in vivo models. For example, analogue **a** (see Figure 12) inhibited CXCL8 induced neutrophil infiltration whereas analogue **b** (see Figure 12) with the reducing end 6-*O*-sulfate GlcN did not, and analogue **b** inhibited CXCL12 induced macrophage infiltration whereas analogue **a,** which lacked the terminal 6-*O*-sulfate moiety did not. These data indicated that for these chemokines the overall sulfation level of the dodecasaccharide was not the critical feature but rather the single non-reducing end 6-*O*-sulfate GlcN determined the biological behavior. The study authors comment that their findings suggest that, "other significant site-specific sulfation-determined effects await discovery and biomedical exploitation" [122].

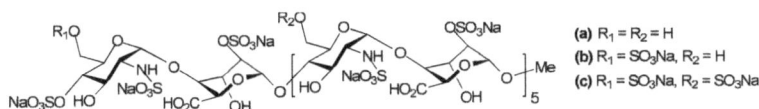

Figure 12. Site-specifically 6-*O*-sulfated dodecasaccharides: (**a**) completely non-6-*O*-sulfated (**b**) site-selectively mono-6-*O*-sulfated (**c**) fully 6-*O*-sulfated.

Homogeneous, discrete GAG-mimetics are proving to be powerful tools for unravelling the structure-specificity issues that have been haunting GAG biology for decades. A glycan array of heparin-like oligosaccharides varying from monomer to hexamer was used to probe the binding specificity of the chemokine, CCL20 [123]. This chemokine bound the un-natural, synthetic monosaccharide 2,4-*O*-sulfated IdoA (Figure 13) with micromolar affinity, and this di-sulfated IdoA interfered with CCL20 heparan sulfate binding in a concentration dependent fashion and it also inhibited the binding of CXCL8 and L-selectin. The in vivo effects of di-sulfated IdoA in a murine model of allergy were intriguing. Injection of di-sulfated IdoA immediately prior to allergen challenge decreased mucus secretion and T lymphocyte recruitment into the lungs. Administering di-sulfated IdoA by inhalation before allergen challenge decreased CCL20 staining on lung endothelial cells and lymphocyte recruitment, as measured by lymphocyte numbers in bronchi alveolar lavage fluid (BALF). These data were interpreted as suggesting that CCL20-mediated recruitment of Th17 and Th2 lymphocytes were critical for the early stages of the asthmatic response. The di-sulfated IdoA was said to act by binding to CCL20, thereby preventing CCL20 from accumulating on HS on the airway endothelium and from binding its receptor CCR6 on the lymphocytes and triggering their recruitment. Importantly, other chemokines (CCL19, CCL21, CCL25, CCL28, CXCL12, CXCL13 and CXCL16) did not bind 2,4-O-sulfated IdoA indicating the specificity of the response [124].

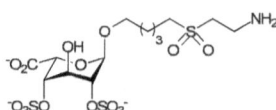

Figure 13. The unnatural synthetic monosaccharide, Di-S-IdoA containing two axial sulfate groups.

Abraham and co-workers similarly tested a disaccharide heparin analogue in an animal asthma model. They first described, what in their view is, a minimal chain length and structural sequence of the anti-allergic domain of heparin. In this study, it was demonstrated that the anti-allergic activity of heparin resided in a tetrasccharide sequence and that the domain responsible for anticoagulant and anti-allergic activity of heparin were distinctly different (Figure 14a) [125]. Later, Abraham and co-workers also demonstrated that "supersulfation" of an anticoagulation inactive disaccharide fragment conferred anti-allergic activity. The disaccharide Hep-SSD (Figure 14b) was prepared by nitrous acid depolymerization of porcine intestinal heparin followed by size exclusion chromatography. The disaccharide fragment was then sulfated to obtain supersulfated Hep-SSD. This disaccharide, Hep-SSD was shown to inhibit allergic airway responses in sheep model of asthma and it displayed activity by both aerosol and oral routes [126]. There has been considerable interest over a number of years in the possibility that non-anticoagulant heparin derivatives may be useful anti-inflammatories for the management of asthma and a number of small clinical trials have examined this notion (see review: [127]). However, to our knowledge this interest has yet to extend to testing heparin mimetics in clinical trials as anti-asthmatics despite the promising data from animal studies.

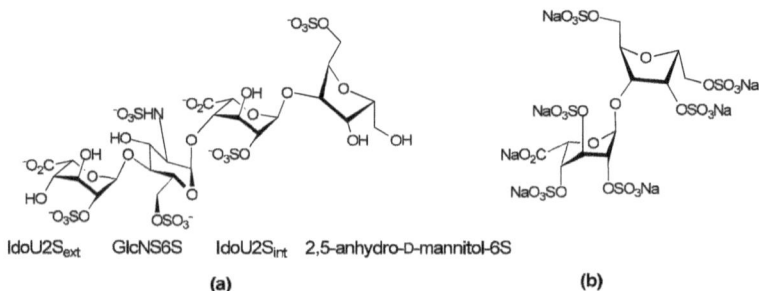

IdoU2S$_{ext}$ GlcNS6S   IdoU2S$_{int}$ 2,5-anhydro-D-mannitol-6S

(a)   (b)

Figure 14. (a) Heparin tetrasaccharide which possess the minimal chain length for anti-allergic and anti-inflammatory properties (b) Supersulfated heparin derived disaccharide, Hep-SSD.

Another lung disease in which heparin mimetics may exert useful anti-inflammatory effects is chronic obstructive pulmonary disease (COPD). This is a disease of neutrophil infiltration and much of the tissue damage is caused by serine proteases released from neutrophil granules. These include neutrophil elastase, cathepsin G and proteinase 3, enzymes known to be inhibited by heparin.

Against this background Craciun et al. synthesized, structurally characterized, and tested a panel of of *N*-arylacyl *O*-sulfonated aminoglycosides to identify inhibitors of these neutrophil serine proteases [128]. This work identified a kanamycin- and a neomycin-based compound as compounds of interest; the kanamycin-based compound (Figure 15a) inhibited all three enzymes whereas the neomycin-based compound (Figure 15b) inhibited neutrophil elastase and cathepsin G. Further functional optimization of the kanamycin-based compound is continuing with the view of developing an inhaled drug for attenuation of protease-mediated lung disease. Others have produced promising compounds using heparin as the starting material. For example, Fryer et al. reported the modification of unfractionated heparin to yield a 2,3-*O*-desulfated heparin (ODSH) that lacks anticoagulant activity, but retains the anti-inflammatory characteristics of the parent molecule [129]. ODSH was developed by selective desulfation of unmodified heparin under extreme alkaline conditions [130]. In preclinical studies, ODSH has shown promising anti-inflammatory activity by inhibiting airway hyperactivity and airway smooth muscle proliferation in mammals. Clinical trials of ODSH in patients with exacerbations of COPD are ongoing [131].

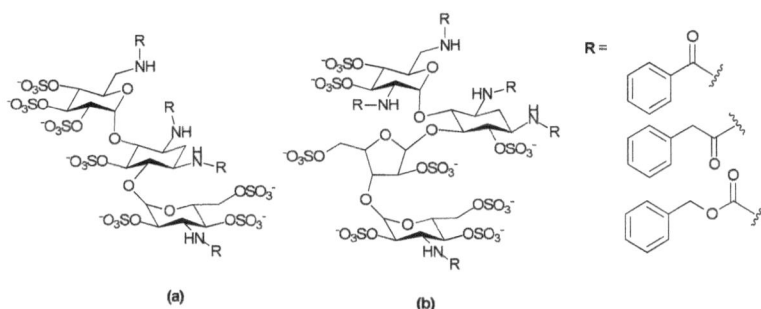

Figure 15. Structure and degree of sulfation of *N*-arylacyl *O*-sulfonated aminoglycosides (**a**) Kanamycin core derivatives (**b**) Neomycin core derivatives.

Clearly, heparin mimetics could be a novel class of therapeutic compounds for a range of inflammatory diseases. However, further work is required to unravel the mechanisms of action that give rise to the anti-inflammatory effects of these molecules. The protein-binding specificities of the mimetics studied to date suggest that different mimetic structures will be optimal for inflammatory diseases with different etiologies. However, it is also likely that the pleiotropic effects of heparin mimetics is a factor in their in vivo efficacy as anti-inflammatory agents. The optimization of drug candidates by increasing their binding affinities for particular protein targets should take into account the likely requirement for pleiotropic activities in an effective anti-inflammation drug. Nevertheless, the results of an increasing number of studies support the likelihood that it will be possible to design agents, mimicking heparin, that exploit the anti-inflammatory actions of the parent molecule but lack its anticoagulation activity.

6. Heparin Mimetics: Potential Toxicities

The therapeutic potential of heparin mimetics is dependent on any drug induced adverse effects, and there are well known molecular interactions that could be undesirable depending on the disease indication and the proteins being targeted. Although in animal studies these types of molecules are generally well tolerated there are some exceptions. For example, at high concentrations (25 and 75 mg/kg intraperitoneally twice a week) pentosan polysulfate, a sulfated xylan polymer, caused immediate mortality in 60% of the mice under study [132]. Anticoagulation was assumed to be a contributor to the adverse effect of pentosan polysulfate in this study, and it is the most obvious possible undesirable effect, if the mimetic is targeting a disease which does not have coagulation as a component of its etiology.

A number of different approaches have been taken to reduce the anticoagulant activities of heparin derivatives and heparin mimetics. Casu and his colleagues pioneered the "glycol-splitting" of heparin chains, where the C(2)-C(3) bond of an un-sulfated uronic acid is split by periodate oxidation with subsequent borohydride reduction [133]. The glucuronic acid in the antithrombin III binding motif is cleaved by this reaction and as this residue is essential for high affinity antithrombin III binding these glycol-split heparin chains have very low anticoagulant activity, but retain the other main activities of heparin. The extent of glycol-splitting can be varied by controlled partial 2-*O*-desulfation followed by periodate oxidation/borohydride reduction to give regions of pentasulfated trisaccharides adjacent to a glycol-split uronic acid. Through this approach some activities of heparin such as FGF-2 binding were retained, whereas others were reduced (e.g., induction of FGF-2 dimerization [134]), and the pattern of activities was found to vary depending on the extent of glycol-splitting. The increased conformational flexibility that is introduced by the more freely-rotating glycol-split uronic acids contributes to the variability in activity. A number of different non-anticoagulant, glycol-split heparins have been produced that differ in molecular weight, extent of glycol-splitting and activities (see the recent review [135]).

Although heparin mimetics that do not resemble the pentasaccharide motif in heparin that is required for high affinity binding to antithrombin III may not be expected to have anticoagulant activity, or to have very low anticoagulant activity, this may not always be the case. For example, sulfate glycans from some marine organisms have anticoagulant activity and their mode of action is enhancement of the antithrombin III and heparin cofactor II inhibitory activities, but the major glycosylation and sulfation structures of these glycans were found not to resemble the antithrombin III motif that is present in heparin [136]. There are numerous examples of non-mammalian sulfated glycan structures with anticoagulant activity that can be primarily attributed to antithrombin III and /or heparin cofactor II inhibition of thrombin, such that it has been possible to propose the types of sulfated glycan structures that are required for anticoagulant activity [137]. Moreover, as well as pentosan polysulfate other synthetic heparin mimetics have been produced that interact with antithrombin III or heparin cofactor II and hence act as anticoagulants, these include a polysulfated trehalose [138] and a sulfated mannogalactan [139]. The interaction of heparin cofactor II with heparin is considered to resemble the interaction of antithrombin III with low affinity heparin (i.e., heparin that does not have the antithrombin III-binding pentasaccharide), with affinity being determined by ionic strength and heparin size [140]. Given this, it is not surprising that heparin mimetics may interact with one or both of these proteins and inhibit thrombin. Thus, anticoagulation testing should be included in the toxicity analyses of all heparin mimetics designed for non-anticoagulation indications. It is also conceivable that a heparin mimetic could contribute to anticoagulation by displacing tissue factor pathway inhibitor (TFPI) from the vascular endothelium and into the circulation. Thus, an in vivo assessment of anticoagulation effects of heparin mimetics in an animal model where TFPI is produced by endothelial cells and is bound by the vascular endothelium, as it is in humans [141], should be part of the toxicity package of a mimetic with planned intravenous delivery.

Other factors in the coagulation cascade may also react with heparin mimetics and of particular interest is the serine protease factor XII (FXII). When FXII comes into contact with negatively charged surfaces this triggers a conformational change in the protein to give activated FXII (FXIIa). FXIIa triggers the proinflammatory and procoagulant pathways of the contact system (the reader is referred to recent reviews for details, [142]). Briefly, FXIIa cleavage of plasma prekallikrein gives plasma kallikrein which reciprocally activates FXII, and results in vastly more FXIIa than originally produced by the negatively charged surface. Plasma kallikrein cleaves high molecular weight kininogen to release bradykinin, a potent proinflammatory peptide. Plasma kallikrein also converts plasminogen into plasmin which is involved in fibrin degradation. FXIIa activates the classical complement pathway (via C1r and C1s) resulting in production of the anaphyatoxins C3a and C5a which stimulate inflammation.

Finally, the intrinsic coagulation cascade is activated by FXIIa cleavage of FXI giving FXIa, which initiates a series of cleavage reactions that generate thrombin, fibrin formation and fibrin clots.

A number of natural negatively charged substances have the potential to trigger FXII activation, these include heparin, heparan sulfate, chondroitin sulfates, dermatan sulfates, lipoproteins, platelet polyphosphate, L-homocysteine and so on [142,143], but some artificial substances including 500 kDa dextran sulfate and chemically over sulfated glycosaminoglycans are particularly potent FXII activators [144]. A comparison of the various oversulfated glycosaminoglycans suggested that activation of the contact system is "pattern-dependent" rather than "structure-dependent" and the degree of chemical sulfation is a key determinant as to whether kallikrein activity is induced in human plasma. The importance of assessing if a heparin mimetic designed for therapeutic application activates the contact system is highlighted by what became known as the "heparin contamination crisis" that occurred in 2007 and 2008. Over sulfated chondroitin sulfate (OSCS) contamination of heparin was discovered to be the main causative agent. Activation of both the kinin-kallikrein system and the complement pathway (evident by the levels of C3a and C5a generated), via activation of FXIIa, were deemed responsible for the adverse effects suffered by patients [145], and which potentially led to the 246 recorded deaths of patients receiving heparin during that period [146]. The enhanced production of bradykinin is believed to be responsible for the hypotension and angioedema experienced by around 50% of patients who suffered adverse events. It is likely that route of delivery, and the dose of the contaminated heparin delivered were factors contributing to the severity of the adverse events. These conclusions are supported by a rat study in which the hypotensive effects experienced by patients could be replicated in rats by intravenous delivery of OSCS-contaminated heparin, whereas subcutaneous administration was not effective, moreover, the hypotensive effect was dependent upon the concentration of the contaminating OSCS [147].

Further studies revealed OSCS interacts with some contact system and coagulation system components in different ways from heparin [148]. Firstly, the anticoagulant activity of OSCS is primarily through heparin cofactor II mediated inhibition of thrombin. Although OSCS binds tightly to antithrombin III, this binding does not cause the conformational change in antithrombin III that is required for its inactivation of thrombin and FXa, moreover, OSCS does not compete with heparin for binding to antithrombin III. Secondly, unlike heparin, OSCS binds tightly to FXIIa. These activity differences may be useful indicators for distinguishing whether a heparin mimetic has OSCS-like toxicology. The generation of the complement pathway anaphylatoxins C3a and C5a by OSCS was particularly intriguing as this appeared to occur via a mechanism that did not involve C3 and C5 convertases. Rather kallikrein induced by FXIIa appeared to be the key initiating factor [145]. When screening for contact system activation and high kallikrein activities the choice of plasma is important as animal plasmas have been reported to differ according to species in their capacity to give rise to the high kallikrein activities seen with human plasma following stimulation with OSCS [145,147]. Curiously a veterinary drug, polysulfated glycosaminoglycan (PSGAG) marketed as Adequan®, also an oversulfated chondroitin sulfate, is administered intramuscularly for animal (dog and horse) osteoarthritis. The mode of delivery is likely to limit FXIIa levels and the kallikrein effect in the animals treated, but this drug has been shown to resemble OSCS in its reactivity with some complement pathway proteins and may activate FXII if delivered by an intravascular route [149].

An adverse event that could be triggered by heparin mimetics is that of drug induced thrombocytopenia. By analogy with heparin induced thrombocytopenia (HIT), this could occur if the mimetic binds PF4 and so exposes antigenic epitopes on PF4 which triggers an antibody response to the mimetic-PF4 complex and the formation of large immune complexes. Antibodies in these complexes bind Fc-receptors on platelets and monocytes triggering platelet aggregation, activation and the release of pro-thrombotic mediators which markedly increase the risk of thrombosis. Thrombocytopenia (a drop in platelet count of around 50% or more) results from the clearance of platelet aggregates. In most HIT patients thrombotic complications and thrombocytopenia occur concurrently, although thrombosis is the main contributor to disease and mortality [150]. Clinical reports have indicated pentosan polysulfate can induce thrombocytopenia and thrombosis at least to the same degree as heparin [151], and in vitro studies have shown that polyphosphates form antigenic complexes with PF4 which are recognized by anti-PF4 antibodies [48]. Thus, neither the monosaccharide composition nor the structure of the anion are determining features for PF4 binding. Studies with heparin showed that ≥10 saccharides and >13 sulfate groups are required for heparin fragments to bind PF4, trigger neoepitope exposure and HIT antibody binding, and it was concluded that charge density and oligosaccharide size were more important than a specific sulfation pattern for PF4 binding [152]. Given these findings it is probable heparin mimetics that broadly fit the criteria of ≥10 saccharides and >13 anions have the potential to bind PF4 in such a way so as to trigger drug induced thrombocytopenia. However, the clinical data obtained with PI-88 indicated that heparin mimetics smaller than 10 saccharides may also trigger immune mediated thrombocytopenia with some patients developing HIT-like disease [69]. Clearly PF4 binding should be included in the off-target screening program for heparin mimetics.

7. Conclusions

Decades of research have highlighted the enormous potential of heparin mimetics as drugs. The rationale for developing heparin mimetic drugs as opposed to using native heparin, or heparin oligosaccharides as drugs, in part depends on the disease being targeted. However, regardless of disease indication, there is a move away from heterogeneous natural product drugs derived from animal tissues, towards homogeneous, synthetic or semi-synthetic, structurally defined entities. The heparin contamination crisis of 2007 and 2008 highlighted potential problems that can arise with heterogeneous natural product drugs, and served to provide an additional impetus to heparin mimetic development. As with all drug discovery programs increased potency, increased selectivity and better pharmacokinetics are also goals of heparin mimetic development. Although the LMWHs have improved bioavailability and pharmacokinetic profiles over that of the parent product, they retain the issues associated with heterogeneity and natural product origins. Heparin oligosaccharides of uniform length and structure isolated from heparin are not viable drugs in our view. It is possible, using the appropriate purification strategies, to obtain pure oligosaccharide structures [14,15], but the final yields are so poor as to be prohibitive for a drug. An alternative would be the production of synthetic heparin oligosaccharides of defined structure; the marketing of Fondaparinux indicates this is possible. However, as Fondaparinux synthesis requires around 50 chemical steps other avenues to achieve heparin structures with less steps are being explored, and encouraging advances in chemoenzymatic methods are being achieved [153].

The heparin mimetic approach is different, in that exact copies of natural heparin oligosaccharides are not the goal, rather ease of synthesis, homogeneity (usually) and a reduction in the promiscuity of heparin's protein binding behavior are the usual goals. In the examples discussed here the structural diversity of heparin mimetics is evident; some display only very minor differences from the natural product, whereas other mimetics bear no resemblance to heparin other than that they are polyanionic and they inhibit heparin from binding to their protein target(s). In the design of heparin mimetics there is the opportunity to tailor the mimetic structure to favor some of heparin's functions and eliminate others. For example, many of the mimetics targeting cancer or inflammation have been designed so they cannot bind antithrombin III, and so anticoagulation activity can only occur by other pathways. In contrast, anticoagulant mimetics can be designed to bind antithrombin III but not PF4, thereby removing drug induced thrombocytopenia as a potential side-effect (see this review). Heparin mimetics generally are less heterogeneous than heparin, or are homogeneous, and thus they may be expected to display a greater specificity and potency of action than heparin. Detailed structural studies of heparin/GAG-protein interactions using NMR spectroscopy, X-ray crystallography and molecular modelling techniques have greatly aided the design of heparin mimetics. However, to be effective the conditions of these in vitro binding studies should mirror, as much as possible, the conditions likely to be encountered in vivo, as the tissue microenvironment pH and cation composition may contribute to the strength of mimetic binding and position on the protein where the mimetic binds.

The consequences of possible pleiotropic effects of heparin mimetics will vary depending on the disease indication. The three disease areas discussed here ranged from the effects of a clear biochemical pathway (blood coagulation and thrombosis), to complex disease processes (cancer and inflammation) that involve a multitude of different molecular pathways, or binding events, a number of which involve heparin/HS-protein interactions. Exquisite specificity of anti-coagulant heparin mimetics would be advantageous, whereas exquisite specificity for one protein target may not provide the therapeutic outcome that is desired in the other two disease indications. In inflammatory diseases and cancers, the molecular redundancy of the pathology is such that although one pathway may be blocked the disease can still progress. There is also considerable overlap in the disease processes, for example thrombogenicity is often associated with cancer or inflammation. Hence, mimetics that display a degree of polypharmacy are likely to be of more therapeutic benefit than a mimetic that is directed towards a single target. The challenge will be to maximize the benefits of polypharmacy whilst managing any adverse effects that could arise from pleiotropic binding behavior. Drug delivery regimes that largely restrict the drug to the site of disease is one way of managing this issue, although this may not always be possible in the case of cancers. Nevertheless, this field is advancing rapidly as new synthetic approaches are explored alongside the advances in structural analysis techniques that have occurred in recent years. As a consequence, we believe heparin mimetics with superior absorption, distribution, metabolism and excretion properties will be developed and for at least some of these mimetics significant therapeutic benefits will result from their ability to act in multiple molecular pathways.

Acknowledgments: This work was supported by grants from Glycan Biosciences LLC, Philadelphia, PA, USA, to Deirdre R. Coombe.

Author Contributions: Both S.M. and D.R.C. provided intellectual input and both drafted sections of the manuscript and S.M. prepared the figures. Both authors vetted and approved the final manuscript.

Conflicts of Interest: The authors declare no conflict of interest.

References

1. Parish, C.R. The role of heparan sulfate in inflammation. *Nat. Rev. Immunol.* **2006**, *6*, 633–643. [CrossRef] [PubMed]
2. Iozzo, R.V.; San Antonio, J.D. Heparan sulfate proteoglycans: Heavy hitters in the angiogenesis arena. *J. Clin. Investig.* **2001**, *108*, 349–355. [CrossRef] [PubMed]
3. Diaz-Nido, J.; Wandosell, F.; Avila, J. Glycosaminoglycans and β-amyloid, prion and tau peptides in neurodegenerative diseases. *Peptides* **2002**, *23*, 1323–1332. [CrossRef]
4. Rosenberg, R.D.; Shworak, N.W.; Liu, J.; Schwartz, J.J.; Zhang, L. Heparan sulfate proteoglycans of the cardiovascular system. Specific structures emerge but how is synthesis regulated? *J. Clin. Investig.* **1997**, *99*, 2062–2070. [CrossRef] [PubMed]
5. Yip, G.W.; Smollich, M.; Goette, M. Therapeutic value of glycosaminoglycans in cancer. *Mol. Cancer Ther.* **2006**, *5*, 2139–2148. [CrossRef] [PubMed]
6. Rostand, K.S.; Esko, J.D. Microbial adherence to and invasion through proteoglycans. *Infect. Immun.* **1997**, *65*, 1–8. [PubMed]
7. Kolset, S.O.; Tveit, H. Serglycin—Structure and biology. *Cell. Mol. Life Sci.* **2008**, *65*, 1073–1085. [CrossRef] [PubMed]
8. Linhardt, R.J. 2003 Claude S. Hudson award address in carbohydrate chemistry. Heparin: Structure and activity. *J. Med. Chem.* **2003**, *46*, 2551–2564. [CrossRef] [PubMed]
9. Wardrop, D.; Keeling, D. The story of the discovery of heparin and warfarin. *Br. J. Haematol.* **2008**, *141*, 757–763. [CrossRef] [PubMed]
10. Mulloy, B.; Hogwood, J.; Gray, E.; Lever, R.; Page Clive, P. Pharmacology of heparin and related drugs. *Pharmacol. Rev.* **2016**, *68*, 76–141. [CrossRef] [PubMed]

11. Iqbal, Z.; Cohen, M. Enoxaparin: A pharmacologic and clinical review. *Expert Opin. Pharmacother.* **2011**, *12*, 1157–1170. [CrossRef] [PubMed]
12. Rabenstein, D.L. Heparin and heparan sulfate: Structure and function. *Nat. Prod. Rep.* **2002**, *19*, 312–331. [CrossRef] [PubMed]
13. El Masri, R.; Seffouh, A.; Lortat-Jacob, H.; Vives, R.R. The "in and out" of glucosamine 6-*O*-sulfation: The 6th sense of heparan sulfate. *Glycoconj. J.* **2017**, *34*, 285–298. [CrossRef] [PubMed]
14. Kett, W.C.; Coombe, D.R. A structural analysis of heparin-like glycosaminoglycans using MALDI-TOF mass spectrometry. *Spectroscopy* **2004**, *18*, 185–201. [CrossRef]
15. Singh, A.; Kett, W.C.; Severin, I.C.; Agyekum, I.; Duan, J.; Amster, I.J.; Proudfoot, A.E.I.; Coombe, D.R.; Woods, R.J. The interaction of heparin tetrasaccharides with chemokine CCL5 is modulated by sulfation pattern and pH. *J. Biol. Chem.* **2015**, *290*, 15421–15436. [CrossRef] [PubMed]
16. Paulsen, H. Advances in selective chemical syntheses of complex oligosaccharides. *Angew. Chem. Int. Ed. Engl.* **1982**, *21*, 155–173. [CrossRef]
17. Dulaney, S.B.; Huang, X. Strategies in synthesis of heparin/heparan sulfate oligosaccharides: 2000–present. *Adv. Carbohydr. Chem. Biochem.* **2012**, *67*, 95–136. [PubMed]
18. Hu, Y.-P.; Zhong, Y.-Q.; Chen, Z.-G.; Chen, C.-Y.; Shi, Z.; Zulueta, M.M.L.; Ku, C.-C.; Lee, P.-Y.; Wang, C.-C.; Hung, S.-C. Divergent synthesis of 48 heparan sulfate-based disaccharides and probing the specific sugar-fibroblast growth factor-1 interaction. *J. Am. Chem. Soc.* **2012**, *134*, 20722–20727. [CrossRef] [PubMed]
19. Arungundram, S.; Al-Mafraji, K.; Asong, J.; Leach, F.E., III; Amster, I.J.; Venot, A.; Turnbull, J.E.; Boons, G.-J. Modular synthesis of heparan sulfate oligosaccharides for structure activity relationship studies. *J. Am. Chem. Soc.* **2009**, *131*, 17394–17405. [CrossRef] [PubMed]
20. Mohamed, S.; Ferro, V. Synthetic approaches to L-iduronic acid and L-idose: Key building blocks for the preparation of glycosaminoglycan oligosaccharides. *Adv. Carbohydr. Chem. Biochem.* **2015**, *72*, 21–61. [PubMed]
21. Coombe, D.; Kett, W.C. Heparin mimetics. *Handb. Exp. Pharmacol.* **2012**, *207*, 361–383.
22. Kreuger, J.; Salmivirta, M.; Sturiale, L.; Gimenez-Gallego, G.; Lindahl, U. Sequence analysis of heparan sulfate epitopes with graded affinities for fibroblast growth factors 1 and 2. *J. Biol. Chem.* **2001**, *276*, 30744–30752. [CrossRef] [PubMed]
23. Khan, S.; Fung Ka, W.; Rodriguez, E.; Patel, R.; Gor, J.; Mulloy, B.; Perkins Stephen, J. The solution structure of heparan sulfate differs from that of heparin: Implications for function. *J. Biol. Chem.* **2013**, *288*, 27737–27751. [CrossRef] [PubMed]
24. Sarrazin, S.; Bonnaffe, D.; Lubineau, A.; Lortat-Jacob, H. Heparan sulfate mimicry: A synthetic glycoconjugate that recognizes the heparin binding domain of interferon-γ inhibits the cytokine activity. *J. Biol. Chem.* **2005**, *280*, 37558–37564. [CrossRef] [PubMed]
25. Blossom, D.B.; Kallen, A.J.; Patel, P.R.; Elward, A.; Robinson, L.; Gao, G.; Langer, R.; Perkins, K.M.; Jaeger, J.L.; Kurkjian, K.M.; et al. Outbreak of adverse reactions associated with contaminated heparin. *N. Engl. J. Med.* **2008**, *359*, 2674–2684. [CrossRef] [PubMed]
26. Chess, E.K.; Bairstow, S.; Donovan, S.; Havel, K.; Hu, P.; Johnson, R.J.; Lee, S.; McKee, J.; Miller, R.; Moore, E.; et al. Case study: Contamination of heparin with oversulfated chondroitin sulfate. *Handb. Exp. Pharmacol.* **2012**, *207*, 99–125.
27. Hirsh, J.; Warkentin, T.E.; Raschke, R.; Granger, C.; Ohman, E.M.; Dalen, J.E. Heparin and low molecular weight heparin: Mechanisms of action, pharmacokinetics, dosing considerations, monitoring, efficacy, and safety. *Chest* **1998**, *114*, 489S–510S. [CrossRef] [PubMed]
28. Warkentin, T.E.; Levine, M.N.; Hirsh, J.; Horsewood, P.; Roberts, R.S.; Gent, M.; Kelton, J.G. Heparin-induced thrombocytopenia in patients treated with low-molecular-weight heparin or unfractionated heparin. *N. Engl. J. Med.* **1995**, *332*, 1330–1335. [CrossRef] [PubMed]
29. Petitou, M.; van Boeckel Constant, A.A. A synthetic antithrombin III binding pentasaccharide is now a Drug! What comes next? *Angew. Chem. Int. Ed. Engl.* **2004**, *43*, 3118–3133. [CrossRef] [PubMed]
30. Klement, P.; Rak, J. Emerging anticoagulants: Mechanism of action and future potential. *Vnitr. Lek.* **2006**, *52*, 119–122. [PubMed]
31. Bauer, K.A. Selective inhibition of coagulation factors: Advances in antithrombotic therapy. *Semin. Thromb. Hemostasis* **2002**, *28*, 15–24. [CrossRef] [PubMed]

32. Herbert, J.M.; Petitou, M.; Lormeau, J.C.; Cariou, R.; Necciari, J.; Magnani, H.N.; Zandberg, P.; van Amsterdam, R.G.M.; van Boeckel, C.A.A.; Meuleman, D.G. SR 90107 A/Org 31540, A novel anti-factor Xa antithrombotic agent. *Cardiovasc. Drug Rev.* **1997**, *15*, 1–26. [CrossRef]
33. Van Boeckel Constant, A.A.; Petitou, M. The unique antithrombin III binding domain of heparin: A lead to new synthetic antithrombotics. *Angew. Chem. Int. Ed. Engl.* **1993**, *32*, 1671–1818. [CrossRef]
34. Herbert, J.M.; Herault, J.P.; Bernat, A.; Van Amsterdam, R.G.M.; Lormeau, J.C.; Petitou, M.; Van Boeckel, C.; Hoffmann, P.; Meuleman, D.G. Biochemical and pharmacological properties of SANORG 34006, a potent and long-acting synthetic pentasaccharide. *Blood* **1998**, *91*, 4197–4205. [PubMed]
35. Westerduin, P.; van Boeckel, C.A.A.; Basten, J.E.M.; Broekhoven, M.A.; Lucas, H.; Rood, A.; van der Heijden, H.; van Amsterdam, R.G.M.; van Dinther, T.G.; et al. Feasible synthesis and biological properties of Six 'non-glycosamino' glycan analogs of the antithrombin III binding heparin pentasaccharide. *Bioorg. Med. Chem.* **1994**, *2*, 1267–1280. [CrossRef]
36. Prandoni, P.; Tormene, D.; Perlati, M.; Brandolin, B.; Spiezia, L. Idraparinux: Review of its clinical efficacy and safety for prevention and treatment of thromboembolic disorders. *Expert Opin. Investig. Drugs* **2008**, *17*, 773–777. [CrossRef] [PubMed]
37. Paty, I.; Trellu, M.; Destors, J.M.; Cortez, P.; Boelle, E.; Sanderink, G. Reversibility of the anti-FXa activity of idrabiotaparinux (biotinylated idraparinux) by intravenous avidin infusion. *J. Thromb. Haemost.* **2010**, *8*, 722–729. [CrossRef] [PubMed]
38. Savi, P.; Herault, J.P.; Duchaussoy, P.; Millet, L.; Schaeffer, P.; Petitou, M.; Bono, F.; Herbert, J.M. Reversible biotinylated oligosaccharides: A new approach for a better management of anticoagulant therapy. *J. Thromb. Haemost.* **2008**, *6*, 1697–1706. [CrossRef] [PubMed]
39. Song, Y.; Li, X.; Pavithra, S.; Li, D. Idraparinux or idrabiotaparinux for long-term venous thromboembolism treatment: A systematic review and meta-analysis of randomized controlled trials. *PLoS ONE* **2013**, *8*, e78972. [CrossRef] [PubMed]
40. Petitou, M.; Herault, J.-P.; Bernat, A.; Driguez, P.-A.; Duchaussoy, P.; Lormeau, J.-C.; Herbert, J.-M. Synthesis of thrombin-inhibiting heparin mimetics without side effects. *Nature* **1999**, *398*, 417–422. [PubMed]
41. Casu, B. Structure and biological activity of heparin. *Adv. Carbohydr. Chem. Biochem.* **1985**, *43*, 51–134. [PubMed]
42. Herbert, J.M.; Herault, J.P.; Bernat, A.; Savi, P.; Schaeffer, P.; Driguez, P.A.; Duchaussoy, P.; Petitou, M. SR123781A, A synthetic heparin mimetic. *Thromb. Haemost.* **2001**, *85*, 852–860. [PubMed]
43. Bal dit Sollier, C.; Kang, C.; Berge, N.; Herault, J.P.; Bonneau, M.; Herbert, J.M.; Drouet, L. Activity of a synthetic hexadecasaccharide (SanOrg123781A) in a pig model of arterial thrombosis. *J. Thromb. Haemost.* **2004**, *2*, 925–930. [CrossRef] [PubMed]
44. Hoppensteadt, D.; Cunanan, J.; Geniaux, E.; Lorenz, M.; Viskov, C.; Ythier-Moury, P.; Brin, J.-F.; Jeske, W. AVE5026: A novel, extractive heparinoid with enriched anti-Xa activity and enhanced antithrombotic activity. *Blood* **2007**, *110*, 1881.
45. Viskov, C.; Just, M.; Laux, V.; Mourier, P.; Lorenz, M. Description of the chemical and pharmacological characteristics of a new hemisynthetic ultra-low-molecular-weight heparin, AVE5026. *J. Thromb. Haemost.* **2009**, *7*, 1143–1151. [CrossRef] [PubMed]
46. Lassen, M.R.; Dahl, O.E.; Mismetti, P.; Destree, D.; Turpie, A.G.G. AVE5026, A new hemisynthetic ultra-low-molecular-weight heparin for the prevention of venous thromboembolism in patients after total knee replacement surgery—TREK: A dose-ranging study. *J. Thromb. Haemost.* **2009**, *7*, 566–572. [CrossRef] [PubMed]
47. Oh Young, I.; Sheng Gloria, J.; Chang, S.-K.; Hsieh-Wilson Linda, C. Tailored glycopolymers as anticoagulant heparin mimetics. *Angew. Chem. Int. Ed. Engl.* **2013**, *52*, 11796–11799.
48. Brandt, S.; Krauel, K.; Jaax, M.; Renne, T.; Helm Christiane, A.; Hammerschmidt, S.; Delcea, M.; Greinacher, A. Polyphosphates form antigenic complexes with platelet factor 4 (PF4) and enhance PF4-binding to bacteria. *Thromb. Haemost.* **2015**, *114*, 1189–1198. [CrossRef] [PubMed]
49. Jaax, M.E.; Krauel, K.; Marschall, T.; Brandt, S.; Gansler, J.; Fuerll, B.; Appel, B.; Fischer, S.; Block, S.; Helm, C.A.; et al. Complex formation with nucleic acids and aptamers alters the antigenic properties of platelet factor 4. *Blood* **2013**, *122*, 272–281. [CrossRef] [PubMed]
50. Zacharski, L.R.; Ornstein, D.L.; Mamourian, A.C. Low-molecular-weight heparin and cancer. *Semin. Thromb. Hemost.* **2000**, *26*, 69–77. [CrossRef] [PubMed]

51. Casu, B.; Vlodavsky, I.; Sanderson, R.D. Non-anticoagulant heparins and inhibition of cancer. *Pathophysiol. Haemost. Thromb.* **2008**, *36*, 195–203. [CrossRef] [PubMed]

52. Lee, D.Y.; Lee, S.W.; Kim, S.K.; Lee, M.; Chang, H.W.; Moon, H.T.; Byun, Y.; Kim, S.Y. Antiangiogenic activity of orally absorbable heparin derivative in different types of cancer cells. *Pharm. Res.* **2009**, *26*, 2667–2676. [CrossRef] [PubMed]

53. Mousa, S.A.; Linhardt, R.; Francis, J.L.; Amirkhosravi, A. Anti-metastatic effect of a non-anticoagulant low-molecular-weight heparin versus the standard low-molecular-weight heparin, Enoxaparin. *Thromb. Haemost.* **2006**, *96*, 816–821. [CrossRef] [PubMed]

54. Kakkar, A.K.; Levine, M.N.; Kadziola, Z.; Lemoine, N.R.; Low, V.; Patel, H.K.; Rustin, G.; Thomas, M.; Quigley, M.; Williamson, R.C.N. Low molecular weight heparin, therapy with dalteparin, and survival in advanced cancer: The Fragmin Advanced Malignancy Outcome Study (FAMOUS). *J. Clin. Oncol.* **2004**, *22*, 1944–1948. [CrossRef] [PubMed]

55. Kuderer, N.M.; Ortel, T.L.; Francis, C.W. Impact of venous thromboembolism and anticoagulation on cancer and cancer survival. *J. Clin. Oncol.* **2009**, *27*, 4902–4911. [CrossRef] [PubMed]

56. Vlodavsky, I.; Ilan, N.; Naggi, A.; Casu, B. Heparanase: Structure, biological functions, and inhibition by heparin-derived mimetics of heparan sulfate. *Curr. Pharm. Des.* **2007**, *13*, 2057–2073. [CrossRef] [PubMed]

57. Miao, H.-Q.; Liu, H.; Navarro, E.; Kussie, P.; Zhu, Z. Development of heparanase inhibitors for anti-cancer therapy. *Curr. Med. Chem.* **2006**, *13*, 2101–2111. [PubMed]

58. Kilarski, W.W.; Bikfalvi, A. Recent developments in tumor angiogenesis. *Curr. Pharm. Biotechnol.* **2007**, *8*, 3–9. [CrossRef] [PubMed]

59. Rusnati, M.; Presta, M. Fibroblast growth factors/fibroblast growth factor receptors as targets for the development of anti-angiogenesis strategies. *Curr. Pharm. Des.* **2007**, *13*, 2025–2044. [CrossRef] [PubMed]

60. Kessler, T.; Fehrmann, F.; Bieker, R.; Berdel, W.E.; Mesters, R.M. Vascular endothelial growth factor and its receptor as drug targets in hematological malignancies. *Curr. Drug Targets* **2007**, *8*, 257–268. [CrossRef] [PubMed]

61. Ellis, L.M.; Hicklin, D.J. VEGF-targeted therapy: Mechanisms of anti-tumour activity. *Nat. Rev. Cancer* **2008**, *8*, 579–591. [CrossRef] [PubMed]

62. Ferro, V.; Fewings, K.; Palermo, M.C.; Li, C. Large-scale preparation of the oligosaccharide phosphate fraction of Pichia holstii NRRL Y-2448 phosphomannan for use in the manufacture of PI-88. *Carbohydr. Res.* **2001**, *332*, 183–189. [CrossRef]

63. Ferro, V.; Li, C.; Fewings, K.; Palermo, M.C.; Linhardt, R.J.; Toida, T. Determination of the composition of the oligosaccharide phosphate fraction of Pichia (Hansenula) holstii NRRL Y-2448 phosphomannan by capillary electrophoresis and HPLC. *Carbohydr. Res.* **2002**, *337*, 139–146. [CrossRef]

64. Khachigian, L.M.; Parish, C.R. Phosphomannopentaose sulfate (PI-88): Heparan sulfate mimetic with clinical potential in multiple vascular pathologies. *Cardiovasc. Drug Rev.* **2004**, *22*, 1–6. [CrossRef] [PubMed]

65. Handley, P.N.; Carroll, A.; Ferro, V. New structural insights into the oligosaccharide phosphate fraction of Pichia (Hansenula) holstii NRRL Y2448 phosphomannan. *Carbohydr. Res.* **2017**, *446–447*, 68–75. [CrossRef] [PubMed]

66. Kudchadkar, R.; Gonzalez, R.; Lewis, K.D. PI-88: A novel inhibitor of angiogenesis. *Expert Opin. Investig. Drugs* **2008**, *17*, 1769–1776. [CrossRef] [PubMed]

67. Liao, B.-Y.; Wang, Z.; Hu, J.; Liu, W.-F.; Shen, Z.-Z.; Zhang, X.; Yu, L.; Fan, J.; Zhou, J. PI-88 inhibits postoperative recurrence of hepatocellular carcinoma via disrupting the surge of heparanase after liver resection. *Tumor Biol.* **2016**, *37*, 2987–2998. [CrossRef] [PubMed]

68. Liu, C.-J.; Lee, P.-H.; Lin, D.-Y.; Wu, C.-C.; Jeng, L.-B.; Lin, P.-W.; Mok, K.-T.; Lee, W.-C.; Yeh, H.-Z.; Ho, M.-C.; et al. Heparanase inhibitor PI-88 as adjuvant therapy for hepatocellular carcinoma after curative resection: A randomized phase II trial for safety and optimal dosage. *J. Hepatol.* **2009**, *50*, 958–968. [CrossRef] [PubMed]

69. Lewis, K.D.; Robinson, W.A.; Millward, M.J.; Powell, A.; Price, T.J.; Thomson, D.B.; Walpole, E.T.; Haydon, A.M.; Creese, B.R.; Roberts, K.L.; et al. A phase II study of the heparanase inhibitor PI-88 in patients with advanced melanoma. *Investig. New Drugs* **2008**, *26*, 89–94. [CrossRef] [PubMed]

70. Karoli, T.; Liu, L.; Fairweather, J.K.; Hammond, E.; Li, C.P.; Cochran, S.; Bergefall, K.; Trybala, E.; Addison, R.S.; Ferro, V. Synthesis, biological activity, and preliminary pharmacokinetic evaluation of analogs of a phosphosulfomannan angiogenesis inhibitor (PI-88). *J. Med. Chem.* **2005**, *48*, 8229–8236. [CrossRef] [PubMed]
71. Johnstone, K.D.; Karoli, T.; Liu, L.; Dredge, K.; Copeman, E.; Li, C.P.; Davis, K.; Hammond, E.; Bytheway, I.; Kostewicz, E.; et al. Synthesis and biological evaluation of polysulfated oligosaccharide glycosides as inhibitors of angiogenesis and tumor growth. *J. Med. Chem.* **2010**, *53*, 1686–1699. [CrossRef] [PubMed]
72. Ferro, V.; Dredge, K.; Liu, L.; Hammond, E.; Bytheway, I.; Li, C.; Johnstone, K.; Karoli, T.; Davis, K.; Copeman, E.; et al. PI-88 and novel heparan sulfate mimetics inhibit angiogenesis. *Semin. Thromb. Hemost.* **2007**, *33*, 557–562. [CrossRef] [PubMed]
73. Dredge, K.; Hammond, E.; Davis, K.; Li, C.P.; Liu, L.; Johnstone, K.; Handley, P.; Wimmer, N.; Gonda, T.J.; Gautam, A.; et al. The PG500 series: Novel heparan sulfate mimetics as potent angiogenesis and heparanase inhibitors for cancer therapy. *Investig. New Drugs* **2010**, *28*, 276–283. [CrossRef] [PubMed]
74. Ferro, V.; Liu, L.; Johnstone, K.D.; Wimmer, N.; Karoli, T.; Handley, P.; Rowley, J.; Dredge, K.; Li, C.P.; Hammond, E.; et al. Discovery of PG545: A highly potent and simultaneous inhibitor of angiogenesis, tumor growth, and metastasis. *J. Med. Chem.* **2012**, *55*, 3804–3813. [CrossRef] [PubMed]
75. Dredge, K.; Hammond, E.; Handley, P.; Gonda, T.J.; Smith, M.T.; Vincent, C.; Brandt, R.; Ferro, V.; Bytheway, I. PG545, A dual heparanase and angiogenesis inhibitor, induces potent anti-tumour and anti-metastatic efficacy in preclinical models. *Br. J. Cancer* **2011**, *104*, 635–642. [CrossRef] [PubMed]
76. Hammond, E.; Handley, P.; Dredge, K.; Bytheway, I. Mechanisms of heparanase inhibition by the heparan sulfate mimetic PG545 and three structural analogues. *FEBS Open Bio* **2013**, *3*, 346–351. [CrossRef] [PubMed]
77. Brennan Todd, V.; Lin, L.; Brandstadter Joshua, D.; Rendell Victoria, R.; Dredge, K.; Huang, X.; Yang, Y. Heparan sulfate mimetic PG545-mediated antilymphoma effects require TLR9-dependent NK cell activation. *J. Clin. Investig.* **2016**, *126*, 207–219. [CrossRef] [PubMed]
78. Jung, D.-B.; Yun, M.; Kim, E.-O.; Kim, J.; Kim, B.; Jung Ji, H.; Kim, S.-H.; Kim, E.-O.; Wang, E.; Mukhopadhyay, D.; et al. The heparan sulfate mimetic PG545 interferes with Wnt/β-catenin signaling and significantly suppresses pancreatic tumorigenesis alone and in combination with gemcitabine. *Oncotarget* **2015**, *6*, 4992–5004. [CrossRef] [PubMed]
79. Rudd, T.R.; Uniewicz, K.A.; Ori, A.; Guimond, S.E.; Skidmore, M.A.; Gaudesi, D.; Xu, R.; Turnbull, J.E.; Guerrini, M.; Torri, G.; et al. Comparable stabilization, structural changes and activities can be induced in FGF by a variety of HS and non-GAG analogues: Implications for sequence-activity relationships. *Org. Biomol. Chem.* **2010**, *8*, 5390–5397. [CrossRef] [PubMed]
80. Freeman, C.; Liu, L.; Banwell, M.G.; Brown, K.J.; Bezos, A.; Ferro, V.; Parish, C.R. Use of sulfated linked cyclitols as heparan sulfate mimetics to probe the heparin/heparan sulfate binding specificity of proteins. *J. Biol. Chem.* **2005**, *280*, 8842–8849. [CrossRef] [PubMed]
81. Liu, L.; Li, C.; Cochran, S.; Feder, D.; Guddat, L.W.; Ferro, V. A focused sulfated glycoconjugate ugi library for probing heparan sulfate-binding angiogenic growth factors. *Bioorg. Med. Chem. Lett.* **2012**, *22*, 6190–6194. [CrossRef] [PubMed]
82. Huang, L.; Fernandez, C.; Kerns, R.J. Different protein-binding selectivities for *N*-acyl heparin derivatives having *N*-phenylacetyl and heterocycle analogs of *N*-phenylacetyl substituted in place of *N*-sulfo groups. *Bioorg. Med. Chem.* **2007**, *17*, 419–423. [CrossRef] [PubMed]
83. Liu, L.; Li, C.; Cochran, S.; Jimmink, S.; Ferro, V. Synthesis of a heparan sulfate mimetic library targeting FGF and VEGF via click chemistry on a monosaccharide template. *ChemMedChem* **2012**, *7*, 1267–1275. [CrossRef] [PubMed]
84. Nancy-Portebois, V.; Cabannes, E.; Petitou, M.; Serin, G.; Mirjolet, J.-F. Antitumor Activity of EP80061, a Small-Glyco Drug in Preclinical Studies. In Proceedings of the 101st Annual Meeting of the American Association for Cancer Research, Washington, DC, USA, 17–21 April 2010; Cancer Research: Washington, DC, USA, 2010; p. 5459.
85. Naggi, A.; Casu, B.; Perez, M.; Torri, G.; Cassinelli, G.; Penco, S.; Pisano, C.; Giannini, G.; Ishai-Michaeli, R.; Vlodavsky, I. Modulation of the heparanase-inhibiting activity of heparin through selective desulfation, graded *N*-acetylation, and glycol splitting. *J. Biol. Chem.* **2005**, *280*, 12103–12113. [CrossRef] [PubMed]

86. Ritchie, J.P.; Ramani, V.C.; Ren, Y.; Naggi, A.; Torri, G.; Casu, B.; Penco, S.; Pisano, C.; Carminati, P.; Tortoreto, M.; et al. SST0001, A chemically modified heparin, inhibits myeloma growth and angiogenesis via disruption of the heparanase/syndecan-1 axis. *Clin. Cancer Res.* **2011**, *17*, 1382–1393. [CrossRef] [PubMed]

87. Cassinelli, G.; Favini, E.; Dal Bo, L.; Tortoreto, M.; Zunino, F.; Zaffaroni, N.; Lanzi, C.; De Maglie, M.; De Maglie, M.; Dagrada, G.; et al. Antitumor efficacy of the heparan sulfate mimic roneparstat (SST0001) against sarcoma models involves multi-target inhibition of receptor tyrosine kinases. *Oncotarget* **2016**, *7*, 47848–47863. [CrossRef] [PubMed]

88. Zhou, H.; Roy, S.; Cochran, E.; Zouaoui, R.; Chu, C.L.; Duffner, J.; Zhao, G.; Smith, S.; Galcheva-Gargova, Z.; Karlgren, J.; et al. M402, A novel heparan sulfate mimetic, targets multiple pathways implicated in tumor progression and metastasis. *PLoS ONE* **2011**, *6*, e21106. [CrossRef] [PubMed]

89. Ni, M.; Elli, S.; Naggi, A.; Guerrini, M.; Torri, G.; Petitou, M. Investigating glycol-split-heparin-derived inhibitors of heparanase: A study of synthetic trisaccharides. *Molecules* **2016**, *21*, 1602. [CrossRef] [PubMed]

90. Cabannes, E.; Caravano, A.; Lewandowski, D.; Motte, V.; Nancy-Portebois, V.; Petitou, M.; Pierdet, P. Oligosaccharide compounds for use in mobilising stem cells. Patent No. WO2010029185 A1, 18 March 2010.

91. Kuhnast, B.; El Hadri, A.; Boisgard, R.; Hinnen, F.; Richard, S.; Caravano, A.; Nancy-Portebois, V.; Petitou, M.; Tavitian, B.; Dolle, F. Synthesis, radiolabeling with fluorine-18 and preliminary in vivo evaluation of a heparan sulfate mimetic as potent angiogenesis and heparanase inhibitor for cancer applications. *Org. Biomol. Chem.* **2016**, *14*, 1915–1920. [CrossRef] [PubMed]

92. Capila, I.; Linhardt Robert, J. Heparin-protein interactions. *Angew. Chem. Int. Ed. Engl.* **2002**, *41*, 391–412. [CrossRef]

93. Yan, Y.; Ji, Y.; Su, N.; Mei, X.; Wang, Y.; Du, S.; Zhu, W.; Zhang, C.; Lu, Y.; Xing, X.-H. Non-anticoagulant effects of low molecular weight heparins in inflammatory disorders: A review. *Carbohydr. Polym.* **2017**, *160*, 71–81. [CrossRef] [PubMed]

94. Chande, N.; MacDonald John, K.; Wang Josh, J.; McDonald John, W.D. Unfractionated or low molecular weight heparin for induction of remission in ulcerative colitis: A Cochrane inflammatory bowel disease and functional bowel disorders systematic review of randomized trials. *Inflamm. Bowel. Dis.* **2011**, *17*, 1979–1986. [CrossRef] [PubMed]

95. Reimann, S.; Groeger, D.; Kuehne, C.; Riese, S.B.; Dernedde, J.; Haag, R. Shell cleavable dendritic polyglycerol sulfates show high anti-inflammatory properties by inhibiting L-selectin binding and complement activation. *Adv. Healthcare Mater.* **2015**, *4*, 2154–2162. [CrossRef] [PubMed]

96. Severin India, C.; Soares, A.; Hantson, J.; Teixeira, M.; Sachs, D.; Valognes, D.; Scheer, A.; Schwarz Matthias, K.; Wells Timothy, N.C.; Proudfoot Amanda, E.I.; et al. Glycosaminoglycan analogs as a novel anti-inflammatory strategy. *Front. Immunol.* **2012**, *3*, 293. [CrossRef] [PubMed]

97. Zaferani, A.; Talsma, D.; Richter, M.K.S.; Daha, M.R.; Navis, G.J.; Seelen, M.A.; van den Born, J. Heparin/heparan sulphate interactions with complement-A possible target for reduction of renal function loss? *Nephrol. Dial. Transplant.* **2014**, *29*, 515–522. [CrossRef] [PubMed]

98. Gaffney, A.; Gaffney, P. Rheumatoid arthritis and heparin. *Br. J. Rheumatol.* **1996**, *35*, 808–809. [CrossRef] [PubMed]

99. Gaffney, P.R.; Doyle, C.T.; Gaffney, A.; Hogan, J.; Hayes, D.P.; Annis, P. Paradoxical response to heparin in 10 patients with ulcerative colitis. *Am. J. Gastroenterol.* **1995**, *90*, 220–223. [PubMed]

100. Evans, R.C.; Shim Wong, V.; Morris, A.I.; Rhodes, J.M. Treatment of corticosteroid-resistant ulcerative colitis with heparin-A report of 16 cases. *Aliment. Pharmacol. Ther.* **1997**, *11*, 1037–1040. [CrossRef] [PubMed]

101. Vancheri, C.; Mastruzzo, C.; Armato, F.; Tomaselli, V.; Magri, S.; Pistorio, P.; LaMicela, M.; D'Amico, L.; Crimi, N. Intranasal heparin reduces eosinophil recruitment after nasal allergen challenge in patients with allergic rhinitis. *J. Allergy Clin. Immunol.* **2001**, *108*, 703–708. [CrossRef] [PubMed]

102. Bendstrup, K.E.; Jensen, J.I. Inhaled heparin is effective in exacerbations of asthma. *Respir. Med.* **2000**, *94*, 174–175. [CrossRef] [PubMed]

103. Ahmed, T.; Gonzalez, B.J.; Danta, I. Prevention of a exercise-induced bronchoconstriction by inhaled low-molecular-weight heparin. *Am. J. Respir. Crit. Care. Med.* **1999**, *160*, 576–581. [CrossRef] [PubMed]

104. Simanek, E.E.; McGarvey, G.J.; Jablonowski, J.A.; Wong, C.-H. Selectin-carbohydrate interactions: From natural ligands to designed mimics. *Chem. Rev.* **1998**, *98*, 833–862. [CrossRef] [PubMed]

105. Nimrichter, L.; Burdick, M.M.; Aoki, K.; Laroy, W.; Fierro, M.A.; Hudson, S.A.; Von Seggern, C.E.; Cotter, R.J.; Bochner, B.S.; Tiemeyer, M.; et al. E-selectin receptors on human leukocytes. *Blood* **2008**, *112*, 3744–3752. [CrossRef] [PubMed]

106. Chang, J.; Patton, J.T.; Sarkar, A.; Ernst, B.; Magnani, J.L.; Frenette, P.S. GMI-1070, A novel pan-selectin antagonist, reverses acute vascular occlusions in sickle cell mice. *Blood* **2010**, *116*, 1779–1786. [CrossRef] [PubMed]

107. Magnani, J.L.; Patton, J.T.; Sarkar, A.K.; Svarovsky, S.A.; Ernst, B. Heterobifunctional Pan-Selectin Inhibitors. Patnent No. WO2007028050 A1, 8 March 2007.

108. Wun, T.; Styles, L.; DeCastro, L.; Telen, M.J.; Kuypers, F.; Cheung, A.; Kramer, W.; Flanner, H.; Rhee, S.; Magnani, J.L.; et al. Phase 1 study of the E-selectin inhibitor GMI 1070 in patients with sickle cell anemia. *PLoS ONE* **2014**, *9*, e101301. [CrossRef] [PubMed]

109. Telen, M.J.; Wun, T.; McCavit, T.L.; De Castro, L.M.; Krishnamurti, L.; Lanzkron, S.; Hsu, L.L.; Smith, W.R.; Rhee, S.; Magnani, J.L.; et al. Randomized phase 2 study of GMI-1070 in SCD: Reduction in time to resolution of vaso-occlusive events and decreased opioid use. *Blood* **2015**, *125*, 2656–2664. [CrossRef] [PubMed]

110. Schwizer, D.; Patton, J.T.; Cutting, B.; Smiesko, M.; Wagner, B.; Kato, A.; Weckerle, C.; Binder, F.P.C.; Rabbani, S.; Schwardt, O.; et al. Pre-organization of the core structure of E-selectin antagonists. *Chem. Eur. J.* **2012**, *18*, 1342–1351. [CrossRef] [PubMed]

111. Somers, W.S.; Tang, J.; Shaw, G.D.; Camphausen, R.T. Insights into the molecular basis of leukocyte tethering and rolling revealed by structures of P- and E-selectin bound to SLex and PSGL-1. *Cell* **2000**, *103*, 467–479. [CrossRef]

112. Egger, J.; Weckerle, C.; Cutting, B.; Schwardt, O.; Rabbani, S.; Lemme, K.; Ernst, B. Nano-molar E-selectin antagonists with prolonged half-lives by a fragment-based approach. *J. Am. Chem. Soc.* **2013**, *135*, 9820–9828. [CrossRef] [PubMed]

113. Kansas, G.S. Selectins and their ligands: Current concepts and controversies. *Blood* **1996**, *88*, 3259–3287. [PubMed]

114. Fritzsche, J.; Alban, S.; Ludwig, R.J.; Rubant, S.; Boehncke, W.-H.; Schumacher, G.; Bendas, G. The influence of various structural parameters of semisynthetic sulfated polysaccharides on the P-selectin inhibitory capacity. *Biochem. Pharmacol.* **2006**, *72*, 474–485. [CrossRef] [PubMed]

115. Simonis, D.; Fritzsche, J.; Alban, S.; Bendas, G. Kinetic analysis of heparin and glucan sulfates binding to P-selectin and its impact on the general understanding of selectin inhibition. *Biochemistry* **2007**, *46*, 6156–6164. [CrossRef] [PubMed]

116. Alban, S.; Ludwig, R.J.; Bendas, G.; Schoen, M.P.; Oostingh, G.J.; Radeke, H.H.; Fritzsche, J.; Pfeilschifter, J.; Kaufmann, R.; Boehncke, W.-H. PS3, A semisynthetic β-1,3-glucan sulfate, diminishes contact hypersensitivity responses through inhibition of L- and P-selectin functions. *J. Investig. Dermatol.* **2009**, *129*, 1192–1202. [CrossRef] [PubMed]

117. Weinhart, M.; Groger, D.; Enders, S.; Dernedde, J.; Haag, R. Synthesis of dendritic polyglycerol anions and their efficiency toward L-selectin inhibition. *Biomacromolecules* **2011**, *12*, 2502–2511. [CrossRef] [PubMed]

118. Pant, K.; Groeger, D.; Bergmann, R.; Pietzsch, J.; Steinbach, J.; Graham, B.; Spiccia, L.; Berthon, F.; Czarny, B.; Devel, L.; et al. Synthesis and biodistribution studies of ^{3}H- and ^{64}Cu-labeled dendritic polyglycerol and dendritic polyglycerol sulfate. *Bioconjugate Chem.* **2015**, *26*, 906–918. [CrossRef] [PubMed]

119. Schoenfeld, A.-K.; Lahrsen, E.; Alban, S. Regulation of complement and contact system activation via C1 inhibitor potentiation and factor XIIa activity modulation by sulfated glycans - structure-activity relationships. *PLoS ONE* **2016**, *11*, e0165493. [CrossRef] [PubMed]

120. Beinrohr, L.; Harmat, V.; Dobó, J.; Löerincz, Z.; Gál, P.; Závodszky, P. C1 inhibitor serpin domain structure reveals the likely mechanism of heparin potentiation and conformational disease. *J. Biol. Chem.* **2007**, *282*, 21100–21109. [CrossRef] [PubMed]

121. Sheng, G.J.; Oh, Y.I.; Chang, S.-K.; Hsieh-Wilson, L.C. Tunable heparan sulfate mimetics for modulating chemokine activity. *J. Am. Chem. Soc.* **2013**, *135*, 10898–10901. [CrossRef] [PubMed]

122. Jayson, G.C.; Hansen, S.U.; Miller, G.J.; Cole, C.L.; Rushton, G.; Avizienyte, E.; Gardiner, J.M. Synthetic heparan sulfate dodecasaccharides reveal single sulfation site inter-converts CXCL8 and CXCL12 chemokine biology. *Chem. Commun.* **2015**, *51*, 13846–13849. [CrossRef] [PubMed]

123. Nonaka, M.; Bao, X.; Matsumura, F.; Götze, S.; Kandasamy, J.; Kononov, A.; Broide, D.H.; Nakayama, J.; Seeberger, P.H.; Fukuda, M. Synthetic di-sulfated iduronic acid attenuates asthmatic response by blocking T-cell recruitment to inflammatory sites. *PNAS* **2014**, *111*, 8173–8178. [CrossRef] [PubMed]

124. De Paz, J.L.; Moseman, E.A.; Noti, C.; Polito, L.; Von Andrian, U.H.; Seeberger, P.H. Profiling heparin-chemokine interactions using synthetic tools. *ACS Chem. Biol.* **2007**, *2*, 735–744. [CrossRef] [PubMed]

125. Ahmed, T.; Smith, G.; Vlahov, I.; Abraham, W.M. Inhibition of allergic airway responses by heparin derived oligosaccharides: Identification of a ietrasaccharide sequence. *Respir. Res.* **2012**, *13*, 6. [CrossRef] [PubMed]

126. Ahmed, T.; Smith, G.; Abraham, W.M. Heparin-derived supersulfated disaccharide inhibits allergic airway responses in sheep. *Pulm. Pharmacol. Ther.* **2014**, *28*, 77–86. [CrossRef] [PubMed]

127. Shastri, M.D.; Peterson, G.M.; Stewart, N.; Sohal, S.S.; Patel, R.P. Non-anticoagulant derivatives of heparin for the management of asthma: Distant dream or close reality? *Expert Opin. Investig. Drugs* **2014**, *23*, 357–373. [CrossRef] [PubMed]

128. Craciun, I.; Fenner, A.M.; Kerns, R.J. *N*-arylacyl *O*-sulfonated aminoglycosides as novel inhibitors of human neutrophil elastase, cathepsin G and proteinase 3. *Glycobiology* **2016**, *26*, 701–709. [CrossRef] [PubMed]

129. Fryer, A.; Huang, Y.-C.; Rao, G.; Jacoby, D.; Mancilla, E.; Whorton, R.; Piantadosi, C.A.; Kennedy, T.; Hoidal, J. Selective *O*-desulfation produces nonanticoagulant heparin that retains pharmacological activity in the lung. *J. Pharmacol. Exp. Ther.* **1997**, *282*, 208–219. [PubMed]

130. Jaseja, M.; Rej, R.N.; Sauriol, F.; Perlin, A.S. Novel regio- and stereoselective modifications of heparin in alkaline solution. Nuclear magnetic resonance spectroscopic evidence. *Can. J. Chem.* **1989**, *67*, 1449–1456. [CrossRef]

131. Kennedy, T.P. Methods of Treating Acute Excerbations of Chronic Obstructive Pulmonary Disease. U.S. Patent No. 2009/0054374 A1, 26 February 2009.

132. Larramendy-Gozalo, C.; Barret, A.; Daudigeos, E.; Mathieu, E.; Antonangeli, L.; Riffet, C.; Petit, E.; Papy-Garcia, D.; Barritault, D.; Brown, P.; et al. Comparison of CR36, a new heparan mimetic, and pentosan polysulfate in the treatment of prion diseases. *J. Gen. Virol.* **2007**, *88*, 1062–1067. [CrossRef] [PubMed]

133. Casu, B.; Diamantini, G.; Fedeli, G.; Mantovani, M.; Oreste, P.; Pescador, R.; Porta, R.; Prino, G.; Torri, G.; Zoppetti, G. Retention of antilipemic activity by periodate-oxidized non-anticoagulant heparins. *Arzneim.-Forsch.* **1986**, *36*, 637–642.

134. Casu, B.; Guerrini, M.; Naggi, A.; Perez, M.; Torri, G.; Ribatti, D.; Carminati, P.; Giannini, G.; Penco, S.; Pisano, C.; et al. Short Heparin Sequences Spaced by Glycol-Split Uronate Residues Are Antagonists of Fibroblast Growth Factor 2 and Angiogenesis Inhibitors. *Biochemistry* **2002**, *41*, 10519–10528. [CrossRef] [PubMed]

135. Cassinelli, G.; Naggi, A. Old and new applications of non-anticoagulant heparin. *Int. J. Cardiol.* **2016**, *212*, S14–S21. [CrossRef]

136. Pomin, V.H. Anticoagulant motifs of marine sulfated glycans. *Glycoconj. J.* **2014**, *31*, 341–344. [CrossRef] [PubMed]

137. Ciancia, M.; Quintana, I.; Cerezo, A.S. Overview of anticoagulant activity of sulfated polysaccharides from seaweeds in relation to their structures, focusing on those of green seaweeds. *Curr. Med. Chem.* **2010**, *17*, 2503–2529. [CrossRef] [PubMed]

138. Rashid, Q.; Abid, M.; Gupta, N.; Tyagi, T.; Ashraf, M.Z.; Jairajpuri, M.A. Polysulfated trehalose as a novel anticoagulant agent with dual mode of action. *BioMed Res. Int.* **2015**, 1–12. [CrossRef] [PubMed]

139. Gracher, A.H.P.; Cipriani, T.R.; Carbonero, E.R.; Gorin, P.A.J.; Iacomini, M. Antithrombin and heparin cofactor II-mediated inactivation of α-thrombin by a synthetic, sulfated mannogalactan. *Thromb. Res.* **2010**, *126*, e180–e187. [CrossRef] [PubMed]

140. O'Keeffe, D.; Olson, S.T.; Gasiunas, N.; Gallagher, J.; Baglin, T.P.; Huntington, J.A. The Heparin Binding Properties of Heparin Cofactor II Suggest an Antithrombin-like Activation Mechanism. *J. Biol. Chem.* **2004**, *279*, 50267–50273. [CrossRef] [PubMed]

141. Mast, A.E. Tissue Factor Pathway Inhibitor: Multiple Anticoagulant Activities for a Single Protein. *Arterioscler. Thromb. Vasc. Biol.* **2016**, *36*, 9–14. [CrossRef] [PubMed]

142. Schmaier, A.H. The contact activation and kallikrein/kinin systems: Pathophysiologic and physiologic activities. *J. Thromb. Haemost.* **2016**, *14*, 28–39. [CrossRef] [PubMed]

143. Long, A.T.; Kenne, E.; Jung, R.; Fuchs, T.A.; Renne, T. Contact system revisited: An interface between inflammation, coagulation, and innate immunity. *J. Thromb. Haemost.* **2016**, *14*, 427–437. [CrossRef] [PubMed]

144. Pan, J.; Qian, Y.; Zhou, X.; Lu, H.; Ramacciotti, E.; Zhang, L. Chemically Oversulfated Glycosaminoglycans Are Potent Modulators of Contact System Activation and Different Cell Signaling Pathways. *J. Biol. Chem.* **2010**, *285*, 22966–22975. [CrossRef] [PubMed]

145. Kishimoto, T.K.; Viswanathan, K.; Ganguly, T.; Elankumaran, S.; Smith, S.; Pelzer, K.; Lansing, J.C.; Sriranganathan, N.; Zhao, G.; Galcheva-Gargova, Z.; et al. Contaminated heparin associated with adverse clinical events and activation of the contact system. *N. Engl. J. Med.* **2008**, *358*, 2457–2467. [CrossRef] [PubMed]

146. Ramacciotti, E.; Clark, M.; Sadeghi, N.; Hoppensteadt, D.; Thethi, I.; Gomes, M.; Fareed, J. Contaminants in heparin: Review of the literature, molecular profiling, and clinical implications. *Clin. Appl. Thromb./Hemost.* **2011**, *17*, 126–135. [CrossRef] [PubMed]

147. Corbier, A.; Le Berre, N.; Rampe, D.; Meng, H.; Lorenz, M.; Vicat, P.; Potdevin, S.; Doubovetzky, M. Oversulfated Chondroitin Sulfate and OSCS-Contaminated Heparin Cause Dose- and Route-Dependent Hemodynamic Effects in the Rat. *Toxicol. Sci.* **2011**, *121*, 417–427. [CrossRef] [PubMed]

148. Li, B.; Suwan, J.; Martin, J.G.; Zhang, F.; Zhang, Z.; Hoppensteadt, D.; Clark, M.; Fareed, J.; Linhardt, R.J. Oversulfated chondroitin sulfate interaction with heparin-binding proteins: New insights into adverse reactions from contaminated heparins. *Biochem. Pharmacol.* **2009**, *78*, 292–300. [CrossRef] [PubMed]

149. Zhou, Z.-H.; Rajabi, M.; Chen, T.; Karnaukhova, E.; Kozlowski, S. Oversulfated chondroitin sulfate inhibits the complement classical pathway by potentiating C1 inhibitor. *PLoS ONE* **2012**, *7*, e47296. [CrossRef] [PubMed]

150. Arepally, G.M. Heparin-induced thrombocytopenia. *Blood* **2017**, *129*, 2864–2872. [CrossRef] [PubMed]

151. Tardy-Poncet, B.; Tardy, B.; Grelac, F.; Reynaud, J.; Mismetti, P.; Bertrand, J.C.; Guyotat, D. Pentosan polysulfate-induced thrombocytopenia and thrombosis. *Am. J. Hematol.* **1994**, *45*, 252–257. [CrossRef] [PubMed]

152. Leroux, D.; Canepa, S.; Viskov, C.; Mourier, P.; Herman, F.; Rollin, J.; Gruel, Y.; Pouplard, C. Binding of heparin-dependent antibodies to PF4 modified by enoxaparin oligosaccharides: Evaluation by surface plasmon resonance and serotonin release assay. *J. Thromb. Haemost.* **2012**, *10*, 430–436. [CrossRef] [PubMed]

153. Xu, Y.; Cai, C.; Chandarajoti, K.; Hsieh, P.-H.; Li, L.; Pham, T.Q.; Sparkenbaugh, E.M.; Sheng, J.; Key, N.S.; Pawlinski, R.; et al. Homogeneous low-molecular-weight heparins with reversible anticoagulant activity. *Nat. Chem. Biol.* **2014**, *10*, 248–250. [CrossRef] [PubMed]

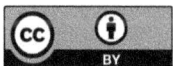

pharmaceuticals

MDPI

Article

Systematic Analysis of Pharmaceutical Preparations of Chondroitin Sulfate Combined with Glucosamine

Gustavo R.C. Santos, Adriana A. Piquet, Bianca F. Glauser, Ana M.F. Tovar, Mariana S. Pereira, Eduardo Vilanova and Paulo A.S. Mourão *

Laboratório de Tecido Conjuntivo, Hospital Universitário Clementino Fraga Filho and Instituto de Bioquímica Médica Leopoldo de Meis, Universidade Federal do Rio de Janeiro (UFRJ), P.O. Box 68041, Rio de Janeiro RJ 21941-913, Brazil; fgugarc@hotmail.com (G.R.C.S.); piquet@hucff.ufrj.br (A.A.P.); biancaglauser@gmail.com (B.F.G.); tovara@gmail.com (A.M.F.T.); marianasa@hucff.ufrj.br (M.S.P.); evilanova@hucff.ufrj.br (E.V.)
* Correspondence: pmourao@hucff.ufrj.br; Tel.: +55-21-3938-2091 Fax: +55-21-3938-2090

Academic Editor: Barbara Mulloy
Received: 26 February 2017; Accepted: 30 March 2017; Published: 1 April 2017

Abstract: Glycosaminoglycans are carbohydrate-based compounds widely employed as nutraceuticals or prescribed drugs. Oral formulations of chondroitin sulfate combined with glucosamine sulfate have been increasingly used to treat the symptoms of osteoarthritis and osteoarthrosis. The chondroitin sulfate of these combinations can be obtained from shark or bovine cartilages and hence presents differences regarding the proportions of 4- and 6-sulfated N-acetyl β-D-galactosamine units. Herein, we proposed a systematic protocol to assess pharmaceutical batches of this combination drug. Chemical analyses on the amounts of chondroitin sulfate and glucosamine in the batches were in accordance with those declared by the manufacturers. Anion-exchange chromatography has proven more effective than electrophoresis to determine the type of chondroitin sulfate present in the combinations and to detect the presence of keratan sulfate, a common contaminant found in batches prepared with shark chondroitin sulfate. 1D NMR spectra revealed the presence of non-sulfated instead of sulfated glucosamine in the formulations and thus in disagreement with the claims declared on the label. Moreover, 1D and 2D NMR analyses allowed a precise determination on the chemical structures of the chondroitin sulfate present in the formulations. The set of analytical tools suggested here could be useful as guidelines to improve the quality of this medication.

Keywords: glycosaminoglycans; glucosamine sulfate; arthritis; arthroses; nuclear magnetic resonance

1. Introduction

Glycosaminoglycans (GAGs) are carbohydrate-based biological compounds widely employed in medicine as therapeutic agents [1]. Currently, heparin stands out as the most exploited GAG drug, being largely used for treatment and prevention of thrombosis and in procedures involving extracorporeal circulation [2]. In recent years, oral formulations of chondroitin sulfate (CS) in combination with glucosamine (GlcN) sulfate have been increasingly employed in therapies for osteoarthritis and osteoarthrosis [3]. The pharmaceutical preparations of CS present in this combination drug are obtained from cartilages of different animals and thus may present structural differences [4], especially regarding to variations in the 4- and 6-sulfation of N-acetyl β-D-galactosamine residues and minor differences in the 2-sulfation of glucuronic acid units (Figure 1A). CS from different animal sources may also present significant differences in their molecular weight [5].

In addition to the structural heterogeneity of CS obtained from different animal sources, some pharmaceutical preparations also present contaminations with other GAGs due to flaws during the purification process [5–7]. A common contaminant is keratan sulfate (KS), a conspicuous component of proteoglycans from cartilages [5–7]. Even the international standards of CS differ in their structures and purities. The CS standard from the United States Pharmacopeia purified from bovine cartilage has galactosamine units predominantly 4-sulfated (CS-A) while the European Pharmacopeia adopts CS obtained from shark cartilage, rich in 6-sulfated galactosamine (CS-C) and contaminated with minor amounts of KS [8,9]. The other pharmacologically active ingredient of these formulations is GlcN sulfate, which alone or in combination with CS ameliorates some symptoms of osteoarthritis [10–12]. The GlcN added in the formulations undergoes to mutarotation equilibrium between α- and β-anomers (~62% and ~38%, respectively) in solution (Figure 1B).

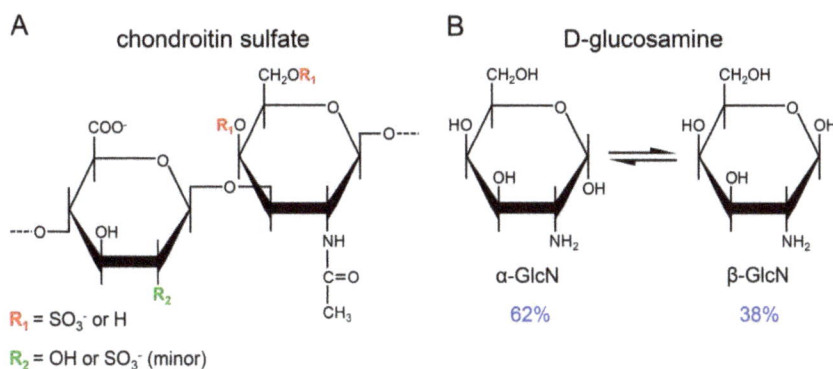

Figure 1. Structure of the active compounds present in the pharmaceutical preparations. (**A**) CS purified from bovine or shark cartilage. The sulfation pattern of the *N*-acetyl β-galactosamine (in red) and β-glucuronic acid (in green) units varies according with the animal source of the CS. Free GlcN (**B**) in solution epimerizes on its α- (62%) and β- (38%) anomers.

Different from heparin, which has a well-known anticoagulant and antithrombotic mechanism of action, the molecular basis of the therapeutic effects of CS and GlcN sulfate in the treatment of osteoarthritis and osteoarthrosis has not been fully determined [13]. Studies performed with chondrocytes undergoing osteoarthritis have been suggesting that CS might act targeting intermediates involved on cell signaling, inflammatory and catabolic pathways and on the oxidative stress [14–17]. Despite that uncertain mechanism of action, several preclinical tests, clinical trials and meta-analysis studies have clearly demonstrated the efficacy of CS combined with GlcN for the management of serious osteoarthritis symptoms such as pain, inflammation and cartilage degradation [18–25].

Since the preparations of CS prescribed for treatment of osteoarthritis and osteoarthrosis present extensive chemical variations depending on their animal source, it is necessary to establish a comprehensive set of analytical protocols to assess the fine structure, physicochemical characteristics and purity of each type of CS present in these pharmaceutical products. In the present study, we employed a systematic set of analytical methodologies to assess two different pharmaceutical products composed of GlcN in combination with CS purified from shark or bovine cartilages. Different batches of these formulations were initially assessed for their CS and GlcN content; afterward, the CS isolated from the batches was analyzed via anion-exchange and size-exclusion chromatography, agarose-gel electrophoresis and one- (1D) and two-dimensional (2D) nuclear magnetic resonance spectroscopy (NMR). We also compared preparations of CS from bovine cartilage in two different pharmaceutical forms (capsule and sachet) using 1D ^{1}H NMR and analyses of the disaccharides formed after digestion with chondroitin AC lyase. The results of this set of analysis clearly demonstrate that the protocol proposed here (Figure 2) is robust enough for a clear and thorough characterization of pharmaceutical preparations of CS in combination with GlcN.

Pharmaceutical preparations

• Content of GlcN and CS	**CS structure**
• Electrophoresis	• 1D H¹ NMR
• Ion-Exchange chromatography	• 2D H¹-H¹ NMR TOCSY
• Gel permeation chromatography	• 2D H¹-C¹³ NMR HSQC
• 1D H¹ NMR	• Disaccharide analyses (HPLC)

GlcN

CS

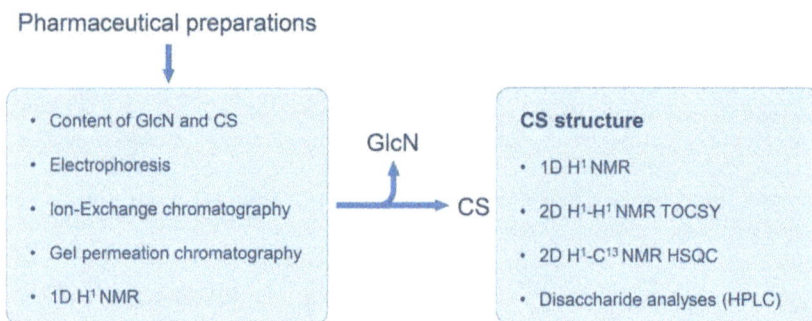

Figure 2. Systematic protocol for analyses of pharmaceutical preparations of CS-GlcN. The whole formulations were assessed via colorimetric reactions for determination of GlcN and CS contents, electrophoresis, chromatography and 1D ^{1}H-NMR. Afterward, the CSs isolated from these formulations were further analyzed via 1D and 2D NMR and SAX-HPLC for determinations of the disaccharides formed after digestion with chondroitin AC lyase.

2. Materials and Methods

2.1. Pharmaceutical Formulations of CS Combined with GlcN and CS Standards

Sixty five batches of pharmaceutical grade preparations of CS (50 containing shark CS and 15 bovine CS) in combination with GlcN commercially available for oral administration as capsules or sachets were obtained from two different Brazilian pharmaceutical companies. The contents of both sachets and capsules were readily soluble in water. The names of the manufacturers were kept anonymous due to ethical principles. Standards of CS were obtained from the US (Rockville, MD, USA; cat. 1133570, Lot HOF184) and the European (Strasbourg, France; code Y0000593, ID. 002SJ4) pharmacopeias. Commercially available CS from whale cartilage (CS-A, mostly 4-sulfated) and shark cartilage (CS-C, mostly 6-sulfated) were purchased from Sigma-Aldrich (St. Louis, MO, USA). Standard of oversulfated CS (Lot No. HOM191) was obtained from US Pharmacopeia.

2.2. Chemical Analyses of the CS and GlcN Contents

The content of uronic acid in the CS from the pharmaceutical preparations was measured using carbazole reaction [26]. Briefly, solutions (200 μL) with different amounts of the preparations (10 → 80 μg) were incubated in 98% sulfuric acid and 0.9% sodium tetraborate (1.0 mL) at 100 °C for 12 min. The reaction was stopped in ice cold bath and then 0.2% carbazole in absolute ethanol (40 μL) was added to the solution and incubated at 100 °C for 5 min. The absorbance was measured at 525 nm in a spectrophotometer (Amershamn Biosciences, Little Chalfont, UK). The concentration of CS was estimated using a standard curve plotted with standard CS. The amount of GlcN in the pharmaceutical preparations was estimated via a colorimetric reaction [27]. Briefly, solutions (200 μL) with different amounts of the preparations (10 → 200 μg) were incubated in acetylacetone (5 mL Na₂CO₃ 1.25 N + 150 μL acetylacetone) at 100 °C for 20 min and cooled in ice cold. Then, Blix reagent (200 μL, 1.6 g p-dimetylaminobenzaldehyde in 30 mL HCl + 30 mL ethanol 96%) were added to the solutions followed for another addition of 200 μL ethanol 96% and kept at room temperature for 1 h. The absorbance was measured at 530 nm in a spectrophotometer (Amersham Biosciences). The concentration of GlcN was estimated using a standard curve plotted with a solution of free GlcN.

2.3. Agarose-Gel Electrophoresis

Solutions containing CS from the pharmaceutical preparations and CS standards (5 μg of each) were applied in an agarose-gel (0.5%). The preparations submitted to enzymatic digestion were incubated with 0.01 units of chondroitin AC lyase from *Flavobacterium heparinum*, recombinant expressed in *E. coli* (Sigma-Aldrich) in 100 μL 0.05 M Tris:HCl (pH 8.0), supplemented with 5 mM EDTA and 15 mM sodium acetate at 37 °C for 12 h. After incubation, the samples were heated at dried-bath at 80 °C for 15 min to stop the reaction through denaturation of the enzyme, cooled in ice cold and applied in the agarose-gel. Electrophoresis run for 1 h at 110 V in 0.05 M 1,3-diaminopropane acetate (pH 9.0). CS in the gel were fixed with 0.1% *N*-cetyl-*N*,*N*,*N*-trimethylammonium bromide solution for 12 h, dried and stained with 0.1% toluidine blue in 0.1:5:5 (*v*/*v*) acetic acid:ethanol:water.

2.4. Anion-Exchange Chromatography

CS from the pharmaceutical formulations and CS standards (1 mg of each) were applied to a anion-exchange column Mono-Q (GE Healthcare, Little Chalfont, UK) pre-equilibrated with 10 mM Tris:HCl containing 0.5 M NaCl, pH 7.4 and connected to a HPLC system (Shimadzu, Kyoto, Japan). The column was eluted at a flow rate of $1.0\ mL \cdot min^{-1}$ using a linear NaCl gradient of 0.5 → 3.0 M NaCl, total volume of 40 mL. The eluent was continuously monitored via UV at 215 nm and conductivity.

2.5. Size-Exclusion Chromatography

The molecular weight of the formulations prepared with CS from shark or bovine cartilages and CS standards (20 μg of each) were evaluated via size-exclusion chromatography using a set of gel filtration columns (TSK gel G4000 SW × 1 and G3000 SW × 1, both 7.5 mm i.d. × 300 mm, Tosoh, Tokyo, Japan) linked to a HPLC system (Shimadzu). The columns were eluted with 0.1 M ammonium acetate, at room temperature with a flow rate of $0.3\ mL \cdot min^{-1}$. The eluent was monitored by refractive index. The columns were calibrated using a low-molecular-weight heparin molecular-weight standard (Lot No. 05/112) from the National Institutes of Biological Standards and Controls (NIBSC) and a heparin sodium molecular-weight calibrant from United States Pharmacopeia (Lot No. FOL4830), as previously described [2].

2.6. NMR Analyses

Spectra were obtained with CSs from shark or bovine cartilages present in the pharmaceutical preparations previously isolated using a syringe HITRAP desalting column (GE Healthcare). Spectra were recorded using a DRX 600 MHz apparatus (Bruker, Billerica, MA, USA) with a triple resonance probe as detailed previously [2]. About 20 mg of each sample was dissolved in 0.6 mL 99.9% deuterium oxide (Cambridge Isotope Laboratory, Cambridge, MA, USA). All spectra were recorded at 35 °C with HOD suppression by presaturation. The 1D ^{1}H-NMR spectra were recorded using 16 scans and inter-scan delay set to 1 s. The 2D ^{1}H–^{1}H TOCSY spectra were recorded using states-time proportion phase incrementation (states-TPPI) for quadrature detection in the indirect dimension. The 2D ^{1}H–^{13}C edited-HSQC spectra was performed with 1024 × 256 points and globally optimized alternating phase rectangular pulses (GARP) for decoupling. Chemical shifts were displayed relative to external trimethylsilylpropionic acid at 0 ppm for ^{1}H and relative to methanol for ^{13}C.

2.7. Analysis of the Disaccharide Composition

The disaccharides were obtained through enzymatic digestion with chondroitin AC lyase as described in the Section 2.3. The disaccharide mixtures obtained from preparations of CS from bovine cartilage formulated as capsules and sachets and the CS standard were lyophilized and then dissolved in 100 μL of distilled water. The disaccharides (20 μL) were analyzed via strong anion-exchange chromatography on a 250 × 5 mm Spherisorb-SAX column (Sigma-Aldrich) linked to a HPLC system (Shimadzu). After the injection, the column was washed with 5 mL of acidified water (pH 3.5) and then the disaccharides were eluted from the column using a linear gradient of 0 → 1 M NaCl (pH 3.5) at a flow rate of $1\ mL \cdot min^{-1}$. The eluent was continuously monitored via UV at 232 nm.

3. Results and Discussion

Pharmaceutical preparations of bovine CS in combination with GlcN (CS-GlcN) for oral administration are available as capsule and sachet formulations. The precise amounts of each active compound present in the formulations was determined through specific colorimetric reactions for hexuronic acid and free GlcN contents. The CS and GlcN contents measured here were very close to those declared by the manufacturers for both formulations (Table 1). Preparations of shark CS-GlcN formulated as capsules presented proportions of the active compounds identical to those of bovine CS-GlcN capsules and in accordance with the declared by the manufacturers as well (data not shown). Both CS and GlcN present pharmacological activities related to the treatment of osteoarthritis symptoms [10–12]; therefore, a precise determination of the amounts of each one of these pharmacologically active ingredients is indispensable to confirm that each preparation is in accordance with the recommended posology.

Table 1. Declared and observed contents of glucosamine (GlcN) and chondroitin sulfate (CS) on pharmaceutical preparations.

Formulation	Component	Declared Content (mg)	Observed Content (mg) [a]
Capsule	GlcN [b]	500	465 ± 20 [b]
	CS [c]	400	376 ± 8 [c]
Sachet	GlcN	1500	1500 ± 60 [b]
	CS	1200	1211 ± 179 [c]

[a] Results as mean ± SD of three determinations; [b] Content of free GlcN determined by a colorimetric reaction [27]; [c] Content of CS determined by the carbazole reaction [26] using standard curves obtained with the international standard of CS from US Pharmacopeia.

After the determination of the active compounds contents, we analyzed in further detail the CS from the different preparations. The first analytical steps toward determining the characteristics of the CS present in the different pharmacological preparations were analyses via agarose-gel electrophoresis and ion-exchange chromatography (Figure 3). The electrophoresis revealed that different batches of bovine and shark CS present electrophoretic mobility identical to the standard of CS (Figure 3A) and that both bovine and shark CS from the formulations are completely susceptible to digestion with chondroitin AC lyase (Figure 3B).

Despite this apparent homogeneity, we further investigated different batches containing shark or bovine CS using anion-exchange chromatography. The two compounds were clearly distinguishable in the chromatograms, with shark CS eluting at higher concentrations of NaCl than bovine CS (Figure 3C,D). Furthermore, the batches of shark CS presented small amounts (~16% of total) of another GAG, which was previously identified as keratan sulfate [5]. As expected, the international standards of CS from different animal sources also showed different chromatographic profiles. The standard of European Pharmacopeia, prepared from shark cartilage [8], elutes at higher concentration of NaCl and presents minor contamination with KS while the standard of US pharmacopeia purified from bovine cartilage [9] elutes at lower NaCl concentration and showed no contamination with other GAGs (Figure 3E). Therefore, the purity and homogeneity of the CSs from different animal sources present in the pharmaceutical preparations prescribed for treatment of osteoarthritis and osteoarthrosis are in strict accordance with the international standards.

Both the US and European pharmacopeias recommend cellulose-acetate electrophoresis stained with toluidine blue to assess the purity of pharmaceutical or nutraceutical preparations of CS [8,9]. This analysis is extremely important to detect the presence of other GAGs such as oversulfated chondroitin sulfate in the preparations. However, this technique has not enough resolution to differentiate neither CS with different chemical structure such as those from shark and bovine cartilage enriched with 6- or 4-sulfated galactosamine units, respectively, nor to detect minor contaminations with KS, even with samples previously digested with chondroitin AC lyase.

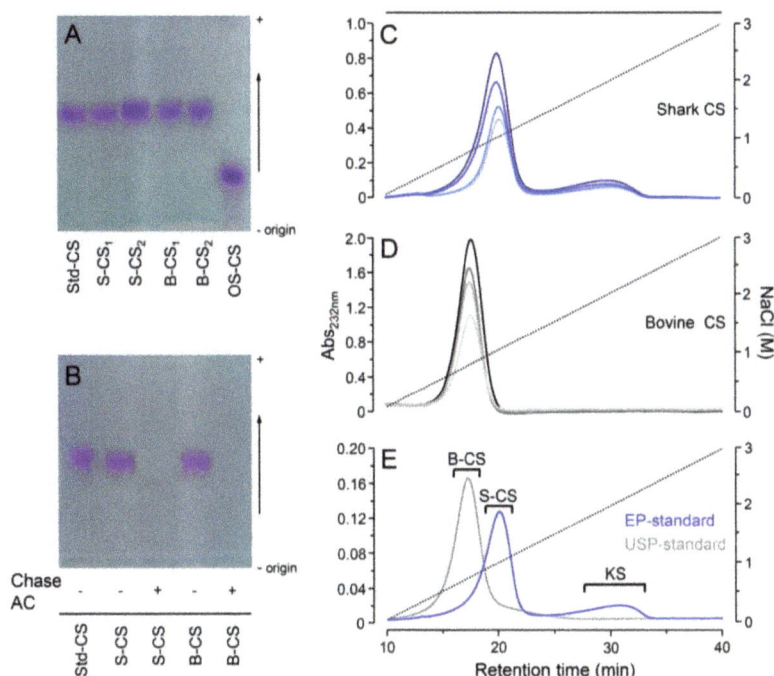

Figure 3. Agarose-gel electrophoresis and anion-exchange chromatography of pharmaceutical preparation of CS-GlcN. Agarose-gel electrophoresis of: (**A**) representative batches containing shark CS (S-CS in all panels) and bovine CS (B-CS in all panels) and standards of CS-A (Std-CS) and oversulfated CS (OS-CS) and (**B**) shark CS and bovine CS before (−) and after (+) digestion with chondroitin AC lyase. Anion-exchange chromatography of representative batches (50 → 200 µg) containing shark CS (panel (**C**), bluish lines), bovine CS (panel (**D**), greyish lines) and standards of CS (200 µg) from the European (in blue) and US (in grey) pharmacopeias (**E**), the peak containing keratan sulfate is also indicated (KS). Chromatography were performed using a Mono-Q column linked to a HPLC system through a linear gradient of 0.5 → 3.0 M NaCl (dotted lines). The eluents were monitored via UV (A_{215nm}).

The inability of electrophoretic techniques to differentiate CS-A from CS-C and to detect small amounts of KS has already shown in analyses of pharmacological preparations of CS [5,28] and in studies on GAGs from other animal sources [29]. Otherwise, the anion-exchange chromatography analyses performed here and elsewhere [5,28] were plainly able to distinguish different CSs and to detect contaminations with KS. Therefore, we can affirm that anion-exchange chromatography is a robust analytical tool to perform evaluations on the source, homogeneity and purity of pharmaceutical preparations of CS.

We also compared the molecular weight of the different pharmaceutical preparations of CS-GlcN using a set of size-exclusion chromatography columns (Figure 4). Shark CS had markedly higher molecular weight than bovine CS (~50 KDa and ~23 KDa, respectively) and the GlcN of both preparations co-eluted as low-molecular weight components at the V_t of the columns (Figure 4A). As expected, the retention time of shark and bovine CS from the pharmaceutical preparations were similar to those of the standards of CS from European (shark) and US (bovine) pharmacopeias, respectively (Figure 4B). We also noticed a high molecular weight component in the standard of CS from the European Pharmacopeia eluting at the void volume of the columns (Figure 4B). This component probably consists of CS polymers with higher molecular weight, denoting a higher polydispersity of this standard in relation to the shark CS from the pharmaceutical preparation. Although the size-exclusion chromatography presents a good resolution to distinguish the different CSs, this technique has proven here and elsewhere [5] unable to detect KS contaminations in CS preparations from shark cartilage because the chromatograms yield a single and polydisperse peak.

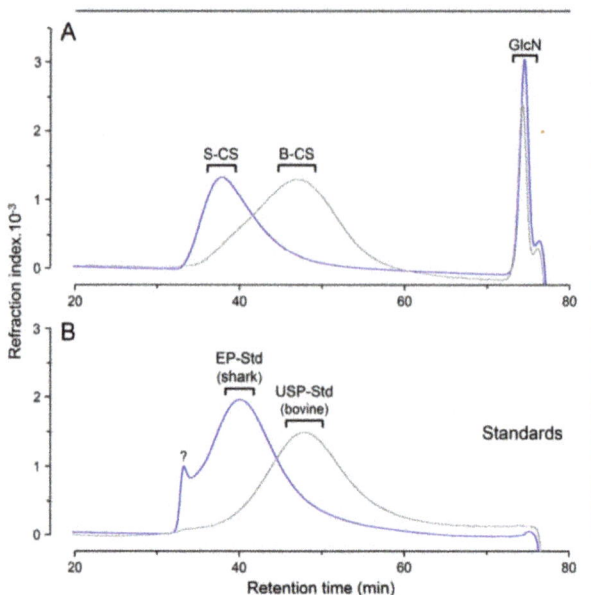

Figure 4. Size-exclusion chromatography of pharmaceutical preparation of CS-GlcN. (**A**) CS from preparations containing shark (S-CS) and bovine (B-CS) cartilages (blue and gray lines, respectively). (**B**) International standards from European and United State pharmacopeia (EP-Std in blue and USP-Std in gray, respectively). Chromatography were performed using a set of TSK gel G4000 SW/G3000 SW columns. The eluents were monitored via differential refractive index. GlcN in panel A indicates the elution of the glucosamine from the preparations and the ? in panel B depicts a non-identified component found in the standard from the European pharmacopeia.

After the assessments on the purity and homogeneity of the different pharmaceutical preparations of CS-GlcN, we proceeded with the determination of the fine structures of their components using 1D and 2D NMR analysis. We first analyzed preparations of bovine CS-GlcN formulated as capsule or sachet via 1D ^{1}H-NMR (Figure 5A). The spectra revealed two preponderant signals assigned to GlcN after mutarotation equilibrium. The proportions of α- (59%) and β-anomers (41%). were close to the expected values depicted in the panel B of Figure 1. Surprisingly, these α- and β-anomers had chemical shifts of their anomeric (α-H1 at 5.48 and β-H1 at 4.98 ppm) and ring protons coincident with those of non-sulfated instead of sulfated GlcN. No shifts indicating sulfation were noticed because the spectra were strictly coincident with that of standard non-sulfated GlcN (not shown). This finding could have pharmacological implications because the active compound present in these formulations (non-sulfated GlcN) differs from that approved for use by the regulatory agencies (viz. glucosamine sulfate sodium). Signals ascribed to CS are wide and discrete in the spectra, except for the clear CH_3 signal from *N*-acetyl β-galactosamine at ~2.1 ppm. A signal of residual solvent (ethanol) was observed at 1.2 ppm. Formulations in capsule and sachet have the same active compounds, but present different excipients such as polyethylene glycol, which was easily identified by the multiplets at 2.6–2.8 ppm present in the spectrum of the sachet formulation. We were unable to compare the integrals of GlcN and CS in the spectra due to differences in relaxation properties of spins of sugars free in solutions and linked as polysaccharides.

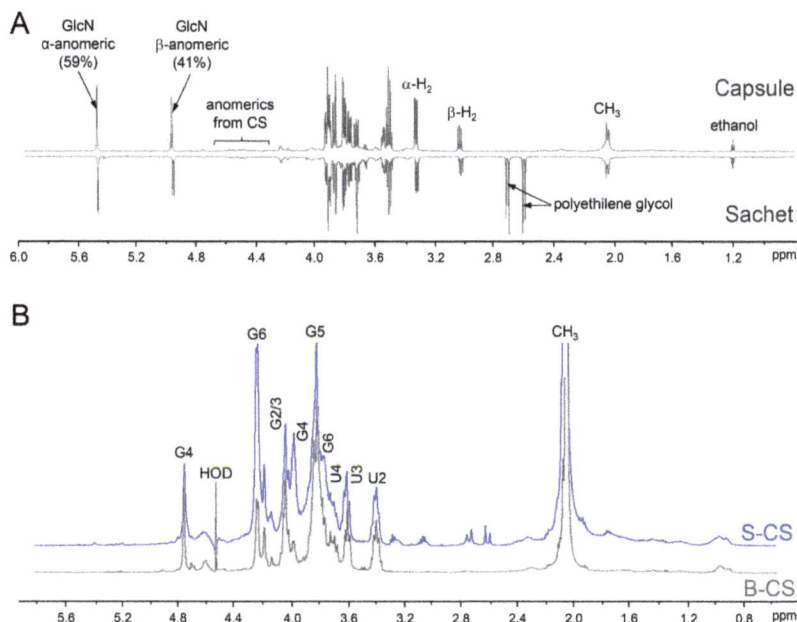

Figure 5. 1D ^{1}H NMR of the pharmaceutical preparation of CS-GlcN. (**A**) Wide range spectra of the preparations containing CS from bovine cartilage formulated as capsules and sachets; (**B**) Spectra of the CSs from shark (S-CS, in blue) and bovine (B-CS, in grey) cartilages isolated from the pharmaceutical preparations. The samples were dissolved on 0.4 mL of D$_2$O and analyzed using a 600 MHz NMR spectrometer at 35 °C.

To perform a precise analysis of the two types of CS present in the formulations we removed the GlcN and other excipients using a desalting column. The 1D ^{1}H-NMR spectra of the purified CSs yielded well-defined signals (Figure 5B). CSs from shark and bovine cartilages (in blue and gray, respectively) showed the same set of signals but some of them present different intensities; notably, the signal at 4.74 ppm, ascribed to H4 of 4-sulfated *N*-acetyl β-galactosamine is more prominent in bovine than in shark CS. In contrast, signal from H6 of 6-sulfated *N*-acetyl β-galactosamine at 4.21 ppm is more intense in the shark CS. These observations indicate that the hexosamine residues of bovine CS are preponderantly 4-sulfated while those from shark CS are mostly 6-sulfated.

Shark and bovine CSs also showed similar 2D ^{1}H-^{1}H TOCSY spectra with two preponderant spin systems (Figure 6), one assigned to 4- and 6-sulfated *N*-acetyl β-galactosamine units (signals indicated as G and G′, respectively, and connected by red lines) and the other assigned to β-glucuronic acid residues (signals indicated as U, connected by green lines). As expected, the spectrum of shark CS showed additional signals assigned to KS (Figure 6A). The spin system of the constituent units of KS, 6-sulfated *N*-acetyl β-glucosamine (assigned as KG) and 6-sulfated β-galactose (assigned as KGal) are connected by purple and yellow lines, respectively, in the spectrum (Figure 6A). The values of ^{1}H chemical shifts of the constituent units of these GAGs are shown in Table 2.

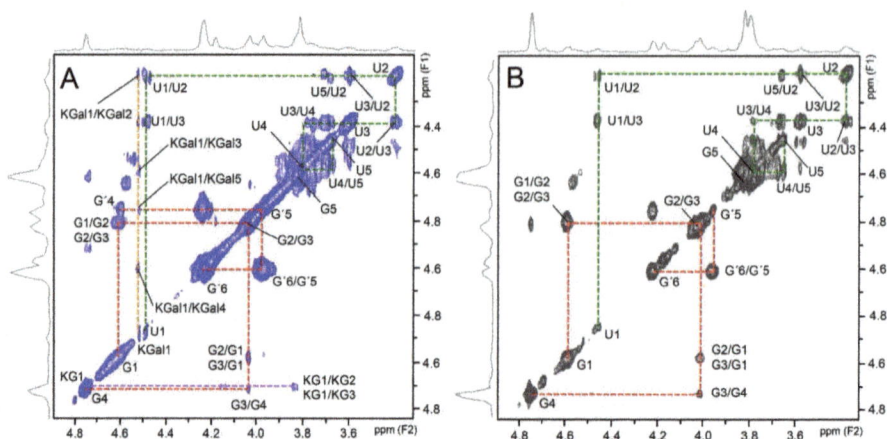

Figure 6. ^{1}H–^{1}H TOCSY NMR spectrum of shark (**A**) and bovine (**B**) CS from the pharmaceutical preparations. Red and green lines in the panels represent the spin systems of *N*-acetyl β-galactosamine and of β-glucuronic acid of the CS, respectively. Note that the β-galactosamine have two distinct spin systems assigned to 4-sulfated residues (signals indicated as G) and 6-sulfated units (signals indicated as G′). Glucuronic acid has a single spin system (signals indicated as U). Shark CS has two additional spin systems assigned to 6-sulfated *N*-acetyl β-glucosamine (KG) and 6-sulfated β-galactose (KGal) units of keratan sulfate, represented by the purple and yellow lines, respectively.

Table 2. ^{1}H- and ^{13}C-NMR chemical shifts of the constituent units of chondroitin sulfate (CS) and keratan sulfate (KS) found in the pharmaceutical preparations.

Signal	Chemical Shifts (ppm)				
	CS			KS	
	GalNAc-4S	GalNAc-6S	GlcA	GalNAc-6S	Gal-6S
H1/C1	4.58/103.6	4.58/103.6	4.46/106.5	4.74/105.2	4.56/105.3
H2/C2	4.02/54.0	4.02/53.4	3.37/75.2	3.85/57.6	3.62/72.3
H3/C3	*4.00/78.5* [a]	3.98/81.7	3.57/76.2	3.83/75.3	3.78/84.6
H4/C4	**4.76/79.2** [a]	4.20/70.3	3.77/83.8	3.87/82.5	4.22/70.6
H5/C5	3.83/77.4	3.97/75.1	3.66/79.5	3.81/74.7	3.97/75.0
H6/C6	3.77/63.8	**4.24/70.1**	-	**4.41–4.33/69.0**	**4.24/69.0**

[a] Sulfation and glycosylation sites are indicated in bold and italic, respectively.

2D ^{1}H–^{13}C HSQC spectra of the two types of CSs yielded well-resolved and similar signals (Figure 7). The spectrum of bovine CS is more homogenous (Figure 7B) while the spectrum of shark CS also shows some additional but less intense signals assigned to KS (Figure 7A) The signals attributed to KS (KG and KGal in the Figure 7A) were assigned by comparison with literature data [30]. The values of ^{13}C chemical shifts of CS and KS present in the pharmaceutical preparations are shown in the Table 2. The integrals of H4/C4 and H6/C6 from 4-sulfated and 6-sulfated *N*-acetyl β-galactosamine, at 4.74/79.2 and 4.21/70.2 ppm, respectively, showed that shark CS is mostly 6-sulfated while bovine CS is preponderantly 4-sulfated (Table 3) and thus in strict accordance with the structure expected for these compounds [5].

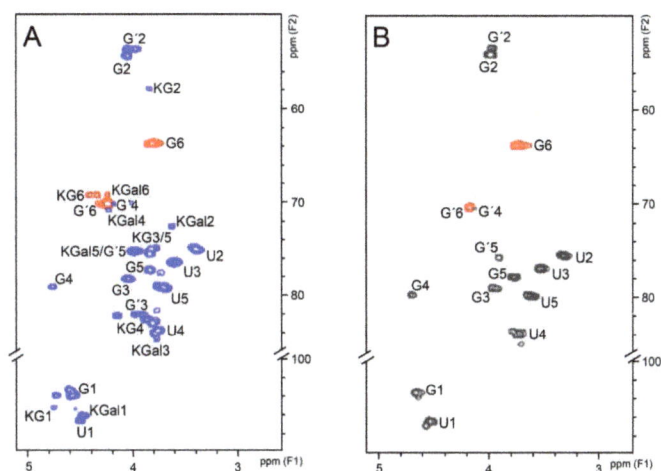

Figure 7. ^{1}H–^{13}C HSQC spectra of shark (**A**) and bovine (**B**) CS from the pharmaceutical preparations. Blue (panel **A**) and gray (panel **B**) signals are in-phase and belong to CH groups whereas red signals are in antiphase and belong to CH$_2$ groups. Signals assigned to 4-sulfated and 6-sulfated N-acetyl β-galactosamine are indicated as G and G′, respectively. Signals from β-glucuronic acid are indicated as U. Signals from N-acetyl β-glucosamine and β-galactose of keratan sulfate are indicated as KG and KGal, respectively.

Table 3. Proportions of 4- and 6-sulfated N-acetil β-galactosamine in bovine and shark chondroitin sulfates (CS) based on signals of 2D ^{1}H–^{13}C HSQC spectra (see Figure 5).

	Bovine CS	Shark CS
4-sulfated β-GalNAc [a]	68%	16%
6-sulfated β-GalNAc [b]	32%	84%

[a] Signal at 4.74/79.2 ppm in the 2D ^{1}H–^{13}C HSQC spectra (see Figure 5); [b] Signal at 4.21/70.2 ppm in the 2D ^{1}H–^{13}C HSQC spectra (see Figure 5).

These results have consistently demonstrated that 1D ^{1}H and 2D ^{1}H–^{1}H TOCSY and ^{1}H–^{13}C HSQC NMR spectra of the preparations of GlcN-CS from different animal sources are informative enough to assess qualitatively and quantitatively the structures of the pharmacologically active ingredients (CS and GlcN) and excipients (polyethylene glycol and ethanol) present in the different formulations. Structural analyses via 1D and 2D NMR have been widely used to determine the chemical differences between porcine and bovine heparins and are routinely employed in the quality control of pharmaceutical grade unfractionated and low-molecular weight heparins [2,31]. Therefore, solution NMR can also be considered an effective analytical tool for structural determinations of the active ingredients of pharmaceutical formulations of GlcN-CS.

Additionally, we analyzed the disaccharide composition of the bovine CS present in the capsule or sachet formulation via SAX-HPLC chromatography (Figure 8). The disaccharides were prepared through enzymatic digestion of the CS isolated from the formulations with chondroitin AC lyase. We observed in both capsule and sachet formulations a preponderance of disaccharides containing 4-sulfate N-acetyl β-galactosamine, followed by units sulfated at position 6 and minor amounts of non-sulfated disaccharides. Only trace amounts di-sulfated disaccharides were detected in the chromatograms. CS from both capsule and sachet formulations presented chromatographic profiles similar to the CS-A standard (Figure 8A) and the quantification of their disaccharides are in accordance with literature data [32] (Table 4). We also include in the Table 4 the disaccharide composition of shark CS available in the literature [33], which were consistent with the NMR data obtained here.

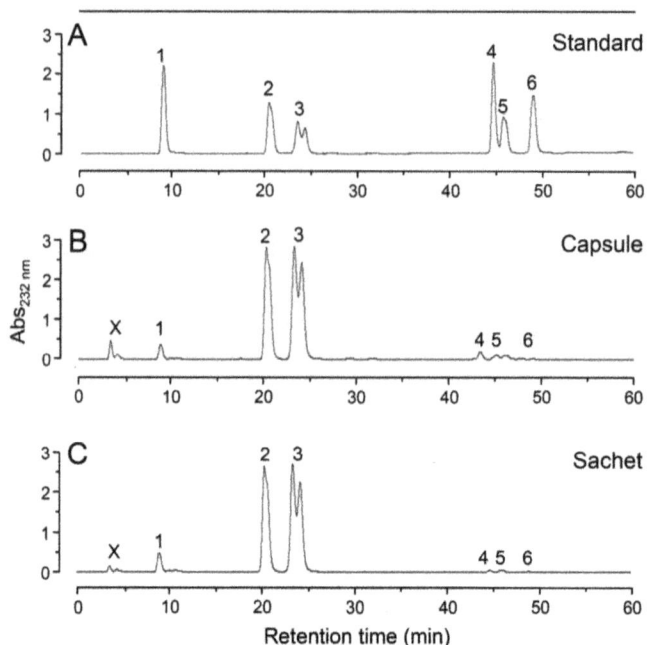

Figure 8. SAX-HPLC analyses of the disaccharides of different formulations containing bovine CS. Disaccharides were prepared through digestion with chondroitin AC lyase of standard of CS-A (**A**) and the bovine CS from capsule (**B**) and sachet (**C**) formulations. The mixtures of disaccharides were applied in a Spherisorb-SAX column linked to an HPLC system and eluted with a gradient of $0 \rightarrow 1$ M NaCl. The eluent was monitored for UV absorbance at 232 nm. The numbered peaks correspond to the elution positions of known disaccharide standards as follows: 1, $\Delta UA \rightarrow GalNAc$; 2, $\Delta UA \rightarrow GalNAc$ ($6SO_4$); 3, $\Delta UA \rightarrow GalNAc$ ($4SO_4$); 4, ΔUA ($2SO_4$) $\rightarrow GalNAc$ ($6SO_4$); 5, $\Delta UA \rightarrow GalNAc$ ($4,6$-diSO_4); 6, $\Delta UA(2SO_4) \rightarrow GalNAc$ ($4SO_4$). X indicates a non-identified product. $\Delta UA \rightarrow GalNAc$ ($4SO_4$) shows two overlapped peaks assigned to the α- and β-anomers.

Table 4. Proportions of the disaccharides (% of total) produced through cleavage of chondroitin sulfate (CS) with chondroitin AC lyase.

Dissacharides	Bovine CS			Shark CS
	Capsule	Sachet	Literature Data [a]	Literature Data [b]
ΔUA-GalNAc	3	2	2	2
ΔUA-GalNAc-$6SO_4$	36	36	41	76
ΔUA-GalNAc-$4SO_4$	59	59	67	15
ΔUA-$2SO_4$-GalNAc-$6SO_4$	1	1	<1	7
ΔUA-GalNAc-$4,6$diSO_4	1	2	<1	<1
ΔUA-$2SO_4$-GalNAc-$6SO_4$	<1	<1	<1	<1
4-sulfation of β-GalNAc	60	58	49	15
6-sulfation of β-GalNAc	38	39	35	83
2-sulfation of β-GlcA	1	1	<1	7

[a] Data derived from Lauder et al. [32] [b] Data from de Waard et al. [33].

4. Conclusions

Herein, we have performed a systematic assessment on the compositions, physicochemical characteristics and chemical structures of pharmaceutical formulations of CS in combination with GlcN prescribed to treat the symptoms of osteoarthritis and osteoarthrosis. Anion-exchange chromatography was proven more effective than agarose-gel electrophoresis to determine the type of CS present in the formulations (CS-A from bovine or CS-C from shark cartilages) as well as to detect contaminations with KS. However, electrophoretic analyses still relevant because they are able to readily detect contaminations with other GAGs, specially, oversulfated CS, a contaminant found in pharmaceutical preparations of heparin that provoked serious adverse effects and some deaths in the late 2000 years [34]. As demonstrated previously [5], size-exclusion chromatography is also unable to detect KS contaminations and thus ineffective to evaluate the purity of these pharmacological preparations.

Structural analysis via 1D ^{1}H-NMR of the pharmacologically active ingredients revealed the presence of non-sulfated instead of sulfated GlcN in both capsule and sachet formulations. This finding is worrying because all the preclinical and clinical tests on the safety and efficacy of GlcN aiming the treatment of osteoarthritis were carried on with the sulfated compound [10–12]. The US pharmacopeia monograph recommends infrared absorption and dosage of sulfate content to assess the chemical characteristics of GlcN [35]; however, these techniques are not precise and/or specific enough to determine the presence and proportions of sulfated and non-sulfated GlcN in the pharmaceutical preparations. In contrast, the 1D ^{1}H NMR analysis performed here was able to determine precisely whether the GlcN is sulfated or non-sulfated through the specific chemical shifts of their α- and β-anomers and, furthermore, it is potentially useful to quantify mixtures of these different sugars in pharmaceutical formulations by integrating their specific signals. Moreover, both 1D and 2D NMR spectra were useful for a precise determination of the chemical structure of the CS-A from bovine and CS-C from shark cartilages and the contaminant KS.

CS and GlcN alone or in combination have been massively marketed worldwide as over the counter dietary supplement or prescribed as a symptomatic slow-acting drug for osteoarthritis [11,36]. Both the US and European pharmacopeias monographs on these active compounds recommend only infrared spectroscopy and/or electrophoresis as analytical techniques to assess their purity and chemical compositions [8,9,35]. However, these techniques are not robust enough to determine: (1) the type of CS (CS-A or CS-C) present in the formulations; (2) the presence and quantity of contaminant KS and (3) the chemical composition of the GlcN (proportion of sulfated and non-sulfated sugars) present in the combinations. A recent update in the US pharmacopeia monograph on CS includes the analysis of disaccharide composition after digestion with chondroitim AC lyase [8]. In this update was recommended a ratio of 4-sulfated/6-sulfated disaccharides above one, this requirement cannot be fulfilled by preparations containing CS from shark cartilage, rich in 6-sulfated *N*-acetyl galactosamine units. Therefore, even this recently improved monograph is not comprehensive enough to evaluate the different types of CS adopted by the manufacturers.

Taking into consideration that the pharmaceutical preparations of CS-GlcN analyzed here presented extensive variations in their compositions such as different CS types, contamination with another GAG and GlcN with incorrect composition, more comprehensive and in-depth guidelines contemplating different CS types and inconsistent GlcN composition must be urgently drafted by the regulatory agencies. Besides the analytical techniques currently recommended by the pharmacopeias, we further suggest anion-exchange chromatography to evaluate the homogeneity and purity of the CS present in the pharmaceutical formulations. We also recommend the use of 1D ^{1}H NMR instead of infrared spectroscopy to assess the chemical structure of both CS and GlcN present in this combination drug. The full implementation of the set of analytical protocols proposed here certainly will yields pharmaceutical preparations of CS-GlcN with more precise composition and hence with improved quality.

The mechanisms of action of neither CS nor GlcN in cartilage and subchondral bone tissues affected with osteoarthritis still not fully determined [14–17]. However, several in vivo studies with experimental animals and clinical trials already showed the effectiveness of these GAG-based compounds to ameliorate serious symptoms of osteoarthritis such as pain and cartilage degradation [18–25]. Nevertheless, it is a challenging task to understand how a carbohydrate-based compound with high molecular weight like CS (20–50 kDa) could be absorbed after oral administration and then remain sufficiently undegraded, even with the action of bacteria and enzymes of the gastrointestinal tract, to exert its therapeutic effects in the cartilages and bones. This lack of information reinforces the necessity of a precise and detailed determination of the chemical structures of the CS and GlcN present in these pharmaceutical preparations to support clinical and preclinical studies on their route of administration and mechanism of action.

Acknowledgments: This work was supported by grants from Conselho Nacional de Desenvolvimento Científico e Tecnológico (CNPq), Coordenação de Aperfeiçoamento do Pessoal de Nível Superior (CAPES), and Fundação de Amparo à Pesquisa do Estado do Rio de Janeiro (FAPERJ). We thank the Centro Nacional de Biologia Estrutural e Bioimagem (CENABIO) for the access to the NMR spectrometers.

Author Contributions: G.R.C.S., A.A.P., B.F.G. and A.M.F.T. performed the experiments; A.M.F.T., E.V., M.S.P. and P.A.S.M. analyzed the data and E.V. and P.A.S.M. wrote the paper.

Conflicts of Interest: The authors declare no conflict of interest.

References

1. Mulloy, B.; Hogwood, J.; Gray, E.; Lever, R.; Page, C.P. Pharmacology of heparin and related drugs. *Pharmacol. Rev.* **2016**, *68*, 76–141. [CrossRef] [PubMed]
2. Tovar, A.M.; Santos, G.R.; Capillé, N.V.; Piquet, A.A.; Glauser, B.F.; Pereira, M.S.; Vilanova, E.; Mourão, P.A. Structural and haemostatic features of pharmaceutical heparins from different animal sources: Challenges to define thresholds separating distinct drugs. *Sci. Rep.* **2016**, *6*, 35619. [CrossRef] [PubMed]
3. Bishnoi, M.; Jain, A.; Hurkat, P.; Jain, S.K. Chondroitin sulphate: A focus on osteoarthritis. *Glycoconj. J.* **2016**, *5*, 693–705. [CrossRef] [PubMed]
4. Garnjanagoonchorn, W.; Wongekalak, L.; Engkagul, A. Determination of chondroitin sulfate from different sources of cartilage. *Chem. Eng. Process.* **2007**, *46*, 465–471. [CrossRef]
5. Pomin, V.H.; Piquet, A.A.; Pereira, M.S.; Mourão, P.A. Residual keratan sulfate in chondroitin sulfate formulations for oral administration. *Carbohydr. Polym.* **2012**, *90*, 839–846. [CrossRef] [PubMed]
6. Nakano, T.; Ozimek, L. Detection of keratan sulfate by immunological methods in commercial chondroitin sulfate preparations. *Carbohydr. Polym.* **2014**, *99*, 547–552. [CrossRef] [PubMed]
7. Restaino, O.F.; Finamore, R.; Diana, P.; Marseglia, M.; Vitiello, M.; Casillo, A.; Bedini, E.; Parrilli, M.; Corsaro, M.M.; Trifuoggi, M.; et al. A multi-analytical approach to better assess the keratan sulfate contamination in animal origin chondroitin sulfate. *Anal. Chim. Acta* **2017**, *958*, 59–70. [CrossRef] [PubMed]
8. European Pharmacopeia. Chondroitin sulfate sodium monograph. In *European Pharmacopeia*, 7th ed.; European Directorate for the Quality of Medicines: Strasbourg, France, 2007; pp. 1681–1683.
9. United States Pharmacopoeia. Chondroitin sulfate sodium monograph [Revision Bulletin, 2015]. In *United States Pharmacopoeia*, 39th ed.; United States Pharmacopeial Convention: Rockville, MD, USA, 2016; pp. 1–3.
10. Reginster, J.Y.; Neuprez, A.; Lecart, M.P.; Sarlet, N.; Bruyere, O. Role of glucosamine in the treatment for osteoarthritis. *Rheumatol. Int.* **2012**, *10*, 2959–2967. [CrossRef] [PubMed]
11. Henrotin, Y.; Mobasheri, A.; Marty, M. Is there any scientific evidence for the use of glucosamine in the management of human osteoarthritis? *Arthritis Res. Ther.* **2012**, *14*, 201. [CrossRef] [PubMed]
12. Clegg, D.O.; Reda, D.J.; Harris, C.L.; Klein, M.A.; O'Dell, J.R.; Hooper, M.M.; Bradley, J.D.; Bingham, C.O., 3rd; Weisman, M.H.; Jackson, C.G.; et al. Glucosamine, chondroitin sulfate, and the two in combination for painful knee osteoarthritis. *N. Engl. J. Med.* **2006**, *354*, 795–808. [CrossRef] [PubMed]
13. Henrotin, Y.; Mathy, M.; Sanchez, C.; Lambert, C. Chondroitin sulfate in the treatment of osteoarthritis: From in vitro studies to clinical recommendations. *Ther. Adv. Musculoskelet. Dis.* **2010**, *6*, 335–348. [CrossRef] [PubMed]

14. Campo, G.M.; Avenoso, A.; Campo, S.; D'ascola, A.; Traina, P.; Sama, D.; Calatroni, A. Glycosaminoglycans modulate inflammation and apoptosis in LPS-treated chondrocytes. *J. Cell. Biochem.* **2009**, *106*, 83–92. [CrossRef] [PubMed]
15. Campo, G.M.; Avenoso, A.; Campo, S.; Traina, P.; D'ascola, A.; Calatroni, A. Glycosaminoglycans reduced inflammatory response by modulating toll-like receptor-4 in LPS-stimulated chondrocytes. *Arch. Biochem. Biophys.* **2009**, *497*, 7–15. [CrossRef] [PubMed]
16. Bian, L.; Kaplun, M.; Williams, D.Y.; Xu, D.; Ateshian, G.A.; Hung, C.T. Influence of chondroitin sulfate on the biochemical, mechanical and frictional properties of cartilage explants in longterm culture. *J. Biomech.* **2009**, *42*, 286–290. [CrossRef] [PubMed]
17. Imada, K.; Oka, H.; Kawasaki, D.; Miura, N.; Sato, T.; Ito, A. Anti-arthritic action mechanisms of natural chondroitin sulfate in human articular chondrocytes and synovial fibroblasts. *Biol. Pharm. Bull.* **2010**, *33*, 410–414. [CrossRef] [PubMed]
18. Cho, S.Y.; Sim, J.S.; Jeong, C.S.; Chang, S.Y.; Choi, D.W.; Toida, T.; Kim, Y.S. Effects of low molecular weight chondroitin sulfate on type II collagen-induced arthritis in DBA/1J mice. *Biol. Pharm. Bull.* **2004**, *27*, 47–51. [CrossRef] [PubMed]
19. Chou, M.M.; Vergnolle, N.; McDougall, J.J.; Wallace, J.L.; Marty, S.; Teskey, V.; Buret, A.G. Effects of chondroitin and glucosamine sulfate in a dietary bar formulation on inflammation, interleukin-1β, matrix metalloprotease-9, and cartilage damage in arthritis. *Exp. Biol. Med.* **2005**, *230*, 255–262.
20. Campo, G.M.; Avenoso, A.; Campo, S.; D'ascola, A.; Traina, P.; Calatroni, A. Chondroitin-4-sulphate inhibits NF-kB translocation and caspase activation in collagen-induced arthritis in mice. *Osteoarthr. Cartil.* **2008**, *16*, 1474–1483. [CrossRef] [PubMed]
21. Wandel, S.; Jüni, P.; Tendal, B.; Nüesch, E.; Villiger, P.M.; Welton, N.J.; Reichenbach, S.; Trelle, S. Effects of glucosamine, chondroitin, or placebo in patients with osteoarthritis of hip or knee: Network meta-analysis. *BMJ* **2010**, *4*, 255–262. [CrossRef] [PubMed]
22. Reginster, J.Y.; Deroisy, R.; Rovati, L.C.; Lee, R.L.; Lejeune, E.; Bruyere, O.; Giacovelli, G.; Henrotin, Y.; Dacre, J.E.; Gossett, C. Long-term effects of glucosamine sulphate on osteoarthritis progression: A randomised, placebo-controlled clinical trial. *Lancet* **2001**, *357*, 251–256. [CrossRef]
23. McAlindon, T.; Formica, M.; LaValley, M.; Lehmer, M.; Kabbara, K. Effectiveness of glucosamine for symptoms of knee osteoarthritis: Results from an internet-based randomized double-bind controlled trial. *Am. J. Med.* **2004**, *117*, 643–649. [CrossRef] [PubMed]
24. Michel, B.A.; Stucki, G.; Frey, D.; De Vathaire, F.; Vignon, E.; Bruehlmann, P.; Uebelhart, D. Chondroitins 4 and 6 sulfate in osteoarthritis of the knee: A randomized, controlled trial. *Arthritis Rheum.* **2005**, *52*, 779–786. [CrossRef] [PubMed]
25. Mazières, B.; Hucher, M.; Zaïm, M.; Garnero, P. Effect of chondroitin sulphate in symptomatic knee osteoarthritis: A multicentre, randomised, double-blind, placebo-controlled study. *Ann. Rheum. Dis.* **2007**, *66*, 639–645. [CrossRef] [PubMed]
26. Bitter, T.; Muir, H.M. A modified uronic acid carbazole reaction. *Anal. Biochem.* **1962**, *4*, 330–334. [CrossRef]
27. Gardell, S. Determination of Hexosamines. In *Methods of Biochemical Analysis*; Glick, D., Ed.; John Wiley & Sons Inc.: Hoboken, NJ, USA, 1958; Volume 6, pp. 256–288.
28. Volpi, N. Analytical aspects of pharmaceutical grade chondroitin sulfates. *J. Pharm. Sci.* **2007**, *12*, 3168–3180. [CrossRef] [PubMed]
29. Souza, A.R.; Kozlowski, E.O.; Cerqueira, V.R.; Castelo-Branco, M.T.; Costa, M.L.; Pavão, M.S. Chondroitin sulfate and keratan sulfate are the major glycosaminoglycans present in the adult zebrafish Danio rerio (Chordata-Cyprinidae). *Glycoconj. J.* **2007**, *9*, 521–530. [CrossRef] [PubMed]
30. Huckerby, T.N. The keratan sulphates: Structural investigations using NMR spectroscopy. *Progr. Nucl. Magn. Reson. Spectrosc.* **2002**, *40*, 35–110. [CrossRef]
31. Vilanova, E.; Glauser, B.F.; Oliveira, S.M.; Tovar, A.M.; Mourão, P.A. Update on Brazilian biosimilar enoxaparins. *Expert Rev. Hematol.* **2016**, *9*, 1015–1021. [CrossRef] [PubMed]
32. Lauder, R.M.; Huckerby, T.N.; Nieduszynski, I.A. A fingerprinting method for chondroitin/dermatan sulfate and hyaluronan oligosaccharides. *Glycobiology* **2000**, *10*, 393–401. [CrossRef] [PubMed]

33. De Waard, P.; Vliegenthart, J.F.; Harada, T.; Sugahara, K. Structural studies on sulfated oligosaccharides derived from the carbohydrate-protein linkage region of chondroitin 6-sulfate proteoglycans of shark cartilage. II. Seven compounds containing 2 or 3 sulfate residues. *J. Biol. Chem.* **1992**, *267*, 6036–6043. [PubMed]
34. Chess, E.K.; Bairstow, S.; Donovan, S.; Havel, K.; Hu, P.; Johnson, R.J.; Lee, S.; McKee, J.; Miller, R.; Moore, E.; et al. Case study: Contamination of heparin with oversulfated chondroitin sulfate. *Handb. Exp. Pharmacol.* **2012**, *207*, 99–125.
35. United States Pharmacopoeia. Glucosamine sulfate sodium chloride monograph. In *United States Pharmacopoeia*, 29th ed.; United States Pharmacopeial Convention: Rockville, MD, USA, 2006; p. 2342.
36. Adebowale, A.; Cox, D.S.; Liang, Z.; Eddington, N.D. Analysis of Glucosamine and Chondroitin Sulfate Content in Marketed Products and the Caco-2 Permeability of Chondroitin Sulfate Raw Materials. *J. Am. Nutraceut. Assoc.* **2000**, *3*, 37–44.

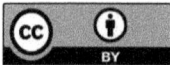

pharmaceuticals

MDPI

Article

Modernization of Enoxaparin Molecular Weight Determination Using Homogeneous Standards

Katelyn M. Arnold [1] (ID), Stephen J. Capuzzi [1] (ID), Yongmei Xu [1], Eugene N. Muratov [1], Kevin Carrick [2], Anita Y. Szajek [2,3], Alexander Tropsha [1] and Jian Liu [1,*]

1   Division of Chemical Biology and Medicinal Chemistry, Eshelman School of Pharmacy,
    University of North Carolina, Chapel Hill, NC 27599, USA; arnoldk2@email.unc.edu (K.M.A.);
    sc464303@email.unc.edu (S.J.C.); yongmeix@email.unc.edu (Y.X.); murik@email.unc.edu (E.N.M.);
    alex_tropsha@unc.edu (A.T.)
2   U.S. Pharmacopeia, Rockville, MD 20852, USA; klc@usp.org (K.C.); anita.szajek@nih.gov (A.Y.S.)
3   Center for Scientific Review, National Institutes of Health, Bethesda, MD 20892, USA
*   Correspondence: liuj@email.unc.edu; Tel.: +01-919-843-6511

Received: 1 May 2017; Accepted: 19 July 2017; Published: 22 July 2017

Abstract: Enoxaparin is a low-molecular weight heparin used to treat thrombotic disorders. Following the fatal contamination of the heparin supply chain in 2007–2008, the U.S. Pharmacopeia (USP) and U.S. Food and Drug Administration (FDA) have worked extensively to modernize the unfractionated heparin and enoxaparin monographs. As a result, the determination of molecular weight (MW) has been added to the monograph as a measure to strengthen the quality testing and to increase the protection of the global supply of this life-saving drug. The current USP calibrant materials used for enoxaparin MW determination are composed of a mixture of oligosaccharides; however, they are difficult to reproduce as the calibrants have ill-defined structures due to the heterogeneity of the heparin parent material. To address this issue, we describe a promising approach consisting of a predictive computational model built from a library of chemoenzymatically synthesized heparin oligosaccharides for enoxaparin MW determination. Here, we demonstrate that this test can be performed with greater efficiency by coupling synthetic oligosaccharides with the power of computational modeling. Our approach is expected to improve the MW measurement for enoxaparin.

Keywords: enoxaparin; USP; MW determination; oligosaccharide calibrants; computational modeling; HPLC; compendial test

1. Introduction

Heparin is a mixture of glycosaminoglycan (GAG) chains originating from porcine intestinal mucosa. It is used therapeutically as an anticoagulant for the treatment and prevention of thrombosis [1]. Heparin's GAG chains are heterogeneous in nature and vary in molecular weight (MW), chain length, degree of sulfation, disaccharide unit composition, and pharmacological effects [2]. The variability in unfractionated heparin's pharmacokinetic properties and pharmacological effects led to the development of low MW heparin (LMWH), which is a degraded product of heparin using chemical or enzymatic cleavage techniques [2]. LMWHs are now considered the standard of care for the clinical management of venous thromboembolism [1,2]. The most common form of LMWH in the U.S. is enoxaparin, which is produced by β-eliminative cleavage of the benzyl esters of porcine mucosal heparin under alkaline conditions [2]. This cleavage process leads to the generation of unnatural structures in enoxaparin (Figure 1A). The majority of the resulting chains have an unsaturated uronate residue at the non-reducing end, which can be utilized for UV detection at 232 nm, and up to 25% of chains have a 1,6-anhydro structure at the reducing end [3].

A.

R₁ = -H or -SO₃⁻Na⁺
R₂ = -COCH₃ or -SO₃⁻Na⁺

B.

C.

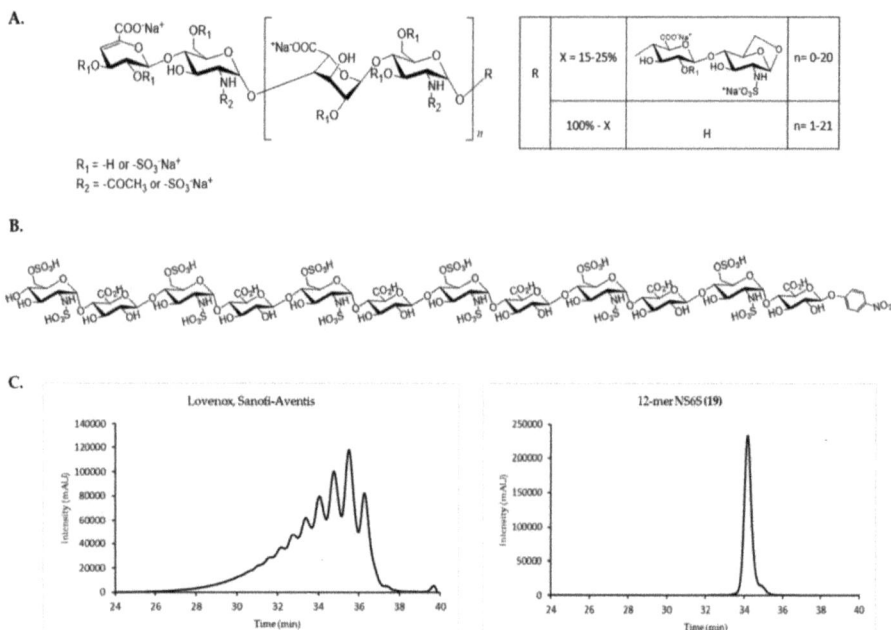

Figure 1. (**A**) Enoxaparin structure. The 1,6-anhydro reducing end is depicted in the box on the right; (**B**) the structure of 12-mer NS6S (**19**); (**C**) representative size exclusion chromatography (SEC) chromatogram of Lovenox and 12-mer NS6S (**19**). Enoxaparin's heterogeneity and complexity is evident from multiple peaks with poor base-line separation.

While heparin drugs have been used extensively in the clinic since the 1930s, the characterization, regulation, and quality control aspects of these materials remain challenging [4]. Since chain length is one of the factors that affects LMWH biological activity [5], an accurate method to determine MW distribution and average weight MW (M_w) is an essential quality control step. However, due to their high degree of structural complexity and acidity, the determination of the M_w and MW distribution of enoxaparin is not readily amenable to analysis by mass spectrometry [6]. An alternative chromatographic method was developed and added to the US Pharmacopeia (USP) monographs [7,8]. The accuracy of this chromatographic analysis relies ultimately on calibration with standards of high purity [8]. Due to the lack of structurally defined calibrants, the evaluation of M_w and MW distribution represents a controversial aspect of LMWH characterization [5].

Ideal standards for analyzing enoxaparin would be oligosaccharides that encompass enoxaparin's MW range in order to determine M_w ~4500 Da [9]. In practice, pure oligosaccharide standards of this size are difficult to isolate. Thus, a mixture of calibrants enriched in particular MW ranges have been used. While the disaccharide composition of these calibrants is known, the precise sequences of the intact oligosaccharide chains are unknown, raising a concern about the reproduction of the calibrants. The goal of this study is to develop a new technique that is reliable and sustainable for the determination of M_w and MW distribution by combining synthetic oligosaccharides and computational modeling. To achieve this goal, the following aims were accomplished; (i) the synthesis of a panel of oligosaccharides covering the enoxaparin MW range between 2226 and 5176 Da; (ii) the development of a predictive computational model for MW analysis; (iii) the development of a system suitability protocol; and (iv) the analysis of commercially available Enoxaparin Sodium from different manufacturers.

2. Results

2.1. Chemoenzymatic Synthesis of Oligosaccharide Panel

A total of 27 oligosaccharides were synthesized by a chemoenzymatic approach, and the MW of each compound was verified by mass spectrometry [10,11]. The compounds are organized into five structural groups (A to E) (see Table 1 and Supplementary Figure S1) based on repeating disaccharide structural units. Group A contains compounds without sulfation; all glucosamine residues are *N*-acetylated. Group B contains compounds with one *N*-sulfo group per disaccharide unit. Group C contains compounds with two sulfo groups per disaccharide unit, with *N*-sulfated glucosamine and 2-*O*-sulfo iduronic acid residues. Group D contains compounds with two sulfo groups per disaccharide unit due to repeating units of *N*, 6-*O*-sulfated glucosamine. Finally, group E contains compounds with three sulfo groups per disaccharide unit due to repeating units of *N*, 6-*O*-sulfated glucosamine and 2-*O*-sulfo iduronic acid.

Table 1. Panel of oligosaccharides and US Pharmacopeia (USP) Enoxaparin MW calibrant A and B materials.

Group	Compound Name	Repeating Unit Structure [1]	MW (Da)
A.	8-mer NAc (1)	GlcNAc-(GlcA-GlcNAc)$_3$-GlcA-pNP	1656
	10-mer NAc (2)	GlcNAc-(GlcA-GlcNAc)$_4$-GlcA-pNP	2036
	12-mer NAc (3)	GlcNAc-(GlcA-GlcNAc)$_5$-GlcA-pNP	2415
	14-mer NAc (4)	GlcNAc-(GlcA-GlcNAc)$_6$-GlcA-pNP	2794
	16-mer NAc (5)	GlcNAc-(GlcA-GlcNAc)$_7$-GlcA-pNP	3174
	18-mer NAc (6)	GlcNAc-(GlcA-GlcNAc)$_8$-GlcA-pNP	3553
B.	8-mer NS (7)	GlcNS-(GlcA-GlcNS)$_3$-GlcA-pNP	1808
	10-mer NS (8)	GlcNS-(GlcA-GlcNS)$_4$-GlcA-pNP	2226
	12-mer NS (9)	GlcNS-(GlcA-GlcNS)$_5$-GlcA-pNP	2643
	14-mer NS (10)	GlcNS-(GlcA-GlcNS)$_6$-GlcA-pNP	3060
	16-mer NS (11)	GlcNS-(GlcA-GlcNS)$_7$-GlcA-pNP	3478
	18-mer NS (12)	GlcNS-(GlcA-GlcNS)$_8$-GlcA-pNP	3895
C.	10-mer NS2S (13)	GlcNS-GlcA-(GlcNS-IdoA2S)$_3$-GlcNS-GlcA-pNP	2466
	12-mer NS2S (14)	GlcNS-GlcA-(GlcNS-IdoA2S)$_4$-GlcNS-GlcA-pNP	2963
	14-mer NS2S (15)	GlcNS-GlcA-(GlcNS-IdoA2S)$_5$-GlcNS-GlcA-pNP	3461
	16-mer NS2S (16)	GlcNS-GlcA-(GlcNS-IdoA2S)$_6$-GlcNS-GlcA-pNP	3958
	18-mer NS2S (17)	GlcNS-GlcA-(GlcNS-IdoA2S)$_7$-GlcNS-GlcA-pNP	4456
D.	10-mer NS6S (18)	GlcNS6S-(GlcA-GlcNS6S)$_4$-GlcA-pNP	2626
	12-mer NS6S (19)	GlcNS6S-(GlcA-GlcNS6S)$_5$-GlcA-pNP	3124
	14-mer NS6S (20)	GlcNS6S-(GlcA-GlcNS6S)$_6$-GlcA-pNP	3621
	16-mer NS6S (21)	GlcNS6S-(GlcA-GlcNS6S)$_7$-GlcA-pNP	4118
	18-mer NS6S (22)	GlcNS6S-(GlcA-GlcNS6S)$_8$-GlcA-pNP	4616
E.	8-mer NS6S2S (23)	GlcNS6S-GlcA-(GlcNS6S-IdoA2S)$_2$-GlcNS6S-GlcA-pNP	2289
	12-mer NS6S2S (24)	GlcNS6S-GlcA-(GlcNS6S-IdoA2S)$_4$-GlcNS6S-GlcA-pNP	3444
	14-mer NS6S2S (25)	GlcNS6S-GlcA-(GlcNS6S-IdoA2S)$_5$-GlcNS6S-GlcA-pNP	4021
	16-mer NS6S2S (26)	GlcNS6S-GlcA-(GlcNS6S-IdoA2S)$_6$-GlcNS6S-GlcA-pNP	4599
	18-mer NS6S2S (27)	GlcNS6S-GlcA-(GlcNS6S-IdoA2S)$_7$-GlcNS6S-GlcA-pNP	5176
F.	dp4 (28)	ΔHexA,2S-GlcNS6S-IdoA2S-GlcNS6S	~1200
	dp6 (29)	ΔHexA,2S-GlcNS6S-(IdoA2S-GlcNS6S)$_2$	~1800
G.	USP A.1		11000
	USP A.2		5200
	USP A.3		2250
	USP A.4		1400
	USP B.1		7750
	USP B.2		3350
	USP B.3		1800

[1] Abbreviations: GlcA (glucuronic acid); GlcN (glucosamine); GlcNAc (*N*-acetylated glucosamine); GlcNS (*N*-sulfo glucosamine); IdoA2S (2-*O*-sulfo iduronic acid); GlcNS6S (6-*O*, *N*-disulfo glucosamine); HexA (hexauronic acid); -pNP (*para*-nitrophenyl).

Additionally, two commercially available heparin oligosaccharides, designated as group F (Iduron, Manchester, UK), were used to address the lower MW range. These oligosaccharides are prepared from partial heparin lyase degradation of heparin, followed by high-resolution gel filtration chromatography purification. The general structure is ΔHexA2S-GlcNS6S-(IdoA2S-GlcNS6S)$_n$, with $n = 1$ for dp4 and $n = 2$ for dp6. Although not homogeneous, the majority (~75%) of structures contain three sulfo groups per disaccharide unit, consisting of *N*, 6-*O*-sulfated glucosamine and 2-*O*-sulfo iduronic acid.

The USP Enoxaparin Sodium MW calibrant A and B materials (USP, Rockville, MD, USA), designated as group G, were included in this study (Table 1 and Figure S2). The reported MW values in the calibrants for each chromatographic peak are 11000, 7750, 5200, 3350, 2250, 1800, and 1400 Da.

Compared to enoxaparin, synthetic oligosaccharides have defined structures, as demonstrated by **19** in Figure 1B. All synthetic oligosaccharides (**1** to **27**) migrated as a single, narrow main peak on size exclusion chromatography (SEC), supporting their homogeneous nature (Figure S1). These oligosaccharides can be reliably reproduced based on the established synthetic schemes with minimal impurities.

2.2. Size Exclusion Chromatography Profiles of Synthetic Oligosaccharides

2.2.1. SEC Characterization of Synthetic Oligosaccharides

The USP compendial method uses size exclusion chromatography (SEC) to relate retention time (RT) to MW. The synthetic oligosaccharides were evaluated for use as reference standards by obtaining a RT via SEC (Figure S1). The analyses were conducted in five groups, group A to E, based on the structural features of these samples. Following the compendial method, a calibration curve for each structural group was generated by plotting log(MW) versus RT and used for nonlinear regression analysis (Figure 2A–E). USP calibrants, as well as the synthetic oligosaccharides in each structural group, exhibited tight correlation between the MW and RT (Figure 2).

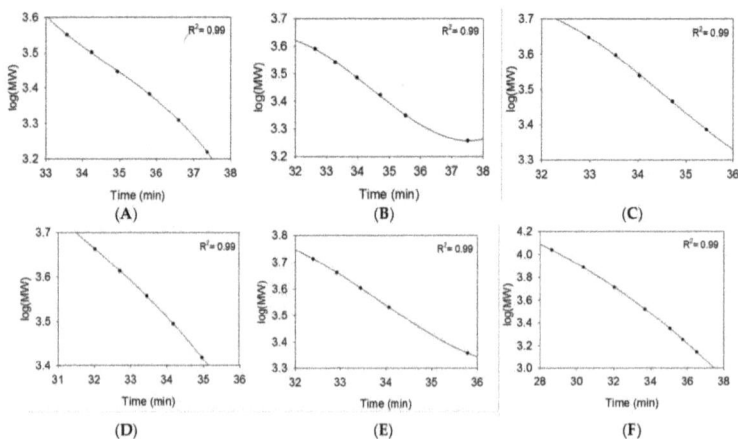

Figure 2. Calibration curves for determining M_w generated from different structural groups: (**A**) NAc series (group A); (**B**) NS series (group B); (**C**) NS2S series (group C); (**D**) NS6S series (group D); (**E**) NS6S2S series (group E); (**F**) USP Calibrant A and B (group G). The nonlinear regression R^2 value is listed in upper right corner of each panel.

2.2.2. SEC RT Depends on Both Oligosaccharide Shape and Size (MW)

We next compared the calibration curves from each structural group to that of the USP calibrants by superimposing the analyses (Figure S3). Two main observations are apparent; (i) the structure of the oligosaccharides affects the RT and (ii) smaller synthetic oligosaccharides do not behave similiarly to enoxaparin-like materials.

Oligosaccharides containing sulfo groups (Figure S3B–E) migrated more closely to the USP calibration curve than group A, the non-sulfated NAc series (Figure S3A), even though each group is comprised of similar MWs. This result suggests that the structures of oligosaccharides impact the RT. This observation raises the possibility that saccharide sequences carrying different sulfo groups or IdoA residues may change the overall oligosaccharide shape and display different SEC migration properties. The assertion is further demonstrated in Figure 3 by comparing group E oligosaccharides (NS6S2S series) with group B oligosaccharides (NS series). Here, the effect on RT becomes noticeable for those oligosaccharides that have a MW greater than 3000 Da. Larger oligosaccharides in group E display similar RT to smaller oliogsaccharides in group B, despite a clear difference in MW. One possible expanation is that group E oligosaccharides contain conformationally flexible IdoA residues, underlining the influence of the molecular shape of oligosaccharides on RT. It is noted that both 1,6-anhydro glucosamine and 1,6-anhydro mannosamine are present at the reducing end of some oligosaccharide chains of enoxaparin [7]. However, the disaccharide building blocks containing 1,6-anhydro residues only represent <2% of the disaccharide building blocks in enoxaparin. At the present time, we were unable to evaluate the impact of 1,6-anhydro residues on the elution behavior during the analysis.

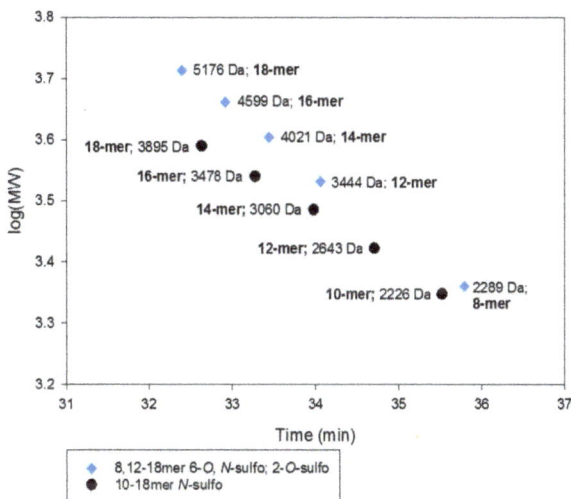

Figure 3. Comparison of two structural series and SEC behavior. Blue diamonds are group E (NS6S2S series). Black circles are group B (NS series).

Another observation is that short oligosaccharides do not have similar RTs to enoxaparin-like materials such as the USP calibrants. We compared all 27 oligosaccharides with to the USP calibrants (Figure 4A) and found that the RT values of the smaller synthetic oligosaccharides deviate the greatest from the USP calibrants. To address this lower MW range deviation, two commerically available heparin oligosaccharides, dp6 (6-mer) and dp4 (4-mer), were included (Figure 4B, blue triangles). dp6 and dp4 both closely align with the USP calibrants. For this reason, three synthetic oligosaccharides, 8-mer NAc (**1**), 10-mer NAc (**2**), and 8-mer NS (**7**), were excluded from further analysis, as described below.

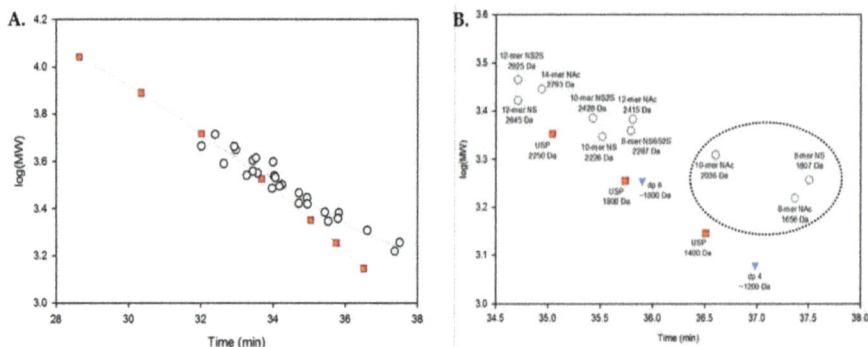

Figure 4. (**A**) USP calibrants (red squares) and all synthetic oligosaccharides (black open circles); (**B**) Correlation of the molecular weight (MW) and retention time (RT) of compounds below 3000 Da annotated. Compounds enclosed in the circle, 8-mer NAc (**1**), 10-mer NAc (**2**), and 8-mer NS (**7**), were the outliers and were excluded from further analysis.

2.3. Using Calibration Curves to Determine M_w of USP Enoxaparin RS

Following the USP compendial method [7], the equation from the nonlinear regression analysis was used to determine the M_w of USP Enoxaparin RS. Using the generated USP calibration curve, the measured M_w is very close to the reported M_w for USP Enoxaparin RS (Table 2, Row 1), suggesting that the procedures were appropriately carried out. However, all of the determined M_w values are outside the USP acceptable range of ±3.4% (Table 2, Rows 2–7). Using all 24 synthesized oligosaccharides, one would expect that the M_w would be accurately determined since the major structural components are accounted for; however, the measured M_w was 3250 Da, which was still 25.6% lower than the anticipated value of 4370 Da.

Table 2. Determination of USP Enoxaparin RS M_w.

Series	USP Enoxaparin RS M_w (4370 ± 150 Da)	Deviation from Acceptability Range (100 ± 3.4%)
USP Calibrants	4300	−1.6%
NAc (group A)	22,300	+410.3%
NS (group B)	3100	−29.1%
NS2S (group C)	3500	−19.9%
NS6S (group D)	3350	−23.3 %
NS6S2S (group E)	3700	−15.3%
All oligosaccharides	3250	−25.6%

The unexpected difference in measured M_w values is likely due to the selection of the calibrants/standards for the analysis. The current USP method was developed using calibrants with heterogeneous structures, while our method uses homogeneous standards. To amend the difference, the relative molar contributions of the disaccharide repeating units of enoxaparin are taken into account. As shown in Table 3, enoxaparin is comprised of a mixture of compounds in which ~89% show similarity to one of our five oligosaccharide structural groups [12]. The remaining 11% of components in enoxaparin includes several structures, each contributing less than 2% to the overall mixture composition and for which we do not have complementary synthetic oligosaccharides. When using all the synthetic oligosaccharides via the nonlinear regression method to determine M_w, each oligosaccharide contributed equally to the overall M_w, even if the structure only accounted for a very small molar percentage. Therefore, we turned to computational tools to allow us to use these homogeneous compounds appropriately as calibrants that account for enoxaparin's heterogeneity during analysis.

Table 3. Major structural components of Enoxaparin.

Disaccharide Structure	Molar %
ΔUA2S-GlcNS6S	~70%
ΔUA-GlcNS6S	~10%
ΔUA2S-GlcNS	~6%
ΔUA-GlcNS	~2%
ΔUA-GlcNAc	~1%

2.4. Method Modernization: SVM Modeling Allows for Synthetic Oligosaccharides to be Used in the Appropriate Proportions to Reflect the Various Quantities of Components in Enoxaparin

We used a Support Vector Machine (SVM) [13] technique for the modeling, in place of the nonlinear regression analysis recommended by the USP. The nonlinear regression assumes that the relationship of MW and RT fits a cubic function. On the other hand, the SVM model learns statistically meaningful relationships between MW and RT, approximates a multidimensional regression function, and optimizes this relationship for predictions. Moreover, unlike the standard nonlinear regression analysis, which treats all data points equally, the SVM model can assign greater statistical importance to specific data points. In our case, several oligosaccharides have nearly identical RTs, yet their MWs are different. If an enoxaparin sample displays a peak at this RT, the MW of the peak is calculated based on the relative abundance of the distinct oligosaccharides.

A total of 33 compounds were included in the training set, including 24 synthetic compounds, seven current USP calibrant data points, and the two purchased oligosaccharides (Table S1). The compounds were represented based on their repeating disaccharide unit to more closely reflect enoxaparin in a process known in statistical modeling as 'weighting'. Group E and F oligosaccharides (NS6S2S, dp4 and dp6) are weighted by a factor of 10, followed by group D oligosaccharides (NS6S series), which were weighted by a factor of four, and group C oligosaccharides (NS2S series), which were weighted by a factor of two. While group A, B, and G (NAc, NS and USP calibrants) remain unweighted in the data set, their inclusion is important in order to adequately capture the low and high ends of the MW range. To visualize how well the model predicts MW, the distribution of the predicted versus observed MW values of the external set compounds is shown in Figure 5. As part of the validation of the model, each compound in the training set is systematically left out of model building and placed into an external set. The resulting model then predicts the compounds in the external set.

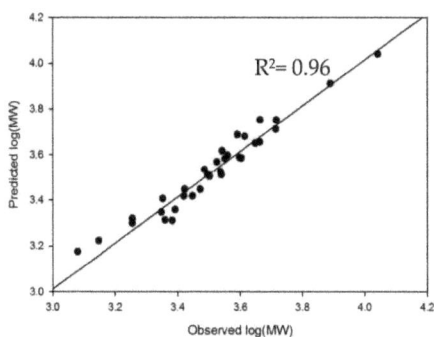

Figure 5. Predicted log(MW) versus observed log(MW) to demonstrate the strength of the model's prediction. For predicted log(MW), only external set MW predictions are used. Observed MW is determined by MS for the pure oligosaccharides. For dp4, dp6, and USP calibrants, the provided MW values were used as the observed MW. The model's predictions highly correlate to the expected results ($R^2 = 0.96$).

The first level of external model validation was performed by determining the M_w of USP Enoxaparin RS. Unlike our nonlinear regression analysis, the SVM model is able to successfully predict M_w within the acceptable range, as seen in Table 4.

Table 4. Validation of oligosaccharide Support Vector Machine (SVM) model.

	USP Calibrants	Oligosaccharide SVM Model
USP Enoxaparin RS (M_w = 4370 ± 150 Da)	4300 Da	4450 Da

The largest oligosaccharide that can currently be synthesized by the chemoenzymatic synthesis approach is 18 residues long (~5000 Da), yet enoxaparin's MW distribution expands beyond 5000 Da. This is not an issue, though, when the SVM model is used for analysis because, in addition, to achieving an acceptable M_w value, the predicted MWs for the largest components in USP Enoxaparin RS are comparable with the results from the USP calibrants up to 11,000 Da (Table S2). The determination of MWs above 11,000 Da requires extrapolation; therefore comparison between the methods at this point must be done with care.

These results demonstrate that the utility of the synthetic oligosaccharides can only be fully realized when coupled with an appropriate computational model. In this way, we are able to reflect the nature of the enoxaparin mixture by weighting oligosaccharides based on their relative molar contribution to the composition of the enoxaparin mixture.

2.5. System Suitability: Applying the SVM Model in a Compendial Technique

The use of the SVM model eliminates the need to run all oligosaccharide standards for analysis, thereby shortening the analysis. Currently the SVM model is a stand-alone tool that only requires RT and peak areas as an input. Ultimately, we envision a software interface that houses this SVM model to facilitate a streamlined analysis process. Any future software development that incorporates the validated SVM model will contain a system suitability assessment before access to the model is granted.

A system suitability test is required in the USP compendial method to ensure that the selected analytical technique offers the adequate resolution to analyze enoxaparin. Using the oligosaccharides coupled with the SVM model, we can accomplish the system suitability test and analysis in one HPLC process by using two detection wavelengths; 232 nm for enoxaparin and 310 nm for the oligosaccharides (Figure 6). To this end, enoxaparin was mixed with three synthetic oligosaccharides, 8-mer NS (**7**), 12-mer NS6S (**19**), and 16–mer NS6S (**21**), for SEC analysis to obtain a chromatogram shown in Figure 6A. A system suitability check was performed by confirming the RTs of the internal oligosaccharide standards at 310 nm (Figure 6B). The 310 nm RTs fell within the acceptable range of ±0.1 min, predetermined by running the oligosaccharides alone. As shown in Figure S4, the overlapped RT values indicated that the system is suitable for use with the SVM model. Next, the peak areas contributed by the oligosaccharides at 232 nm (Figure 6C, blue trace) were subtracted from the chromatogram. The resulting 232 nm chromatogram is used by the SVM model for the determination of the M_w and the MW distribution (Figure 6D).

2.6. Analysis of Commercially Available Enoxaparin Sodium Using Oligosaccharide SVM Model

Using the SVM model and system suitability procedure, three commercially available Enoxaparin Sodium samples, both brand and generic versions, were analyzed. The M_w and MW distribution results are shown in Table 5. The results demonstrate that our approach allows for consistent and adequate testing of M_w. We acknowledge that our UV detection method differs from the refractive index (RI) detection method listed in the monograph. We chose UV detection because the oligosaccharides have a tag that absorbs at 310 nm with very high sensitivity. Although RI detection can be used in principle, large quantities of the oligosaccharide standards will be needed due to the RI's low detection sensitivity. This would unnecessarily increase the cost of analysis. The difference in detection methods may account for the consistently high percentage between 2000–8000 Da. The harmonization of RI and UV detection can be achieved in subsequent studies after analyzing a large set of enoxaparin samples.

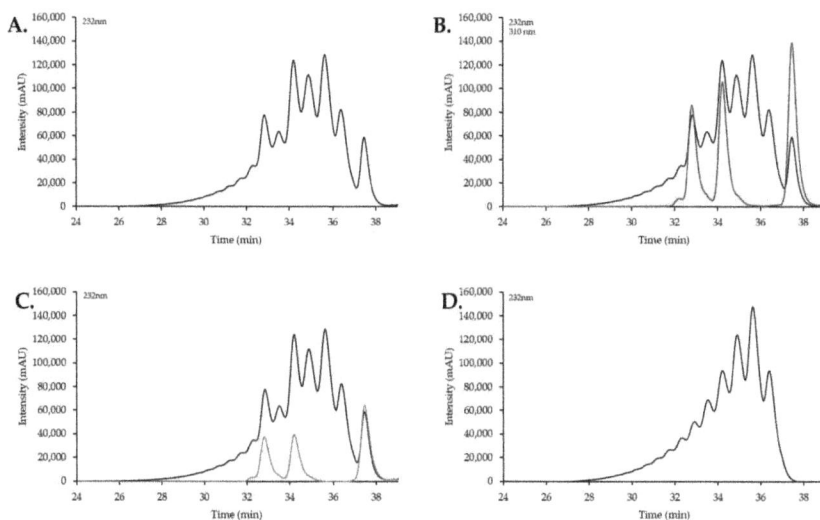

Figure 6. (**A**) 232 nm trace of enoxaparin mixed with three oligosaccharides. Although primary detection of the synthetic oligosaccharides is at 310 nm, there is some residual absorbance also at 232 nm, as evidenced by the abnormal profile compared to Figure 1C; (**B**) Overlay of 310 nm and 232 nm trace from a single run of the enoxaparin/oligosaccharide mixture. 310 nm peak RTs (red trace) were used to determine the suitability of the HPLC system by comparing them with the predetermined 310 nm chromatogram from oligosaccharides alone (Figure S4); (**C**) Overlay of predetermined 232 nm trace (blue trace); (**D**) The resulting 232 nm trace when the oligosaccharide contribution is removed. The peak RTs and area values are input into the model for analysis.

Table 5. Analysis of commercially available Enoxaparin Sodium using SVM model.

Sample	M_w	Distribution
Lovenox	M_w = 4650 ± 35 Da	M_{2000}: 14.0 ± 0.5% $M_{2000–8000}$: 82.0 ± 0.5% M_{8000}: 4.0 ± 0.5%
Enoxaparin Sodium; Sandoz	M_w = 4350 ± 0 Da	M_{2000}: 16.5 ± 1.0% $M_{2000–8000}$: 81.0 ± 1.0% M_{8000}: 2.5 ± 0.0%
Enoxaparin Sodium; Amphastar	M_w = 4350 ± 27 Da	M_{2000}: 13.5 ± 1.0% $M_{2000–8000}$: 83.5 ± 1.0% M_{8000}: 3.5 ± 1.0%

3. Discussion

LMWHs are heterogeneous mixtures of oligosaccharides, the MW distribution of which can be described by M_w and by identifying the percentage of material that falls within specificied MW ranges [6]. The determination of these parameters is an important step in enoxaparin quality control and requires reliable, pure calibrants. Since the RT from SEC is the result of both a molecule's size/weight and shape, the calibrants must closely reflect the structure of enoxaparin [14]. However only a portion of its natural oligosaccharides have been isolated and characterized [15], leaving the rest of the mixture largely unknown. There are several reports on the disaccharide composition of heparin and enoxaparin, which sheds light on proportions of repeating structural units found in these complex mixtures [16–18]. With this in mind, we report the generation of enoxaparin-like oligosaccharides via chemoenzymatic synthesis. The panel of compounds is comprehensive both in the scope of MW and structural class coverage, which is important when considering the influence of both MW and shape on RT.

After SEC characterization, it became evident that the synthetic oligosaccharides cannot be simply substituted for the existing USP calibrants without changing the procedures for data analysis. Surprisingly, although each structural series fits its own regression lines closely, no individual structural group was able to correctly determine the M_w for USP Enoxaparin RS (Table 2, Rows 2–7). For example, using the group A calibration curve, the measured M_w was 22300 Da, 410% above the label value, whereas using the group B calibration curve, the measured M_w was 3100 Da, 29.1% below the anticipated value. The deviation of the calibration curves using synthetic oligosaccharides and USP calibrants (Figure S3) suggests that the homogeneous oligosaccharides did not fully represent the migration properties of the USP calibrants that contain mainly heterogeneously sulfated oligosaccharides. The current compendial method is designed for specific use with the intended USP calibrants, and replacement with synthetic oligosaccharides does not give the correct M_w for USP Enoxaparin RS. Therefore, we needed to amend the analysis method to accommodate our homogeneous compounds.

Using structurally defined oligosaccharides as MW standards for SEC analysis is undoubtedly a superior approach compared to a mixture of oligosaccharides since these homogeneous standards can be accurately re-synthesized. However, implementation of the pure oligosaccharides requires careful consideration. Our study represents an important first step towards using these materials in practice. The key finding from our study is that a combination of a set of synthetic oligosaccharides and a computational model for data processing is essential for predicting the M_w of enoxaparin. SVM modeling techniques allowed us to use the panel of synthetic oligosaccharides in appropriate proportions based on their relative abundance in enoxaparin, with groups E and F weighted the greatest, followed by groups C and D. Groups A, B, and G are included but not weighted in the data set in order to cover a large MW range. Without coverage of the extremes of the range, the extrapolative ability of the SVM model would be hampered. Therefore, these compounds are needed to capture a broad MW range so that this model can be extended to other heterogeneous heparin materials (i.e., bovine sourced preparations) in the future. To further demonstrate the robustness of this method, more enoxaparin lots from different manufacturers will be analyzed in future studies.

Our approach is also more efficient both in terms of time and cost compared to the current method (Table 6). The overall time from injection onto the HPLC to the final result is dramatically reduced since only one analysis (enoxaparin sample mixed with oligosaccharides) needs to be run. In comparison, the current method requires running several individual materials (MW Calibrant A and B, RS, and an enoxaparin sample). With further software development, the process can become automated. For example, the software will house the SVM model in such a way that the M_w and the distribution are automatically reported after input data passes the system suitability check, thereby eliminating operators' subjectivity during the analysis. We envisage that our approach will improve the quality control for enoxaparin production. Given that numerous structurally heterogeneous drugs exist on the marketplace, our strategy, using homogenous standards to calibrate a mixture of heparin, can be potentially expanded to analyze these complex drugs.

Table 6. Comparison of the technical aspects of each method.

	USP Method	Proposed Method
Required materials	USP Enoxaparin MW Calibrant A USP Enoxaparin MW Calibrant B USP Enoxaparin RS Enoxaparin sample	Oligosaccharide Standard Solution Enoxaparin sample
Required HPLC time [1]	~5.3 h	~1.3 h
Analysis	• Create calibration curve • Determine system suitabiltiy: determine M_w for each duplicate USP Enoxaparin RS • Analyze sample: determine M_w and distribution range for each duplicate enoxaparin sample	• Input RT and peak area data from chromatogram into SVM model

[1] Chromatograms should be recorded for a length of time sufficient for complete elution, including salt and solvent peaks. In this work, all samples were recorded for 40 min, and therefore the approximate total HPLC run time is calculated by multiplying the number of samples to be run (accounting for duplicate injections of each) by 40 min.

4. Materials and Methods

4.1. Chemoenzymatic Synthesis

The panel of oligosaccharides, ranging in length from octasaccharide (8-mer) to octadecasaccharide (18-mer), was synthesized using an established chemoenzymatic approach [10]. Briefly, each compound was synthesized from a commercially available glucuronide-*para*-nitrophenyl monosaccharide starting material, followed by a series of elongation steps and subsequent epimerization and sulfation modifications catalyzed by recombinant enzymes. Structural characterization was confirmed by nuclear magnetic resonance (NMR) and electrospray ionization mass spectrometry (ESI-MS), as previously described [10].

4.2. MW Distribution and M_w

The USP compendial method for the determination of enoxaparin M_w and MW distribution utilizes SEC. The reported method is adapted from the compendial method stated in the Enoxaparin Sodium monograph [7]. The apparatus was composed of a Shimadzu LC-20AB pump, a Shimadzu SIL-20A HT auto sampler, a Shimadzu CBM-20A controller, and a Shimadzu SPD-M20A diode array detector (Shimadzu, Kyoto, Japan). The following chromatography columns were connected in series; TSKgel guard column SWxl (6 mm I.D. × 4 cm), TSKgel G2000 SWxl (7.8 mm I.D × 30 cm), and TSKgel G3000 SWxl (7.8 mm I.D. × 30 cm). The mobile phase consisted of 0.1 M ammonium acetate and 0.5 M NaCl, filtered through 0.22 micron membrane, at a flow rate of 0.6 mL/min. Samples were filtered through a 0.22 micron membrane and injected in 20 uL volumes.

USP Enoxaparin MW Calibrant A and B (USP, Rockville, MD, USA) were dissolved in mobile phase and run in duplicate to obtain peak RTs. The provided peak MWs were used to plot log(MW) versus RT. USP Enoxaparin RS (USP, Rockville, MD, USA) was dissolved in mobile phase and run in duplicate. The nonlinear regression analysis of log(MW) versus RT (MS Excel, Sigmaplot, Seattle, WA USA) was used to determine the weight-average MW (Equation (1)), M_w, of the USP Enoxaparin RS, which has a label M_w value of 4370+/−150 Da, in order to demonstrate the system's suitability.

$$M_w = \frac{\sum_i N_i M_i^2}{N_i M_i},$$ (1)

where N_i is the number of molecules at MW M_i. Although refractive index (RI) detection is listed in the USP monograph, using UV signal intensity from the Calibrant A and B materials with Equation (1) resulted in a determination of the M_w of USP Enoxaparin RS within the acceptable range. UV detection is preferred due to the ability to discriminate the oligosaccharides from enoxaparin in a single sample based on their respective λ_{max} values.

The M_w and MW distribution of enoxaparin was determined by dissolving in mobile phase and running in duplicate. The peak areas and total area under the chromatogram, excluding salt and solvent peaks, are used by the model to determine the MW distribution, which is defined by the percentage of enoxaparin with MW less than 2000 Da, M_{2000}, the percentage between 2000 to 8000 Da, $M_{2000-8000}$, and the percentage greater than 8000 Da, M_{8000}.

The total panel of synthesized oligosaccharides was run individually to obtain a RT for each. Collectively, the MWs and RTs were used to subsequently determine the M_w and MW distribution of USP Enoxaparin RS and the enoxaparin samples.

Commercially available heparin oligosaccharides (Iduron, Manchester, UK) with approximate MWs of 1800 Da and 1200 Da were used to address the MW range below 2000 Da. These RTs were included with the oligosaccharide panel in the nonlinear regression analysis and computational model.

For system suitability tests, 8-mer NS, 12-mer NS6S, and 16-mer NS6S were combined and vortexed to mix. 30 µg of this solution (10 µg of each) was injected in duplicate in order to determine the absorbance at 310 and 232 nm. Then an enoxaparin sample (1 mg) was combined with the oligosaccharide solution and vortexed to mix. From the resulting solution, a single injection containing 0.2 mg of enoxaparin and 10ug of each oligosaccharide was injected in duplicate, and chromatograms were recorded at 310 and 232 nm.

The monograph specifications were used as criteria to evaluate the effectiveness of oligosaccharide nonlinear regression and the SVM model:

- The determination of USP Enoxaparin RS within 150 Da of labeled M_w value.
- The determination of an enoxaparin test sample with M_w ~4500 Da, the range being between 3800 and 5000 Da.
- The determination of an enoxaparin test sample MW distribution:

  ○   ~16.0% below 2000 Da, the range being between 12.0 and 20.0%;
  ○   ~74.0% between 2000 and 8000 Da, the range being between 68.0 and 82.0%;
  ○   Not more than 18.0% higher than 8,000 Da.

4.3. Development and External Validation of SVM Model

The training set of the model contains 33 unique samples;–6, 8–29, and the current USP calibrants (seven data points). Based on the relative molar percent contribution to the overall enoxaparin mixture the NS6S2S, NS6S, and NS2S oligosaccharides, as well as the purchased oligosaccharides were weighted. The NS and NAc oligosaccharides and the current USP calibrants were not weighted.

Each of these 33 samples has an experimentally derived RT and an associated MW. Thus, the MW is the endpoint to be predicted by the model, and the RT of each sample is the input descriptor used to establish the statistical relationship. The machine learning algorithm utilized in the model is a Radial-Basis Function Support Vector Machine (RBF-SVM). During the generation and validation of the model, external leave-one-out cross validation (LOO-CV) was performed and the overall q^2 (LOO-CV regression) was calculated and deemed statistically valid [19,20]. Y-randomization [21] was performed to ensure that a statistically meaningful relationship between MW and RT exists.

An additional round of external validation [21] was performed to ensure the predictivity of the model using samples obtained from commercially available Enoxaparin Sodium; Lovenox™, Sanofi-Aventis, Bridgewater, NJ; Enoxaparin Sodium Injection, Sandoz, Princeton, NJ; and Enoxaparin Sodium Injection, Amphastar Pharmaceuticals, Rancho Cucamonga, CA. Each sample was from the same lot and was run five times. Data are presented as an average ± standard deviation of M_w and its distribution. These samples were not used as training set samples during model building, thereby constituting purely external data points. The RTs of these samples were used as model inputs, and a MW prediction was made.

5. Conclusions

The determination of the MW distribution and the M_w of enoxaparin is an essential yet challenging quality control step that relies on calibrants to ensure the quality and consistency of the product. Chemoenzymatic synthesis allows for a reproducible production of pure oligosaccharides that can be used as standards for a MW analysis of enoxaparin. We employed 27 oligosaccharides that vary in MW and structure in order to match the range of possible compounds present in enoxaparin. Following the nonlinear regression analysis, we were unable to achieve accurate results. We addressed this issue by utilizing an SVM computational technique. Using the oligosaccharides and the current USP calibrants as a training set, we succeeded in developing a robust SVM model for efficient analysis by appropriately weighting oligosaccharides based on their relative abundance in enoxaparin. In addition to standard external validation, we have proven the predictive power of the model by analyzing both brand and generic versions of Enoxaparin Sodium. For the most effective use in practice, we recommend first performing a system suitability check, in which three designated oligosaccharides are run to ensure that the HPLC conditions are adequate, before the subsequent use of the developed SVM model.

We recognize that using a different HPLC detection method than what is stated in the monograph is a limitation of this work. The current calibrants, RS materials, and acceptability criteria have been established using RI detection. Therefore, it is not surprising that our results (Table 5) are not in exact agreement with the monograph criteria. In this study, we demonstrate the proof-of-concept that homogenous oligosaccharides can be used for MW determination. To further advance this promising approach, future studies will focus on (i) harmonization between RI and UV detection to ensure accuracy when comparing the results to the established acceptability criteria; (ii) the determination of the limits of SVM model in terms of HPLC variability; (iii) the development of a user-interface software to house the SVM model; and (iv) the extension of the method to compare to other countries' pharmacopeias, namely the European Pharmacopeia. As a result, our work provides a sustainable and efficient method for performing this compendial test for enoxaparin and represents a promising approach that could improve quality testing in the future.

Supplementary Materials: The following are available online at www.mdpi.com/1424-8247/10/3/66/s1. Figure S1: SEC chromatograms of synthetic oligosaccharides, Figure S2: (A) USP MW Calibrant A with provided MW values indicated; (B) USP MW Calibrant B with provided MW values indicated, Figure S3: Comparison of USP Enoxaparin Calibrants (red) and structural series (black) (A) NAc series (B) NS series (C) NS2S series (D) NS6S series (E) NS6S2S series, Figure S4: 310 nm trace from enoxaparin/oligosaccharide mixture (black) overlaid with 310 nm trace from oligosaccharide mixture alone (red). Chromatograms were obtained on different days and under the same HPLC conditions. Overlap of traces indicates that data from this system is suitable for use by the SVM model, Table S1: SVM data set parameters, Table S2: MW determination of largest components in USP Enoxaparin RS.

Acknowledgments: K.M.A. is the recipient of a USP Global Fellowship; S.J.C., E.N.M., and A.T. acknowledge NIH (grants 1U01CA207160 and GM5105946).

Author Contributions: K.M.A. and J.L. designed the experiments. Y.X. synthesized the oligosaccharides. K.M.A. performed the experiments. S.J.C., E.N.M., and A.T. planned and conducted computational modeling. K.C. and A.Y.S. served as mentors and contributed expertise. K.M.A. and J.L wrote the manuscript. All the authors contributed to editing the manuscript.

Conflicts of Interest: The authors declare no conflict of interest. This work was prepared while Anita Szajek was employed at United States Pharmacopeia. The opinions expressed in this article are the author's own and do not reflect the view of the National Institutes of Health, the Department of Health and Human Services, or the United States government.

References

1. Alquwaizani, M.; Buckley, L.; Adams, C.; Fanikos, J. Anticoagulants: A Review of the Pharmacology, Dosing, and Complications. *Curr. Emerg. Hosp. Med. Rep.* **2013**, *1*, 83–97. [CrossRef] [PubMed]
2. Jeske, W.P.; Walenga, J.M.; Hoppensteadt, D.A.; Vandenberg, C.; Brubaker, A.; Adiguzel, C.; Bakhos, M.; Fareed, J. Differentiating low-molecular-weight heparins based on chemical, biological, and pharmacologic properties: Implications for the development of generic versions of low-molecular-weight heparins. *Semin. Thromb. Hemost.* **2008**, *34*, 74–85. [CrossRef] [PubMed]

3. Lee, S.; Raw, A.; Yu, L.; Lionberger, R.; Ya, N.; Verthelyi, D.; Rosenberg, A.; Kozlowski, S.; Webber, K.; Woodcock, J. Scientific considerations in the review and approval of generic enoxaparin in the United States. *Nat. Biotechnol.* **2013**, *31*, 220–226. [CrossRef] [PubMed]

4. Szajek, A.Y.; Chess, E.; Johansen, K.; Gratzl, G.; Gray, E.; Keire, D.; Linhardt, R.J.; Liu, J.; Morris, T.; Mulloy, B.; et al. The US regulatory and pharmacopeia response to the global heparin contamination crisis. *Nat. Biotechnol.* **2016**, *34*, 625–630. [CrossRef] [PubMed]

5. Bisio, A.; Mantegazza, A.; Vecchietti, D.; Bensi, D.; Coppa, A.; Torri, G.; Bertini, S. Determination of the molecular weight of low-molecular-weight heparins by using high-pressure size exclusion chromatography on line with a triple detector array and conventional methods. *Molecules* **2015**, *20*, 5085–5098. [CrossRef] [PubMed]

6. Mulloy, B.; Heath, A.; Shriver, Z.; Jameison, F.; Al Hakim, A.; Morris, T.S.; Szajek, A.Y. USP compendial methods for analysis of heparin: Chromatographic determination of molecular weight distributions for heparin sodium. *Anal. Bioanal. Chem.* **2014**, *406*, 4815–4823. [CrossRef] [PubMed]

7. USP. *Enoxaparin Sodium United States Pharmacopeia*; USP: Rockville, MD, USA, 2016; Volume 39, pp. 3695–3697.

8. Mulloy, B.; Hogwood, J. Chromatographic molecular weight measurements for heparin, its fragments and fractions, and other glycosaminoglycans. *Methods Mol. Biol.* **2015**, *1229*, 105–118. [PubMed]

9. Sommers, C.D.; Ye, H.; Kolinski, R.E.; Nasr, M.; Buhse, L.F.; Al-Hakim, A.; Keire, D.A. Characterization of currently marketed heparin products: Analysis of molecular weight and heparinase-I digest patterns. *Anal. Bioanal. Chem.* **2011**, *401*, 2445–2454. [CrossRef] [PubMed]

10. Xu, Y.; Cai, C.; Chandarajoti, K.; Hsieh, P.H.; Li, L.; Pham, T.Q.; Sparkenbaugh, E.M.; Sheng, J.; Key, N.S.; Pawlinski, R.; et al. Homogeneous low-molecular-weight heparins with reversible anticoagulant activity. *Nat. Chem. Biol.* **2014**, *10*, 248–250. [CrossRef] [PubMed]

11. Xu, Y.; Masuko, S.; Takieddin, M.; Xu, H.; Liu, R.; Jing, J.; Mousa, S.A.; Linhardt, R.J.; Liu, J. Chemoenzymatic Synthesis of Homogeneous Ultralow Molecular Weight Heparins. *Science* **2011**, *334*, 498–501. [CrossRef] [PubMed]

12. Ganesh, V.; Zachary, S.; Malikarjun, S.; Yi-Wei, Q.I.; Ram, S. Analysis of Sulfated Polysaccharides. U.S. Patent 7575886, 18 August 2009.

13. Ivanciuc, O. Applications of Support Vector Machines in Chemistry. In *Reviews in Computational Chemistry*; John Wiley & Sons, Inc.: Hoboken, NJ, USA, 2007; Volume 23, pp. 291–400.

14. Mulloy, B.; Hogwood, J.; Gray, E. Assays and reference materials for current and future applications of heparins. *Biologicals* **2010**, *38*, 459–466. [CrossRef] [PubMed]

15. Shastri, M.D.; Johns, C.; Hutchinson, J.P.; Khandagale, M.; Patel, R.P. Ion exchange chromatographic separation and isolation of oligosaccharides of intact low-molecular-weight heparin for the determination of their anticoagulant and anti-inflammatory properties. *Anal. Bioanal. Chem.* **2013**, *405*, 6043–6052. [CrossRef] [PubMed]

16. Li, G.; Steppich, J.; Wang, Z.; Sun, Y.; Xue, C.; Linhardt, R.J.; Li, L. Bottom-Up Low Molecular Weight Heparin Analysis Using Liquid Chromatography-Fourier Transform Mass Spectrometry for Extensive Characterization. *Anal. Chem.* **2014**, *86*, 6626–6632. [CrossRef] [PubMed]

17. Fu, L.; Li, G.; Yang, B.; Onishi, A.; Li, L.; Sun, P.; Zhang, F.; Linhardt, R.J. Structural Characterization of Pharmaceutical Heparins Prepared from Different Animal Tissues. *J. Pharm. Sci.* **2013**, *102*, 1447–1457. [CrossRef] [PubMed]

18. Zhang, F.; Yang, B.; Ly, M.; Solakyildirim, K.; Xiao, Z.; Wang, Z.; Beaudet, J.M.; Torelli, A.Y.; Dordick, J.S.; Linhardt, R.J. Structural characterization of heparins from different commercial sources. *Anal. Bioanal. Chem.* **2011**, *401*, 2793–2803. [CrossRef] [PubMed]

19. Golbraikh, A.; Tropsha, A. Beware of q2! *J. Mol. Graph. Model.* **2002**, *20*, 269–276. [CrossRef]

20. Cherkasov, A.; Muratov, E.N.; Fourches, D.; Varnek, A.; Baskin, I.I.; Cronin, M.; Dearden, J.; Gramatica, P.; Martin, Y.C.; Todeschini, R.; et al. QSAR Modeling: Where Have You Been? Where Are You Going To? *J. Med. Chem.* **2014**, *57*, 4977–5010. [CrossRef] [PubMed]

21. Tropsha, A. Best Practices for QSAR Model Development, Validation, and Exploitation. *Mol. Inform.* **2010**, *29*, 476–488. [CrossRef] [PubMed]

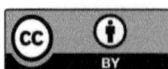

MDPI
St. Alban-Anlage 66
4052 Basel
Switzerland
Tel. +41 61 683 77 34
Fax +41 61 302 89 18
www.mdpi.com

Pharmaceuticals Editorial Office
E-mail: pharmaceuticals@mdpi.com
www.mdpi.com/journal/pharmaceuticals

www.ingramcontent.com/pod-product-compliance
Lightning Source LLC
Chambersburg PA
CBHW051728210326
41597CB00032B/5651